Advances in Orthopedic Surgery of the Knee

E. Carlos Rodríguez-Merchán

Editor

Advances in Orthopedic Surgery of the Knee

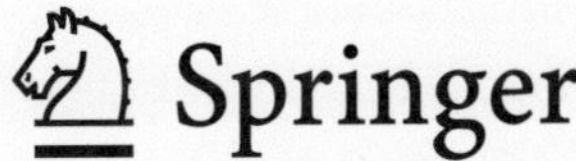

Editor
E. Carlos Rodríguez-Merchán
Department of Orthopaedic Surgery
Hospital Universitario La Paz
Madrid, Spain

ISBN 978-3-031-33063-6   ISBN 978-3-031-33061-2   (eBook)
https://doi.org/10.1007/978-3-031-33061-2

This Springer imprint is published by the registered company Springer Nature Switzerland AG
The registered company address is: Gewerbestrasse 11, 6330 Cham, Switzerland

Preface

Recent advances in orthopedic surgery of the knee allow many people suffering from knee joint problems to improve their quality of life. This book discusses the latest advances in meniscal repair, meniscal allograft transplantation, and the treatment of patellofemoral (PF) osteoarthritis (OA) by arthroplasty, and other methods. Also compares PF arthroplasty to total knee arthroplasty (TKA) for isolated PF OA and reviews unicompartmental arthroplasty (medial and lateral). With respect to TKA, its results have been analyzed after proximal tibia fracture, in patients with severe obesity and in patients younger than 55 years. In addition, the results of unilateral primary TKA have been compared with those of simultaneous bilateral primary TKA, and mobile bearing TKA has been compared to fixed bearing TKA. Finally, fast-track primary and revision TKA, repeat two-stage revision for knee periprosthetic joint infection, revision knee arthroplasty for "pain without loosening" versus "aseptic loosening," and robotic-assisted primary unicompartmental knee arthroplasty and TKA have been analyzed.

In this book, expert authors in the management of knee pathology have presented their knowledge and reviewed the recent literature on all aspects of orthopedic knee surgery previously mentioned. As the editor of this book, my aim has been to concentrate on the most important current topics concerning orthopedic knee surgery in a single volume.

Madrid, Spain

E. Carlos Rodríguez-Merchán

Contents

Meniscal Repair

E. Carlos Rodríguez-Merchán,
Carlos A. Encinas-Ullán, Juan S. Ruiz-Pérez,
and Primitivo Gómez-Cardero

1.1 Introduction

In 2022 Ozeki et al. stated that the meniscus is of great importance for load distribution, shock absorption, and stability of the knee articulation. Also, meniscus tear or meniscectomy causes diminished function of the meniscus and augmented risk of knee osteoarthritis (OA). Figure 1.1 shows the main types of meniscal tears. To maintain the meniscal functions, meniscal repair should be contemplated as the first alternative for meniscus tear. Figure 1.2 shows the main types of meniscal repair. Despite the fact that reoperation rates are more elevated following meniscal repair compared with arthroscopic partial meniscectomy, long-run follow-up of meniscal repair shows better clinical results and less severe degenerative changes of OA compared with partial meniscectomy [1]. In the past, the indication of a meniscal repair was restricted both because of technical reasons and due to the localized vascularity of the meniscus. In the meantime, it spreads today as the development of the idea to maintain the meniscus and the amelioration of meniscal repair techniques. Longitudinal vertical tears in the peripheral third are contemplated the "gold standard" indication in terms of meniscus healing. Techniques for meniscal repair include "inside-out," "outside-in," and "all-inside" approaches. Surgical decision-making depends on the type, size, and location of the meniscus injury. Meniscal root tears mainly impact on meniscal hoop function and speed up cartilage degeneration; therefore, meniscus root repair is needed to preclude the progression of OA change. For symptomatic meniscus defects following meniscectomy, transplantation of allograft or collagen meniscus implant might be indicated, and reasonable clinical outcomes have been achieved. Within the recent past, meniscus extrusion has enticed focus due to augmented interest in early OA. The centralization techniques have been suggested to diminish the meniscus extrusion by suturing the meniscus-capsule complex to the edge of the tibial plateau. Long-run clinical results of this surgical technique might alter the plan of treating meniscus extrusion. When malalignment of the lower leg coexists with meniscus lesions, knee osteotomies are an acceptable alternative to guard the repaired meniscus by unloading the pathological compartment. Progress in biological augmentation such as bone marrow stimulation, fibrin clot, platelet-rich plasma (PRP), stem cell treatment, and scaffolds has also extended the indications for meniscus surgery. Improved repair techniques and biological augmentation have made meniscus repair more appealing to treat [1].

E. C. Rodríguez-Merchán (✉) · C. A. Encinas-Ullán
J. S. Ruiz-Pérez · P. Gómez-Cardero
Department of Orthopedic Surgery, La Paz University Hospital, Madrid, Spain

© The Author(s), under exclusive license to Springer Nature Switzerland AG 2023
E. C. Rodríguez-Merchán (ed.), *Advances in Orthopedic Surgery of the Knee*,
https://doi.org/10.1007/978-3-031-33061-2_1

According to Mahmoud et al., menisci play an essential role in the biomechanics of knee joint function, including loading transmission, joint lubrication, prevention of soft tissue impingement during motion, and articulation stability. Meniscal repair presents a challenge due to an absence of vascularization that restricts the healing capacity of meniscal tissue. Diverse surgical techniques have been created to treat meniscal tears; nevertheless, clinical results are limited. Therefore, many orthopedic surgeons have focused on different therapies such as the application of exogenous and/or autologous growth factors, scaffolds including tissue-derived matrix, cell-based therapy, and microribonucleic acid 210 (miRNA-210) [2].

In 2022 Arner et al. claimed that debate existed regarding the ideal treatment of meniscal tears including debridement, repair, root repair, and transplantation. Also, the tear location and morphology played a fundamental role in the determination of adequate treatment. Repair was usually recommended in tear types with healing potential to preclude meniscal function and joint health [3]. Besides, it has been reported that root radial tears and ramp lesions are the most disregarded or misdiagnosed sources of chronic knee pain [4]. The purpose of this chapter is to review recent developments on meniscal repair.

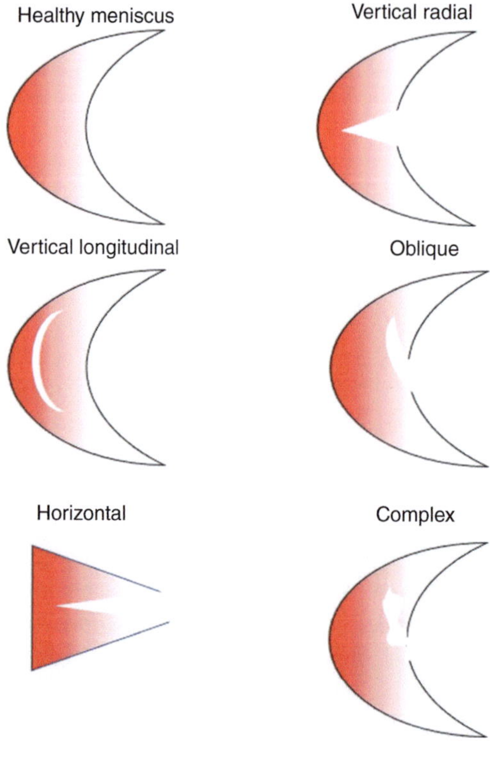

Fig. 1.1 Types of meniscal tears

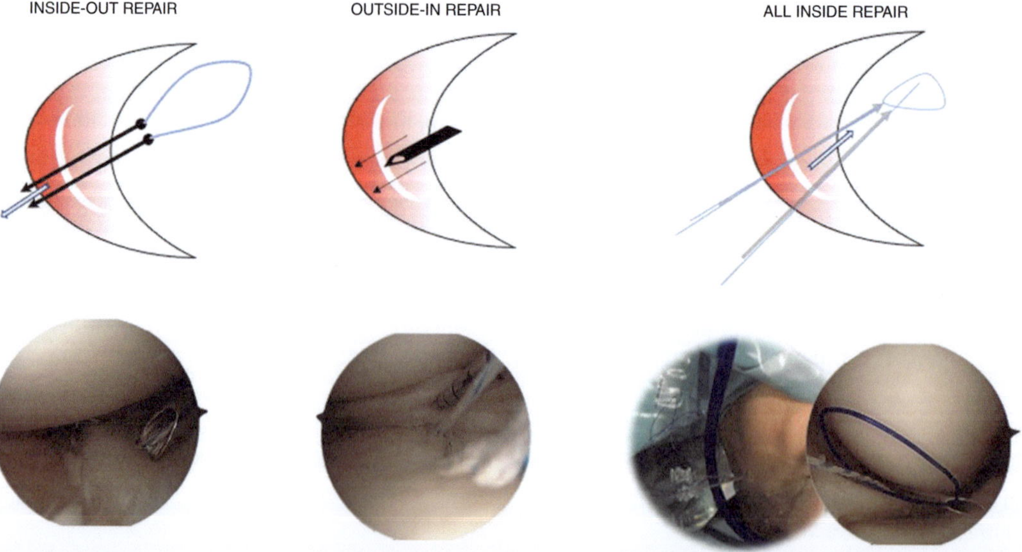

Fig. 1.2 Meniscal repair techniques

1.2   One-Third of Meniscal Tears Are Repairable

Espejo-Reina et al. analyzed, in a case series of individuals with knee injuries (level 4 of evidence), the meniscal tear patterns in both stable and unstable knees to establish the precise percentage of such injuries that could have been repaired [5]. A descriptive cross-sectional study was carried out by reviewing the clinical reports of arthroscopic knee operations performed in one hospital. A total of 2066 consecutive individuals were included in the study. An analysis of clinical and anatomical information of knee injuries, including the shape of the meniscal tears and the surrounding injuries, was carried out. Out of all meniscal tears, 34.9% were discovered to be repairable, a figure that increased to 55.6% in those tears associated with anterior cruciate ligament (ACL) injuries; 37% of meniscal tears in men were repairable, and 28% in their women counterparts; 38.2% of medial meniscal tears were repairable and 30.6% in their lateral counterparts. The most commonly found injury was the complex tear (46.9%) [5].

1.3   Long-Term Results After Meniscus Repair

Petersen et al. performed a systematic review (level 4 of evidence) to analyze long-run results following meniscus refixation with a minimum follow-up of 7 years [6]. Primary result criterion was the failure percentage. Secondary result criteria were radiological signs of OA and clinical scores. There was no statistical difference in the failure percentages between open repair, arthroscopic inside-out repair with posterior incisions, and arthroscopic all-inside repair with flexible non-resorbable implants. In long-run studies that analyzed meniscal repair in children and adolescents, failure percentages were significantly higher than in studies that analyzed adults. The reported clinical scores at follow-up were good to very good. Petersen et al. showed that good long-run results can be achieved in individuals following isolated meniscal repair and in combination with ACL reconstruction (ACLR). With regard to the chondroprotective effect of meniscus repair, the long-run failure percentage was admissible [6].

1.4   Meniscal Tears in Athletes

According to Borque et al., meniscal injuries in elite athletes are a usual source of missed game time and even have the potential to be career shortening. Essential is the differentiation between injuries to the medial and lateral meniscus. Deficiency of the lateral meniscus, as a result of a tear or a meniscectomy, leads to frequent early problems and inevitably to chondral degeneration, by that means having an effect on an athlete's capability to perform. Consequently, it is firmly advised to repair most lateral meniscal tears. Medial meniscal tears create a more defiant treatment difficulty, as the success of partial meniscectomy in accomplishing reproducible, early return to play must be balanced against the long-run degenerative effects. It is important to emphasize that a lot of meniscal tears are correctly treated nonoperatively [7].

1.5   All-Inside Meniscus Repair

According to Golz et al., indications for partial meniscectomy are becoming progressively restricted, and new evidence proposes that the meniscus should be maintained anytime feasible. Because of its multiple suggested pros, all-inside meniscus repairs are turning into more and more usual [8]. Golz et al. claimed that all-inside meniscus repair showed equivalent functional results, healing percentages, and adverse events compared to inside-out repair of vertical longitudinal and bucket-handle tears with the pros of diminished surgical time and quicker postoperative recovery. Besides, they observed that return-to-sport (RTS) and activity levels were elevated after all-inside repair regardless of whether concurrent ACLR was carried out. On the other hand, biomechanical studies have shown pross of all-inside meniscal-based repairs on radial and horizontal tears. All-inside meniscus repair compares well to inside-out repair of vertical longitudinal and bucket-handle tears and persists to rise in acceptance. Both capsular-based and meniscal-based repairs can be utilized to repair a diversity of tear configurations. Golz et al. stated that while biomechanical outcomes were promising, more investigation on the clinical results of meniscal-based repairs was required to clarify the role of these techniques in the time to come [8].

1.6 Inside-Out Meniscal Repair Versus All-Inside Repair

According to Yanke and Dandu, meniscus repairs for vertical, peripheral tears can be troublesome because of bad tissue quality and/or vascularity that can lead to re-rupture and consequent elimination [9]. The gold standard, inside-out repair technique, has been defied by all-inside techniques. While all-inside techniques might have biomechanical properties that are similar to inside-out techniques, it has not been demonstrated in a clinical setting yet. Yanke and Dandu think that the indication must be based on tear pattern while respecting biology, because all fixation will finally fail if the meniscus does not eventually heal. They still utilize inside-out repair techniques for big tears or for high-demand subjects due to its structural integrity and small penetration of the meniscus [9].

1.7 Horizontal Meniscal Tears

A scarcity of evidence exists by which to notify clinical decision-making in the management of repair of horizonal cleavage tears of the meniscus. Available information proposes reasonable results and low failure percentages; however, high-quality investigation is needed to define optimal indications, techniques, and long-run results with respect to function and joint preservation [10].

1.8 Radial Meniscus Tears

In a systematic review, Oosten et al. compared biomechanical characteristics of diverse radial tear repair techniques in the medial and lateral menisci. They found 20 studies that carried out mechanical testing on 21 different radial meniscal tear repair techniques. They encountered that less-invasive all-inside vertical techniques reinforced with suture parallel to the tear instead of standard inside-out horizontal sutures might ameliorate the strength of repair. Besides, transtibial two-tunnel augmentation may also increase the strength of radial meniscus tear repairs. Oosten et al. stated that there might be alternatives to traditional inside-out horizontal repairs for radial meniscus tears [11].

Hamada and Tsujii have expressed that treatment of radial tears of the lateral meniscus is challenging. Previous publications following repairing radial tears demonstrated small healing percentages. Diverse suture techniques are now being developed, and biomechanical and clinical studies utilizing these new techniques are underway. Amid development, the all-inside double vertical cross-suture technique appears to be effective. However, limited assessments following meniscal repair might not entirely demonstrate whether the repaired meniscus can preserve its function [12].

In a systematic review of level 3–4 studies (level 4 of evidence), Milliron et al. tried to quantify healing percentage and patient-reported outcomes (PROMs) following repair of radial meniscus tears [13]. Arthroscopic techniques were utilized in all studies, with one study using an arthroscopic-assisted two-tunnel transtibial pullout technique. The mean patient age was 32 years. The mean follow-up was 35 months. The average time to surgery was 10.9 months. Eight of the 12 studies reported concurrent ACLR, with 64% having concurrent ACL injury. Healing percentages were reported via magnetic resonance imaging (MRI) and second-look arthroscopy. Second-look arthroscopy was carried out for a variety of indications, including removal of screw, washers, or plates, dissatisfaction with original technique, partial healing encountered on MRI, or wish of the subject to know the true healing status prior to RTS. Of those evaluated, 62% had complete healing, 30%

partial healing, and 8% failure to heal. PROMs of radial meniscus repair with and without ACLR were promising, with high PROMs reported at final follow-up when compared with preoperative scores. Among all meniscus repairs evaluated for healing, most of them showed at least some healing with an overall low percentage of failure [13].

1.9   Meniscal Ramp Lesions

In 2022 Brophy et al. claimed that injuries to the medial meniscus meniscocapsular junction, also known as ramp lesions, were usual in the context of ACL injuries with an incidence of 9% to 42%. Anatomically, ramp lesions entail disruption of the posterior meniscocapsular junction and meniscotibial ligaments. MRI is useful in assessing the meniscocapsular junction. The contemporary criterion for diagnosis is arthroscopic visualization of the posterior medial meniscocapsular junction seen through the intercondylar notch. When a ramp lesion is detected, stability should be evaluated by arthroscopic probing to ascertain the grade of anterior displacement. Ideal management has been discussed in the literature, particularly for stable ramp lesions, although good results have been demonstrated with and without repair. Repair is warranted for those lesions that are unstable to probing [14] (Fig. 1.3).

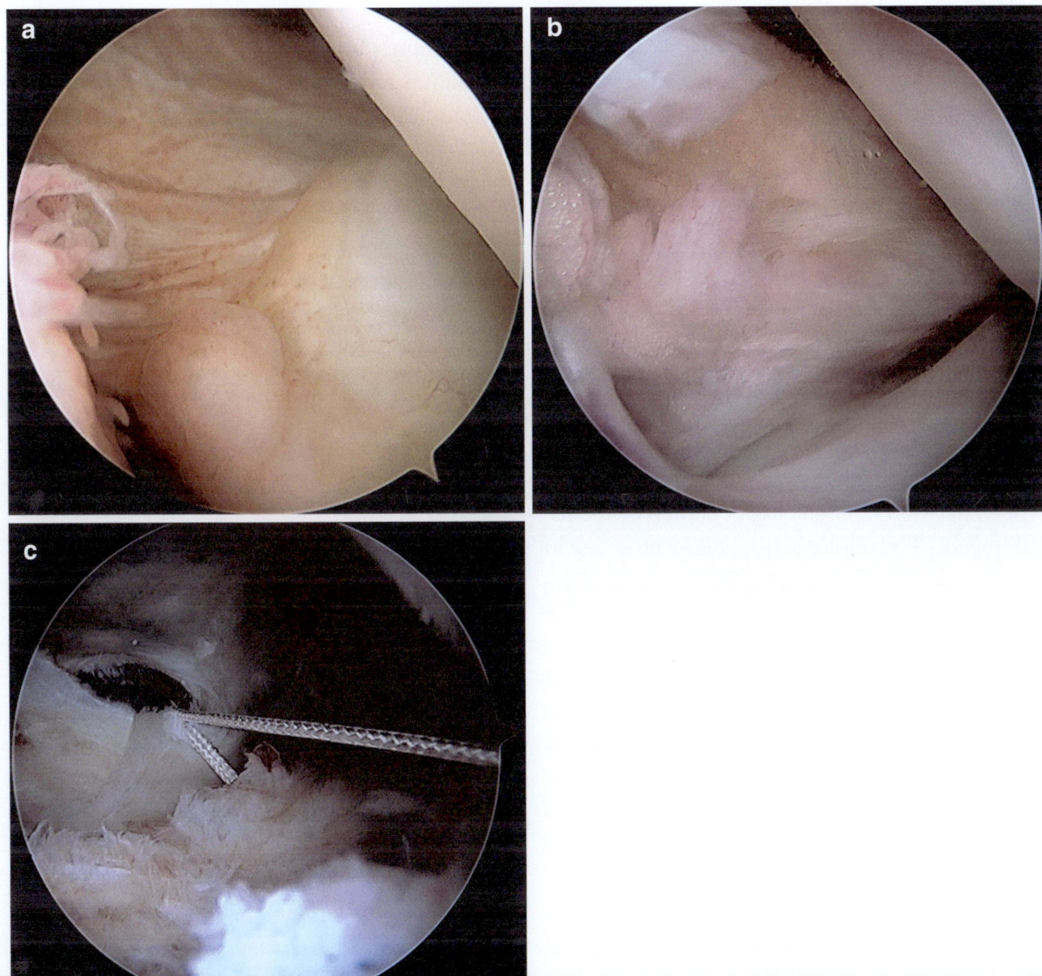

Fig. 1.3 (**a–c**) Tear of the medial meniscal ramp sutured by posteromedial portal: (**a**) arthroscopic image of normal medial meniscal ramp. (**b**) Arthroscopic image of medial meniscal ramp tear. (**c**) Arthroscopic image of medial meniscal ramp tear sutured by posteromedial portal

According to Kaiser et al., the prevalence of ramp lesions is between 16% and 42%. Arthroscopy remains the diagnostic gold standard as MRI has insufficient sensitivity. While there is evidence to propose that ramp lesion repair can restore joint kinematics, contemporary literature fails to suggest that results after repair are better than injuries treated conservatively [15].

Vadhera et al. stated that meniscal ramp lesions can be frequently missed when reviewing standard MRI. Besides, they described an approach to repair a meniscal ramp lesion utilizing a minimally invasive all-inside technique. Vadhera et al. utilized this technique for meniscal tears involving the peripheral and meniscocapsular attachment of the posterior horn causing increased meniscal translation [16].

1.10 Biological Augmentation of Meniscal Repair

According to Keller et al., orthopedic literature remains divided on the utility of biologic augmentation to optimize outcomes after isolated meniscal repair. In a systematic review with level 4 of evidence, they analyzed the clinical outcomes and reoperation rates of biologically augmented meniscal repairs [17]. Of 3794 articles, 18 met inclusion criteria and yielded 537 patients who underwent biologic augmentation of meniscal repair. The biologically augmented repair rates were 5.8–27% with PRP augmentation, 0–28.5% with fibrin clot augmentation, 0–12.9% with marrow stimulation, and 0% with stem cell augmentation. Patients reported substantial improvements in functional result scores following repair with biological augmentation, although the benefit over standard repair controls was dubious. Revision percentages following biologically augmented meniscal repair also seemed similar to standard repair procedures [17].

In a meta-analysis published in 2022, Migliorini et al. compared arthroscopic meniscal repair carried out in solitude or augmented with PRP. The current published scientific evidence did not support PRP augmentation for arthroscopic meniscal repair [18]. In a case series with level 4 of evidence, Hashimoto et al. evaluated the clinical outcome of meniscal repair with a bone marrow aspirate-derived fibrin clot (BMA clot) for isolated meniscal injury in the avascular zone. Avascular meniscal injury was identified as horizontal tear, radial tear, and flap tear. Percentages of clinical failure, anatomic failure, and retear were 10%, 6.7%, and 3.3%, respectively [19].

1.11 Tissue Adhesive Use for Meniscal Repair

According to Maron et al., tissue adhesives (TAs) represent a promising alternative or augmentation method to conventional tissue repair techniques [20]. In a systematic review with level 4 of evidence, they analyzed the current evidence regarding the clinical usage of TAs for meniscal repair. The use of TAs, specifically fibrin-based TAs, for meniscal repair showed good outcomes as either an augmentation or primary repair of various patterns of meniscal tears. However, the study revealed an absence of comparative high-quality information supporting the routine utilization of TAs for meniscal repair and emphasized the lack of an ideal TA designed for that purpose [20].

1.12 Meniscal Cyst Formation Rates After Meniscal Repair

In retrospective cohort study published in 2022, Kinoshita et al. compared the MRI-confirmed cyst formation percentage following meniscal tear repair utilizing a new all-inside suture device (N group) versus the older all-inside suture device (O group) [21]. In a 10-year period (October 2008–July 2019), 94 menisci of 89 subjects were diagnosed with meniscal tears and underwent arthroscopic meniscal repair utilizing the all-inside suture device. Five of these subjects were lost to follow-up within 1 year and were excluded from the study. The remaining 89 menisci were followed up for at least 1 year and were included. Older (O) all-inside suture devices (FasT-Fix, Ultra FasT-Fix) were utilized until December 2012, while the new (N) all-inside suture device (FasT-Fix 360) was utilized from January 2013 onwards. Meniscal cysts were detected on T2-weighted fat-suppressed MRI at 1 year postoperatively. In total, 36 and 53 menisci were included in the N and O groups, respectively. The incidence of meniscal cysts was significantly greater in the O group (14 out of 53, 26.4%) than in the N group (two out of 36, 5.56%). Two subjects in the O group had symptomatic cysts that needed removal. The MRI-confirmed cyst formation percentage following meniscal tear repair was significantly lower utilizing the new than the older all-inside suture devices, indicating that the utilization of a low-profile device may diminish the cyst formation percentage [21].

1.13   Failed Meniscal Repair

In a study with level 3 of evidence, Rönnblad et al. tried to determine the effect of meniscal repair on OA in the knee joint and PROMs [22]. Three-hundred and sixteen meniscal repairs performed between 1999 and 2011 were analyzed. Mean follow-up time was 9.3 years, 162 (51%) subjects answered the questionnaires, and 86 subjects completed the X-ray. The odds ratio for OA with a failed meniscus repair was 5.1 adjusted for gender and age at the time of follow-up. KOOS (Knee Injury and Osteoarthritis Outcome Score) showed a clinically important difference in the sport and recreation subscale. There was an augmented risk for OA in the affected compartment with a failed meniscus fixation. This supported the fact that the meniscus is an important protector of the cartilage in the knee. The meniscus injury affects the long-run health-related quality of life according to KOOS. Rönnblad et al. advised repair of a torn meniscus whenever plausible [22].

1.14   Younger Patients Are More Likely to Undergo Arthroscopic Meniscal Repair and Revision Meniscal Surgery

Bradley et al. assessed recent trends in the management of meniscus tears with arthroscopic repair and debridement as well as evaluated revision surgery within 2 years utilizing a large cross-sectional database [23]. Of the 1,383,161 patients diagnosed with meniscus tears, 53% experienced surgical treatment. Surgical treatment consisted of 96.6% meniscal debridement and 3.4% meniscal repair. The rate of meniscal repairs augmented from 2.7% to 4.4% over those 8 years, while meniscal debridement diminished from 97.3% to 95.6%. Younger subjects were more likely to experience meniscal repair (23% age 10–19 years) than older subjects (<1% age over 60 years). This study found that the percentage of meniscal repair was augmenting over time with subjects under age 30 years most likely to experience repair for a meniscus tear. Revision surgery for meniscal repair or debridement was more usual in adolescents and subjects who experienced an index meniscal repair [23].

1.15   Meniscal Retears After Repair

Considering that accurate diagnosis of meniscal retear can present a clinical challenge, in 2022 Syed et al. carried out a systematic review of literature [24]. They compared the sensitivities, specificities, and accuracies of different diagnostic modalities of diagnosing knee meniscal retears in subjects who had experienced surgical meniscal repair, such as MRI, magnetic resonance arthrography (MRA) with intraarticular contrast (direct MRA), and a combination of MRI and direct MRA. In this analysis, Syed et al. calculated sensitivity to be 78.79%, specificity to be 56.58%, and overall accuracy to be 66.25% for MRI and sensitivity to be 87.84%, specificity to be 88.68%, and overall accuracy to be 87.22%

for direct MRA. Syed et al. advised the utilization of direct MRA for the diagnosis of meniscal retears due to its superior sensitivity, specificity, and accuracy as compared to MRI and its diminished cost and invasive nature as compared to second-look arthroscopy [24].

1.16 Revision Meniscal Repair

In a meta-analysis with level 4 of evidence, Schweizer et al. assessed the overall failure rate of meniscus repair with a minimum follow-up of 5 years. Besides, possible factors affecting meniscus repair result were evaluated [25]. The overall failure percentage of meniscal repair at a mean follow-up of 86 months was 19.1%. There was no significant difference in meniscus repair result when carried out in combination with ACLR compared to isolated meniscus repair (18.7% vs. 28%) or when carried out on the lateral meniscus compared to the medial meniscus (19.5% vs. 24.4%). There was no significant difference of meniscus repair result between vertical/longitudinal tears and bucket-handle tears. Thirty-six percent of meniscus repair failures happened after the second postoperative year. The only significant finding was that inside-out repair resulted in an inferior failure percentage compared to all-inside repair (5.6% vs. 22.3%) at 5 years. The overall meniscus repair failure percentage was 19% in long-run studies. Despite technical advantages of all-inside repair devices, this meta-analysis could not demonstrate better results compared to inside-out or outside-in repair at 5 years [25].

Jackson et al. performed a meta-analysis to determine the results and failure percentages for revision meniscus repairs in subjects with re-tears after primary repair failure. They found a failure rate of 25.3%. Of these failed repairs, 30.95% were of the medial meniscus, and 18.9% were of the lateral meniscus. This study found that revision meniscus repairs in individuals with re-tears after primary repair failure resulted in clinical outcomes similar to that of primary repairs [26].

1.17 Medial Meniscus

1.17.1 Repair of Bucket-Handle Medial Meniscal Tears

Figure 1.4 shows a bucket-handle medial meniscal tear (BHMMT). In a study with level 4 of evidence, Keyhani et al. reported the results of locked BHMMT repairs utilizing an arthroscopic posterior approach during ACLR [27]. They analyzed 48 subjects with BHMMTs and ACL. They used a posterolateral transseptal portal and repaired utilizing a posteromedial portal. Transportal ACLR was carried out using hamstring autograft. Subjects were assessed based on their IKDC (International Knee Documentation Committee) and Lysholm scores and Tegner activity level. After 3–5 years, excellent clinical results were achieved when locked BHMMTs were repaired utilizing an all-inside suture technique that employed posteromedial and posterolateral transseptal portals [27].

Imada et al. claimed that in limited-resource settings (LRS), the majority of meniscal tears are frequently treated with meniscectomy. A simple, low-cost option for meniscal repair was developed by Imada et al. [28]. They assessed PROMs and clinical failure percentages of

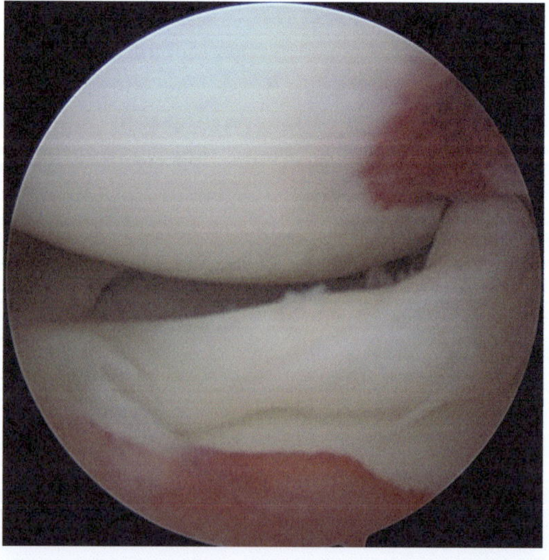

Fig. 1.4 Arthroscopic image of bucket-handle tear

bucket handle meniscus tears (BHMTs) treated with meniscal repair in LRS. In 19 subjects over 18 years (mean age 25.4 years), meniscal repair was primarily performed utilizing an outside-in technique. Two subjects sustained a clinical failure (10.5%). Clinical failure was defined as the need for reoperation or symptoms that prevented the subjects from returning to recreational activities or work responsibilities. At mean follow-up of 40.6 months, there was significant improvement in all PROMs from baseline. The conclusion was that bucket-handle meniscal tears can be repaired utilizing a low-cost technique resulting in satisfactory healing percentages and excellent results [28].

In 2022 Costa et al. published a systematic review and meta-analysis (level 4 of evidence) to determine the failure percentage following arthroscopic repair of BHMTs. The failure rate found was 14.8%. Medial BHMT repairs and isolated repairs had statistically higher risk of failure, but no statistically significant difference was encountered between tears in red-red versus red-white zones. Among the other factors assessed, only the mean number of stitches demonstrated a statistically significant effect on failure percentages. Failure percentage following arthroscopic BHMT repair was 14.8%. Medial tears and isolated repairs were the two main predictors of failure [29].

Ding et al. stated that BHMTs are large longitudinal vertical tears that have an attached fragment flipped into the intercondylar notch [30]. They represent about 10% of all meniscal tears. Meniscectomy frequently results in significant meniscal loss and augmented joint loading. Alternatively, meniscal repair tries to restore the function of the meniscus and intends to maintain articular mechanics. In a case series with level 4 of evidence, Ding et al. assessed the long-run risk of subsequent ipsilateral knee surgery in subjects who experienced a bucket-handle meniscal repair (BHMR). They analyzed 1359 patients with a median age of 24 years who underwent BHMR for a BHMT. During the follow-up period (median, 50.2 months), 495 subsequent ipsilateral procedures were carried out in 274 (20.2%) subjects, and the median time to the first procedure was 10.6 months. One-fifth of subjects experienced subsequent ipsilateral surgery during follow-up, with 4.3% receiving a repeat meniscal repair and 12.1% undergoing a meniscectomy. Risk factors for subsequent surgery of the same knee included younger age and normal or overweight body mass index (BMI). Concomitant ACLR at the time of BHMR diminished the risk of subsequent reoperation [30].

In a retrospective cohort study with level 3 of evidence, Kalifis et al. evaluated long-run follow-up results following repair of bucket-handle meniscal tears [31]. They focused on knee OA development and failure percentage and risk factors associated with failure. They analyzed 66 subjects with bucket-handle tears within 4 mm of the menisco-synovial junction, who experienced meniscal repair, either isolated or combined with ACLR. A combination of all-inside, outside-in, and inside-out repair technique was utilized in all subjects. During the follow-up, a meniscus was considered healed utilizing Barrett's criteria, while knee OA assessment was carried out according to Kellgren-Lawrence (K-L) classification utilizing standing knee radiographs. Median age at the time of operation was 21.9 years. Median follow-up was 114 months. Total failure rate was around 33% at a median time of 19 months. OA was statistically significantly more frequent in subjects with failed repairs (mean K-L score: 2.09) in comparison to subjects with successful repairs (mean K-L score: 0.54). Subjects with medial meniscus repair had 4.8 higher relative likelihood of failure compared to lateral meniscus. Subjects over 16 years old had 5.7 higher relative likelihood of failure. Concurrent ACLR did not have a significant impact on the postoperative results. An elevated percentage of clinical failure was observed following meniscal repair of bucket-handle tears. However, successful treatment led to lower percentages of knee OA development and better knee function, about 10 years postoperatively. Meniscal repair of bucket-handle tears was advised to improve knee function and prevent knee OA in young subjects [31].

1.17.2 Medial Meniscus Posterior Root Repair

According to Chahla and LaPrade, in 2019 meniscus root tears have been reported to account for 10% to 21% of all meniscal tears, affecting around 100,000 subjects per year [32]. Meniscal root tears are defined as either an avulsion of the insertion of the meniscus attachment or complete radial tears that are located within 1 cm of the meniscus insertion. Biomechanical studies have shown that meniscal root injuries disrupt the continuity of the circumferential fibers and consequently lead to failure of the normal meniscal function to convert axial loads into transverse hoop stresses. The most frequent presenting symptoms in meniscal root tears are posterior knee pain and joint line tenderness, particularly with deep squatting. Another frequent symptom is a popping sound heard while participating in light activities such as ascending stairs or squatting. MRI signs of medial meniscus root tears include medial meniscal extrusion of ≥ 3 mm in a coronal view, high signal indicating a disruption of the posterior meniscal root region in an axial plane, and a "ghost sign," which is the lack of an identifiable meniscus in the sagittal view, or augmented signal replacing the normally dark meniscal tissue signal at the posterior root attachment. Active subjects, irrespective of age, should be referred early and considered for a meniscal root repair. Indications for a meniscal root repair include acute, traumatic root tears in subjects with nearly normal or normal cartilage and chronic symptomatic root tears in young or middle-aged subjects without substantial preexisting OA. Meniscal root repair has been shown to have high satisfaction percentages and better results to arthroscopic meniscectomy for root tears. To reestablish the function of the meniscus following medial meniscus root tears, a transosseous meniscal root repair technique is most frequently utilized. The advantage of this technique is the ability to reduce and fix the meniscal root to the broad anatomic footprint to maximize its healing potential. Besides, the transtibial tunnels might contribute to the liberation of biological factors that can augment the healing of the meniscal root repair [32].

In 2022 Furumatsu et al. stated that medial meniscus posterior root repairs led to favorable clinical results in individuals with medial meniscus posterior root tears (MMPRTs). However, there were few comparative studies in assessing the superiority among several pullout repair techniques such as modified Mason-Allen suture, simple stitch, and concomitant posteromedial pullout repair. They compared the clinical usefulness among several types of arthroscopic pullout repair techniques in 83 subjects with MMPRTs [33]. Subjects were divided into three groups utilizing different pullout repair techniques: a modified Mason-Allen suture utilizing FasT-Fix all-inside meniscal repair device (F-MMA, $n = 28$), two simple stitches (TSS, $n = 30$), and TSS concomitant with posteromedial pullout repair utilizing all-inside meniscal repair device (TSS-PM, $n = 25$). Postoperative clinical results and semi-quantitative arthroscopic meniscal healing scores were assessed at second-look arthroscopies. No significant differences among the three groups were found in subject demographics and preoperative clinical scores, except for preoperative Lysholm scores. At second-look arthroscopies, there were no significant differences among the three techniques in postoperative clinical results and meniscal healing scores. The TSS-PM pullout repair technique did not show better scores in postoperative clinical results and meniscal healings compared with the F-MMA and TSS techniques. This study suggested that the concomitant posteromedial pullout suture may have no clinical advantage in the conventional pullout repairs for the subjects with MMPRTs [33].

Repair of medial meniscus posterior root tears is essential in precluding rapid progression of knee OA. There are many repair techniques, and good clinical outcomes have been published.

Ishikawa et al. described arthroscopic medial meniscus posterior root reconstruction and pullout repair combined technique for medial meniscus root tears [34].

According to Chen et al., a meniscal root tear can augment the tibiofemoral contact pressure to approximate that of total meniscectomy and finally lead to degenerative change. An anatomic and stable meniscal root repair is paramount in restoring the tibiofemoral contact pressure back to that of a normal knee. Suture anchor technique and pullout suture technique are the two main arthroscopic root repair procedures with equivalent success; nonetheless, there remains a lack of an optimal technique with a biomechanical property matching that of the intact root. Chen and Lin presented a technically simple, fast, and robust pullout suture construct that incorporated two slipknot locking loops at the meniscus-suture interface. This technique can be utilized for both medial and lateral posterior root repairs, as well as concomitantly with ACLR [35].

Transtibial root repair for medial and lateral posterior meniscal root tears showed significantly improved clinical results at 2 years postoperatively in a case-control study with level 3 of evidence reported by Krych et al. Increased age, increased BMI, cartilage status, and meniscal extrusion did not have a negative influence on short-run functional outcomes (IKDC), but age greater than or equal to 50 years and extrusion negatively impacted subject activity level (Tegner). They analyzed 45 subjects (29 female, 16 male; mean age, 42.3 years; mean BMI, 31.6 kg/m^2) who experienced 47 meniscal root repairs (29 medial and 16 lateral; 2 had both) [36].

In 2022 Wu published a technique for transtibial medial meniscus root repair with centralization using knotless suture anchors. In cases of medial meniscus root tears with meniscal extrusion, centralization may help diminish extrusion and protect the root repair [37].

Perry et al. performed a systematic review of biomechanical results and a meta-analysis of clinical and radiographic results following medial meniscus posterior root (MMPR) repair (level 4 of evidence). MMPR repair generally ameliorated biomechanical outcomes and led to improved PROMs with greater improvements noted in subjects experiencing concomitant high tibial osteotomy (HTO). Repair did not significantly improve meniscal extrusion, while only 5.9% of subjects were noted to progress to low-grade OA [38].

In a study with level 3 of evidence, Hiranaka et al. assessed the impact of tibial rotation on the postoperative healing status of the medial meniscus after pullout repair of the MMPRT. Ninety-one subjects (68 women and 23 men; mean age 63.3 years) who had experienced transtibial pullout repair of MMPRT were analyzed. This study showed that the tibial external rotation angle (ERA) was significantly correlated with the postoperative meniscal healing status. Postoperative tibial rotation could be one of the factors affecting postoperative results of pullout repair of MMPRT. Controlling the tibial rotation might potentially improve meniscal healing [39].

Meniscus extrusion in MMPRT is a consistent MRI finding and correction of extrusion is a principal goal of the meniscal root repair. In a retrospective case series (level 4 of evidence) published in 2022, Sundararajan et al. assessed suitability of correction of extrusion and correlation of diverse factors influencing the postoperative extrusion correction and results in 54 degenerative MMPRTs, including isolated Laprade type 2 root tear with extrusion in MRI [40]. All subjects experienced arthroscopic transtibial tunnel suture pullout repair. The mean follow-up was 34.6 months. A screening MRI was taken at a 6-month follow-up. Mean functional results improved postoperatively IKDC (43.40–78.65) and Lysholm's (65.27–83.16) scores at final follow-up. Moreover, 57.4% (31) had good correction of extrusion, 3.7% (2) no correction, and 38.8% (21) demonstrated increase in extrusion postoperatively. Age, International Cartilage Repair Society (ICRS) (low grade), and knee varus (less 2.5°) influenced extrusion correction. Subjects with healed ($n = 41$), partially healed ($n = 9$), and anatomic tunnel placement ($n = 46$) had better extrusion correction than those with nonhealing ($n = 4$) and nonanatomical tunnel ($n = 8$). Subjects younger than 50 years, with low-grade cartilage damage (ICRS 1, 2), lower KL grade, and varus alignment (<2.5°) had good correction of extrusion. Correction of extrusion/progression did not influence the clinical result in the short run. The progression of meniscal extrusion is unavoidable even following successful repair in elderly and high-risk subjects [40].

In a single-center, retrospective study with level 4 of evidence, Kaplan et al. assessed the mid-run results of 10 MMPRT repairs via evaluation of functional outcome scores and MRI. The technique used was transtibial suture pullout with two locking cinch sutures. The mean age and BMI were 48.4 years and 29.5, respectively, with a mean follow-up of 65.5 months (60% female). Subjects managed with the transtibial suture pullout technique with two locking cinch sutures had preservation of clinical result improvements at 5-year follow-up. However, extrusion was usual, with worsening progression of femoral and tibial chondral disease [41].

According to Hiranaka et al., transtibial pullout repairs utilizing TSS and a combination of TSS PM pullout repair (TSS + PM) utilizing an all-inside meniscal repair device have been published previously for the management of MMPRTs [42]. They investigated the postoperative clinical results of these techniques including medial meniscus extrusion (MME). Fifty-two subjects who experienced transtibial pullout repair were analyzed and divided into TSS ($n = 27$) and TSS + PM ($n = 25$) groups. This study showed that both techniques improved clinical results in the short-run postoperative period. However, MME progressed significantly in the TSS + PM group 1 year postoperatively, which indicated that PM may not be a useful additional procedure for diminishing the postoperative MME [42].

MMPRTs cause abnormal kinematic changes in the knee and may induce pathological external rotation of the tibia during knee flexion. Okazaki et al. investigated changes in the length and inclination of the ACL after MMPR repair utilizing MRI. In a retrospective study, they analyzed 44 subjects who experienced MMPR repair [43]. Clinical results significantly improved 1 year after surgery. The postoperative ACL length (29.7 mm) and proximal angle (47°) at 90° of knee flexion diminished relative to the preoperative values (31.5 mm and 51.8°). The postoperative ACL inclination (64.9°) at 10° of knee flexion diminished relative to the preoperative value (69.7°). Pathologically stretched linear ACL at 90° of knee flexion and a steep ACL inclination at 10° of knee flexion could be reduced following MMPR repair. This suggested that pullout repair could reestablish medial meniscus function as a secondary stabilizer, therefore precluding meniscal and cartilage degeneration [43]. Figure 1.5 shows a meniscal suture of a posteromedial root meniscal tear.

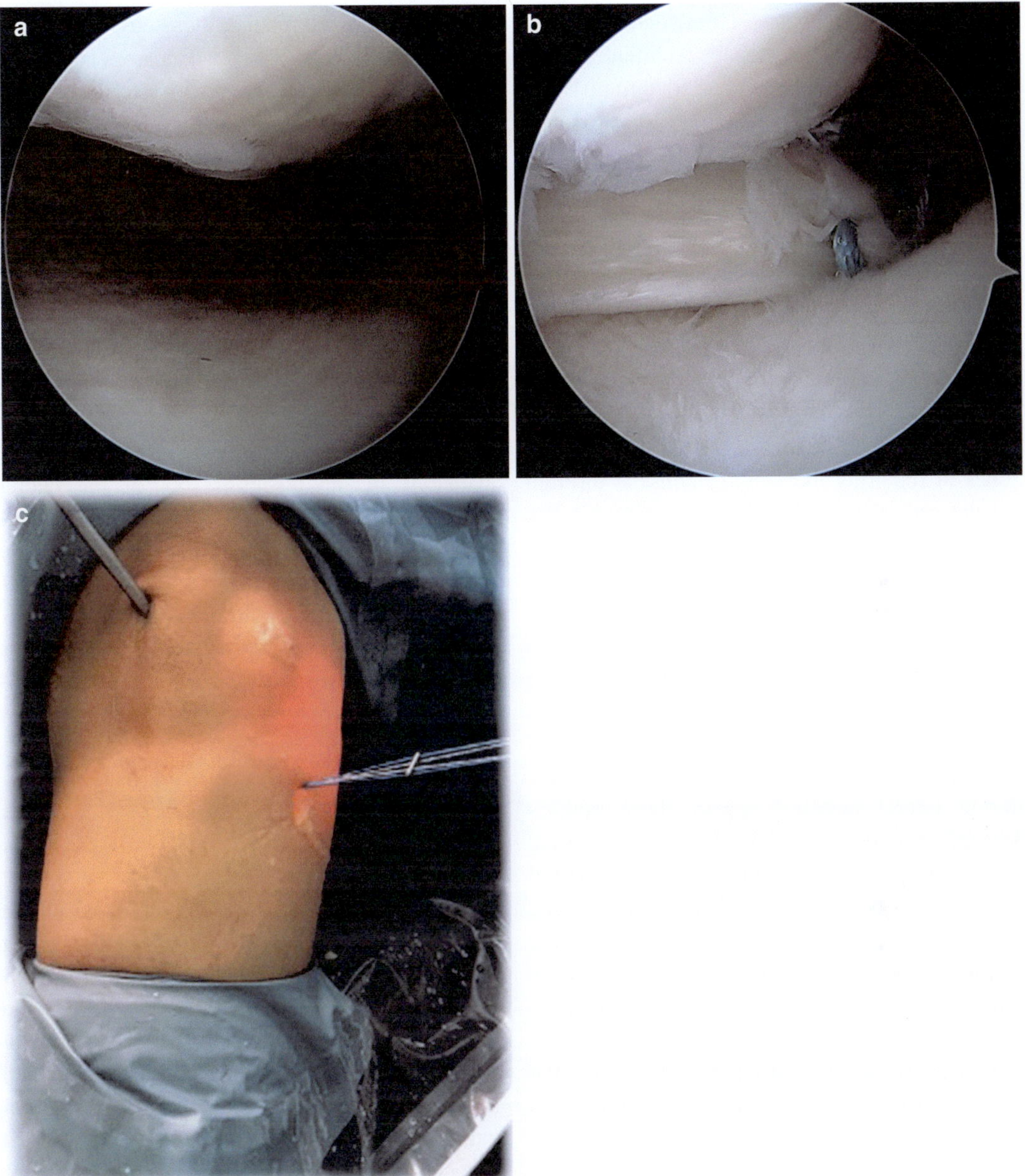

Fig. 1.5 (**a–c**) Posteromedial meniscal root tear: (**a**) arthroscopic image of tear. (**b**) Arthroscopic image of suture passage through posteromedial root and tibial tunnel. (**c**) Fixation of posteromedial root sutures in tibia

1.18 Lateral Meniscal Repair

1.18.1 Lateral Meniscus Posterior Root Repair

In 2022 Familiari et al. reported their preferred method for repair of posterior lateral meniscus root tears (PLMRTs) utilizing an all-suture anchor. They stated that this technique was reproducible, did not require a tunnel, and lessened the bungee effect of the transtibial technique, and the anchor can easily be inserted on the footprint without a need for a guide [44].

Arthroscopic repair of the posterior horn of the lateral meniscus from an anterolateral portal has a risk of popliteal artery injury. In 2022 Ozeki et al. reported an ultrasound-assisted, arthroscopic, all-inside repair technique for a posterior lateral meniscus tear to diminish the risk of neurovascular injury [45].

1.18.2 Risk of Iatrogenic Peroneal Nerve Injury

Lateral meniscal repair using an all-inside meniscal repair device involves a risk of iatrogenic peroneal nerve injury. In 2022 Chuaychoosakoon et al. assessed and compared the risk of peroneal nerve injury and established the safe and danger zones in repairing the lateral meniscus through the anteromedial, anterolateral, or transpatellar portal in relation to the medial and lateral borders of the popliteal tendon (PT) [46]. They found that it was safe to repair the body of the lateral meniscus through the anteromedial portal in the area lateral to the lateral border of the PT or through the anterolateral portal in the area medial to the medial border of the PT. Taking into account that there is a risk of iatrogenic peroneal nerve injury during lateral meniscal repair, these authors advised repairing the lateral meniscal tissue through the anteromedial portal in the area lateral to the lateral border of the PT and utilizing the anterolateral portal in the area medial to the medial border of the PT, as neither of these approaches resulted in peroneal nerve injury. Besides, the orthopedic surgeon can diminish this risk by repairing the meniscal tissue utilizing the all-inside meniscal device in the safe zone area [46].

1.19 Transosseous Meniscus Root Repair in Pediatric Patients

In a case series with level 4 of evidence, Clifton Willimon et al. described meniscus root tear configurations, associated injuries, and results of transosseous meniscus root repair in 20 pediatric subjects (11 male, 9 female) aged <19 years (mean age 15.6 years) with a meniscus posterior root tear managed with transosseous root repair over 4 years [47]. There were 14 lateral meniscus root tears and 6 medial meniscus root tears. Seventeen subjects (85%) had an associated ligament tear: 12 ACL tears and 5 posterior cruciate ligament (PCL) tears. Two root tears occurred in isolation and both were the posterior root of the medial meniscus. Most meniscus root tears ($n = 14$ subjects; 70%) were root avulsions (type 5). The mean follow-up was 42 months. One subject experienced secondary surgery on the affected meniscus after a new injury 4 years postoperatively. Thirteen of 16 subjects (81%) reported returning to the same or higher level of sports after surgery. Meniscus root tears most frequently occurred in pediatric subjects as root avulsions of the posterior root of the lateral meniscus and in association with ACL tears. This is unique compared with the adult population, in which the medial meniscus posterior root is frequently injured in isolation from a radial tear adjacent to the root. In this series, transosseous root repair led to successful results in most subjects, with long-lasting outcomes at the mid-run follow-up [47].

1.20 Conclusions

Meniscal repair should be contemplated as the first alternative for meniscus tear. Despite the fact that reoperation rates are more elevated following meniscal repair compared with arthroscopic partial meniscectomy, long-run follow-up of meniscal repair yields better clinical results and less severe degenerative changes of OA compared with partial meniscectomy. Longitudinal vertical tears in the peripheral third are contemplated the "gold standard" indication in terms of meniscus healing. Techniques for meniscal repair include "inside-out," "outside-in," and "all-inside" approaches. Surgical decision-making will depend on the type, size, and location of the meniscus injury.

Successful healing and excellent patient results have been published with a diversity of all-inside and open techniques. The optimal management of root tears and meniscocapsular separations stays dubious, and definitive suggestions concerning their management are lacking.

Postoperative protocols regarding weight-bearing and range of motion are controversial and need future research. The role of biologics in the augmentation of meniscal repair remains unclear but promising.

References

1. Ozeki N, Seil R, Krych AJ, Koga H. Surgical treatment of complex meniscus tear and disease: state of the art. J ISAKOS. 2021;6:35–45.

2. Mahmoud EE, Mawas AS, Mohamed AA, Noby MA, Abdel-Hady AA, Zayed M. Treatment strategies for meniscal lesions: from past to prospective therapeutics. Regen Med. 2022;17:547–60.

3. Arner JW, Ruzbarsky JJ, Vidal AF, Frank RM. Meniscus repair part 1: biology, function, tear morphology, and special considerations. J Am Acad Orthop Surg. 2022;30:e852–8.

4. Srimongkolpitak S, Chernchujit B. Current concepts on meniscal repairs. J Clin Orthop Trauma. 2022;27:101810.

5. Espejo-Reina A, Aguilera J, Espejo-Reina MJ, Espejo-Reina MP, Espejo-Baena A. One-third of meniscal tears are repairable: an epidemiological study evaluating meniscal tear patterns in stable and unstable knees. Arthroscopy. 2019;35:857–63.

6. Petersen W, Karpinski K, Bierke S, Müller Rath R, Häner M. A systematic review about long-term results after meniscus repair. Arch Orthop Trauma Surg. 2022;142:835–44.

7. Borque KA, Jones M, Cohen M, Johnson D, Williams A. Evidence-based rationale for treatment of meniscal lesions in athletes. Knee Surg Sports Traumatol Arthrosc. 2022;30:1511–9.

8. Golz AG, Mandelbaum B, Pace JL. All-inside meniscus repair. Curr Rev Musculoskelet Med. 2022;15:252–8.

9. Yanke AB, Dandu N. Editorial commentary: moving the needle: traditional inside-out meniscal repair has advantages over all-inside repair. Arthroscopy. 2020;36:3008–9.

10. Khan M. Editorial commentary: repair of horizontal meniscal tears—a need for high-quality research! Arthroscopy. 2020;36:2332–3.

11. Oosten J, Yoder R, DiBartola A, Bowler J, Sparks A, Duerr R, et al. Several techniques exist with favorable biomechanical outcomes in radial meniscus tear repair—a systematic review. Arthroscopy. 2022;38(8):2557–78.

12. Hamada M, Tsujii A. Editorial commentary: all-inside double-vertical cross-suture is an effective technique for knee meniscus radial tear repair, but there is no gold-standard evaluation tool for evaluating healing and function of the repaired meniscus. Arthroscopy. 2022;38:1930–2.

13. Milliron EM, Magnussen RA, Cavendish PA, Quinn JP, DiBartola AC, Flanigan DC. Repair of radial meniscus tears results in improved patient-reported outcome scores: a systematic review. Arthrosc Sports Med Rehabil. 2021;3:e967–80.

14. Brophy RH, Steinmetz RG, Smith MV, Matava MJ. Meniscal ramp lesions: anatomy, epidemiology, diagnosis, and treatment. J Am Acad Orthop Surg. 2022;30:255–62.

15. Kaiser JT, Meeker ZD, Horner NS, Sivasundaram L, Wagner KR, Mazra AF, et al. Meniscal ramp lesions - skillful neglect or routine repair? J Orthop. 2022;32:31–5.

16. Vadhera AS, Parvaresh K, Swindell HW, Verma N, Gursoy S, Evuarherhe A Jr, et al. Arthroscopic all -inside repair of meniscal ramp lesions. J ISAKOS. 2022;7(4):82–3.

17. Keller RE, O'Donnell EA, Medina GIS, Liderman SE, Cheng TTW, Sabbag OD, et al. Biological augmentation of meniscal repair: a systematic review. Knee Surg Sports Traumatol Arthrosc. 2022;30:1915–26.

18. Migliorini F, Cuozzo F, Cipollaro L, Oliva F, Hildebrand F, Maffulli N. Platelet-rich plasma (PRP) augmentation does not result in more favourable outcomes in arthroscopic meniscal repair: a meta-analysis. J Orthop Traumatol. 2022;23(1):8.

19. Hashimoto Y, Nishino K, Orita K, Yamasaki S, Nishida Y, Kinoshita T, et al. Biochemical characteristics and clinical result of bone marrow-derived fibrin clot for repair of isolated meniscal injury in the avascular zone. Arthroscopy. 2022;38:441–9.

20. Marom N, Ode G, Coxe F, Jivanelli B, Rodeo SA. Current concepts on tissue adhesive use for meniscal repair-we are not there yet: a systematic review of the literature. Am J Sports Med. 2022;50:1442–50.

21. Kinoshita T, Hashimoto Y, Nishino K, Nishida Y, Takahashi S, Nakamura H. Comparison of new and old all-inside suture devices in meniscal cyst formation rates after meniscal repair. Int Orthop. 2022;46:1563–71.

22. Rönnblad E, Barenius B, Stålman A, Eriksson K. Failed meniscal repair increases the risk for osteoarthritis and poor knee function at an average of 9 years follow-up. Knee Surg Sports Traumatol Arthrosc. 2022;30:192–9.

23. Bradley K, Cevallos N, Jansson H, Lansdown DA, Pandya NK, Feeley BT, et al. Younger patients are more likely to undergo arthroscopic meniscal repair and revision meniscal surgery in a large cross-sectional cohort. Arthroscopy. 2022;38(10):2875–83.

24. Syed S, Nagdi Zaki M, Lakshmanan J, Kundra R. Knee meniscal retears after repair: a systematic review comparing diagnostic imaging modalities. Libyan J Med. 2022;17(1):2030024.

25. Schweizer C, Hanreich C, Tscholl PM, Ristl R, Apprich S, Windhager R, et al. Nineteen percent of meniscus repairs are being revised and failures frequently occur after the second postoperative year: a systematic review and meta-analysis with a minimum

follow-up of 5 years. Knee Surg Sports Traumatol Arthrosc. 2022;30:2267–76.

26. Jackson GR, Meade J, Yu Z, Young B, Piasecki DP, Fleischli JE, et al. Outcomes and failure rates after revision meniscal repair: a systematic review and meta-analysis. Int Orthop. 2022;46:1557–62.

27. Keyhani S, Soleymanha M, Verdonk R, Amouzadeh F, Movahedinia M, Kazemi SM. Posterior knee arthroscopy facilitates the safe and effective all-inside repair of locked bucket-handle medial meniscal tear using a suture hook technique. Knee Surg Sports Traumatol Arthrosc. 2022;30:1311–5.

28. Imada AO, O'Hara JJ, Proumen IL, Molinari PS, Wascher DC, Richter DL, et al. Bucket handle meniscus tears in low-resource settings can be successfully treated with a cost-effective technique. Int Orthop. 2022;46:43–9.

29. Costa GG, Grassi A, Zocco G, Graceffa A, Lauria M, Fanzone G, et al. What is the failure rate after arthroscopic repair of bucket-handle meniscal tears? A systematic review and meta-analysis. Am J Sports Med. 2022;50:1742–52.

30. Ding DY, Tucker LY, Vieira AL, Freshman RD. Surgical outcomes after bucket-handle meniscal repairs: analysis of a large contained cohort. Am J Sports Med. 2022;50:2390–6.

31. Kalifis G, Raoulis V, Panteliadou F, Liantsis A, D'Ambrosi R, Hantes M. Long-term follow-up of bucket-handle meniscal repairs: chondroprotective effect outweighs high failure risk. Knee Surg Sports Traumatol Arthrosc. 2022;30:2209–14.

32. Chahla J, LaPrade RF. Meniscal root tears. Arthroscopy. 2019;35:1304–5.

33. Furumatsu T, Hiranaka T, Okazaki Y, Kintaka K, Kodama Y, Kamatsuki Y, et al. Medial meniscus posterior root repairs: a comparison among three surgical techniques in short-term clinical outcomes and arthroscopic meniscal healing scores. J Orthop Sci. 2022;27:181–9.

34. Ishikawa H, Okamura H, Ohno T, Fujita S, Akezuma H, Inagaki K. Arthroscopic medial meniscus posterior root reconstruction and pull-out repair combined technique for root tear of medial meniscus. Arthrosc Tech. 2022;11:e109–14.

35. Chen HY, Lin KY. Arthroscopic transtibial pull-out repair for meniscal posterior root tear: the slip knot technique. Arthrosc Tech. 2022;11:e209–15.

36. Krych AJ, Song BM, Nauert RF 3rd, Cook CS, Levy BA, Camp CL, et al. Prospective consecutive clinical outcomes after transtibial root repair for posterior meniscal root tears: a multicenter study. Orthop J Sports Med. 2022;10(2):23259671221079794.

37. Wu TY. Arthroscopic medial meniscus posterior root repair with centralization using knotless suture anchors. Arthrosc Tech. 2022;11:e661–8.

38. Perry AK, Lavoie-Gagne O, Knapik DM, Maheshwer B, Hodakowski A, Gursoy S, et al. Examining the efficacy of medial meniscus posterior root repair: a meta-analysis and systematic review of biomechanical and clinical outcomes. Am J Sports Med. 2022;6:3635465221077271. https://doi.org/10.1177/03635465221077271.

39. Hiranaka T, Furumatsu T, Okazaki Y, Kintaka K, Kamatsuki Y, Zhang X, et al. Postoperative external tibial rotation is correlated with inferior meniscal healing following pullout repair of a medial meniscus posterior root tear. Knee Surg Sports Traumatol Arthrosc. 2022;30:1491–8.

40. Sundararajan SR, Ramakanth R, Sethuraman AS, Kannan M, Rajasekaran S. Correlation of factors affecting correction of meniscal extrusion and outcome after medial meniscus root repair. Arch Orthop Trauma Surg. 2022;142:823–34.

41. Kaplan DJ, Bloom D, Alaia EF, Walter WR, Meislin RJ, Strauss EJ, et al. ICRS scores worsen between 2-year short term and 5-year mid-term follow-up after transtibial medial meniscus root repair despite maintained functional outcomes. Knee Surg Sports Traumatol Arthrosc. 2022;30:2235–43.

42. Hiranaka T, Furumatsu T, Miyazawa S, Okazaki Y, Kintaka K, Kodama Y, et al. Transtibial pull-out repair techniques using two simple stitches for medial meniscus posterior root tear can prevent the progression of medial meniscus extrusion and obtain successful outcomes. Eur J Orthop Surg Traumatol. 2022;32:795–802.

43. Okazaki Y, Furumatsu T, Kodama Y, Hiranaka T, Kintaka K, Kamatsuki Y, et al. Medial meniscus posterior root repair influences sagittal length and coronal inclination of the anterior cruciate ligament: a retrospective study. Eur J Orthop Surg Traumatol. 2022; https://doi.org/10.1007/s00590-022-03285-0.

44. Familiari F, Palco M, Russo R, Moatshe G, Simonetta R. Arthroscopic repair of posterior root tears of the lateral meniscus with all-suture anchor. Arthrosc Tech. 2022;11:e781–7.

45. Ozeki N, Koga H, Nakamura T, Nakagawa Y, Ohara T, An JS, et al. Ultrasound-assisted arthroscopic all-inside repair technique for posterior lateral meniscus tear. Arthrosc Tech. 2022;11:e929–35.

46. Chuaychoosakoon C, Boonsri P, Tanutit P, Laohawiriyakamol T, Boonriong T, Parinyakhup W. The risk of iatrogenic peroneal nerve injury in lateral meniscal repair and safe zone to minimize the risk based on actual arthroscopic position: an MRI study. Am J Sports Med. 2022;50:1858–66.

47. Clifton Willimon S, Busch MT, Murata A, Perkins CA. Transosseous meniscus root repair in pediatric patients and association with durable midterm outcomes and high rates of return to sports. Am J Sports Med. 2022;50:2070–4.

Meniscal Allograft Transplantation

E. Carlos Rodríguez-Merchán,
Carlos A. Encinas-Ullán, Juan S. Ruiz-Pérez,
Primitivo Gómez-Cardero,
and Hortensia De la Corte-Rodríguez

2.1   Introduction

Meniscal allograft transplantation (MAT) is a treatment modality for restoring knee function in subjects with irreversible meniscal injury [1] (Fig. 2.1). MAT is not commonly utilized due to costs and accessibility [2]. Clinical results of MAT are not always consistent with graft status [3]. Anatomic placement of the meniscal allograft is mandatory to accomplish satisfactory results after MAT [4]. The purpose of this chapter is to review recent developments on MAT.

E. C. Rodríguez-Merchán (✉) · C. A. Encinas-Ullán
J. S. Ruiz-Pérez · P. Gómez-Cardero
Department of Orthopedic Surgery, La Paz University
Hospital, Madrid, Spain

H. De la Corte-Rodríguez
Department of Physical and Rehabilitation Medicine,
La Paz University Hospital, Madrid, Spain

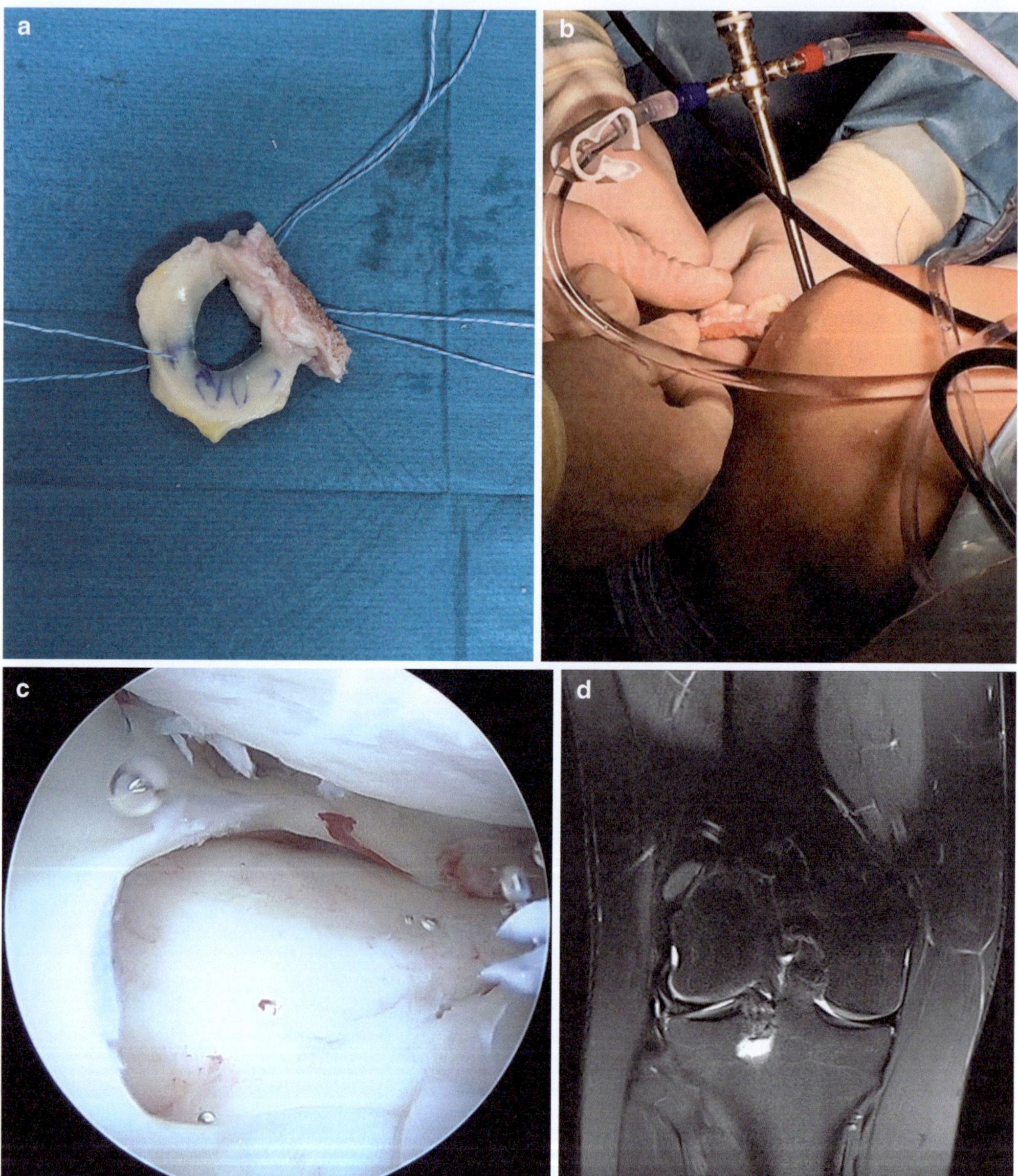

Fig. 2.1 (**a–f**) Images of a lateral meniscal allograft transplantation (MAT): (**a**) preparation of lateral meniscal allograft. (**b**) Introduction of the allograft into the joint. (**c**) Arthroscopic view of the meniscal allograft. (**d**) Postoperative magnetic resonance imaging (MRI) (coronal view). (**e**) Postoperative MRI (sagittal view). (**f**) Postoperative MRI (axial view)

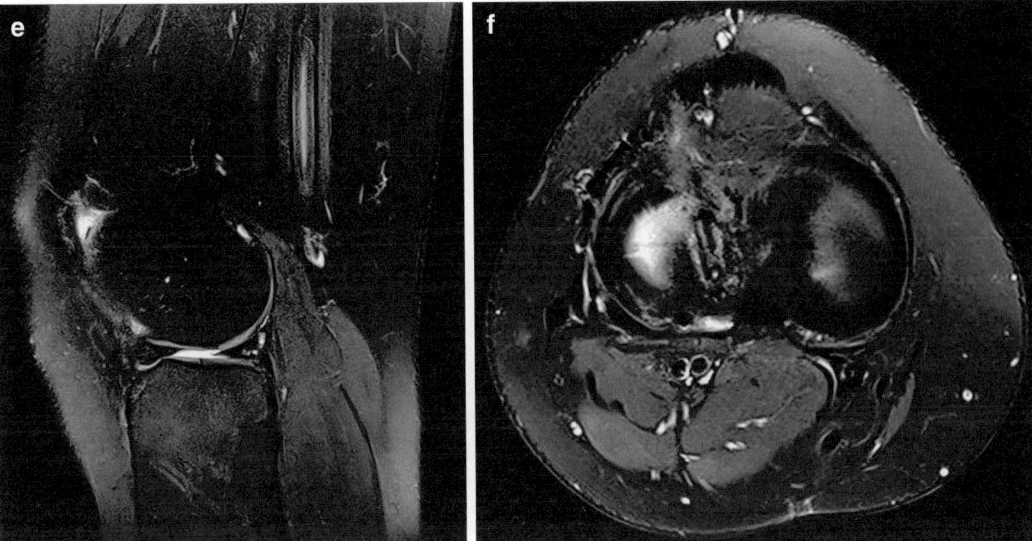

Fig. 2.1 (continued)

2.2 Long-Run Chondroprotective Impact

In a cohort study with level 3 of evidence published in 2022, Wang et al. hypothesized that MAT would diminish osteoarthritis (OA) progression when compared with the meniscus-deficient knee [5]. Graft extrusion distance would highly influence the chondroprotective impact of the MAT. Seventeen knees experiencing MAT were followed up as the MAT group. The MAT group was further divided into the nonextrusion subgroup ($n = 9$) and the meniscal extrusion (ME) subgroup ($n = 8$) according to 3-mm extrusion on the magnetic resonance imaging (MRI) coronal view. A further 26 subjects undergoing meniscectomy in the same period were followed up as the ME group. The healthy control group consisted of healthy contralateral legs selected from the MAT and ME groups ($n = 27$). Joint space width (JSW) narrowing was measured on X-rays. Three-dimensional MRI with a T2 mapping sequence was utilized to quantitatively study cartilage degeneration and meniscal allograft extrusion in five directions (0°, 45°, 90°, 135°, and 180°). The cartilage degeneration index (CDI) was estimated according to the size and grade of the chondral lesions on MRI scans. The correlation between the CDI increase and the extrusion distance was analyzed. The mean follow-up time was 11.3 years. MAT had moderate advantages in chondroprotection compared with meniscectomy in the long run. Graft extrusion distance highly influenced the chondroprotective impact of MAT. The chondroprotective effect of the nonextruded meniscal allograft was close to that of the native meniscus, but the allografts with an extrusion >3 mm entirely lost their function following meniscectomy [5].

2.3 Predictors of Meniscal Allograft Failure

In a retrospective study published in 2022 by Winkler et al., it was hypothesized that young subject age, high posterior tibial slope (PTS), and high-degree OA were predictors of meniscal allograft failure. Seventy-seven subjects experiencing MAT with a minimum follow-up of 2 years were included in this retrospective study (mean age, 25.7 years). After a mean follow-up of 7.6 years, meniscal allograft failure was found in 26 subjects (34%). The median time from MAT to meniscal allograft failure was 1.3 years.

Meniscal allograft tears (88%) were the primary cause of graft failure, followed by high-grade OA (12%). Subjects experiencing meniscal allograft failure were an average of 2.7 years older at the time of MAT than subjects without failure. Subjects with high-degree preoperative OA of the index compartment had 28 times higher odds of undergoing meniscal allograft failure than subjects with low-degree preoperative OA [6].

2.4 Medial MAT with Bone Plugs Utilizing a Three-Tunnel Technique

In 2022 Teo et al. described a modified meniscal allograft transplantation technique utilizing three bone tunnels with allograft fixation through the use of bone plugs. The addition of a third tunnel augmented the strength of fixation, averting ME and ameliorating load distribution [7].

2.5 Outcomes, Complications, and Reoperations

In a case series with level 4 of evidence, Vasta et al. reviewed clinical results in 61 younger, previously active subjects (63 knees) who experienced an isolated MAT or MAT plus any osteotomy. Mean presurgery age was 25.5 years, mean body mass index (BMI) was 26.7, and mean follow-up was 4.8 years. Adverse events (conditions requiring at least one subsequent surgery) affected about one-quarter of the subjects who experienced MAT. Nonetheless, MAT appeared to provide subjects with appropriate pain alleviation and improved function [8].

In 2022 Barlow et al. analyzed 526 subjects to identify factors that impact both functional result and survival of MAT. Their results indicated that baseline KOOS4 (Knee Injury and Osteoarthritis Outcome Score 4) affected functional result at 2 years. The only factor that influenced failure percentage was the presence of cartilage lesions down to bone on both the femur and tibia, diminishing the 5-year survivorship from 95% to 84%.

They stated that factors such as age, BMI, and cartilage lesions down to bone on both the femur and tibia of the affected compartment should not present barriers to offering MAT [9].

In a study with level 4 of evidence, Bonanzinga et al. evaluated the return to sport (RTS) percentage of 13 young professional athletes, analyzed their careers in terms of matches played and league participation over a minimum period of 6 years after MAT, and assessed the long-run clinical subjective results and satisfaction [10]. Their mean age at surgery was 23.4 years. Six MATs were medial, and seven MATs were lateral. At an average follow-up of 9 years, 13 subjects (100%) RTS after an average period of 11.8 months. Nine athletes (69%) RTS at the same preinjury level. Overall, 93%, 85%, 62%, and 55% were active until the third, the fifth, the seventh, and the ninth season following MAT, respectively. Seven subjects (54%) experienced a reoperation after MAT, where only two of them (15%) were related to graft problems (one meniscectomy and one graft suture). Of the ten athletes that completed subjective assessment, the mean Lysholm score was 72 (0% "excellent," 10% "good," 60% "fair," 30% "poor"). Of the athletes with lower scores, one suffered from patellar tendon rupture, one from postoperative infection, and one from a previous femoral fracture. MAT permitted all athletes to return to preinjury sport and in nearly 70% of cases at their preinjury level. After five seasons following MAT, 85% of athletes were still active or playing more than 20–30 matches per season. About 50% experienced at least one reoperation and only 70% of athletes were rated as "good" or "fair" utilizing the Lysholm score [10].

In 2022 Palumbo and Matava stated that MAT is the reconstructive procedure of choice after a total or near-total meniscectomy for the symptomatic subject with a stable, well-aligned knee before the beginning of degenerative OA. Historically, the objectives were to get rid of symptoms with activities of daily living and ameliorate longevity of the articular cartilage. Nonetheless, athletically active subjects were almost never pleased except if they return to their previous level of function, which is dependent on patient-specific, knee-specific, and sports-specific factors. In spite of the fact that subjective patient-reported outcomes (PROMs) were substantially improved in most MAT patients, there is broad variability in the percentage at which athletic subjects are able to RTS, when they return, and their eventual level of performance. Palumbo and Matava recommended active subjects who experience a MAT to undertake "low-impact" activities based on 10-year survivorship of 70% to 80%. Risk of a repetitive meniscal tear was the most frequent adverse event, and the ability of MAT to preclude OA was not established [11].

2.6   Do Outcomes Differ Based on Age and Sex?

Frank et al. analyzed the effect of patient age, sex, and associated preoperative factors on PROM measures and graft survival following primary MAT (therapeutic retrospective comparison study with level 3 of evidence) [12]. A prospectively collected database was retrospectively reviewed to recognize subjects who experienced primary MAT with a minimum of 2 years. Postoperative outcomes were stratified based on age and sex, and comparative statistical analysis was carried out between sexes, both >40 and <40. A total of 238 subject experienced primary MAT, of which 212 subjects (mean age, 28.5 years) met the inclusion criteria with a mean follow-up of 5.1 years. At final follow-up, patients ≥40 and <40 years of age showed statistically significant improvements in nearly all PROM scores. There were no significant differences between either group for accomplishment of minimal clinically important difference for IKDC (International Knee Documentation Committee) or KOOS symptoms. Because of insufficient numbers, a statistically significant difference could not be shown in reoperation percentage (≥40, 1.49 years; <40, 1.87 years), failure rate (≥40, 7/32 [21.9%]; <40, 19/180 [10.6%]), or complication percentage (≥40, 2/32 [6.3%]; <40, 12/180

[6.7%]) based on age. Both sexes demonstrated a significant improvement in PROMs, whereas women were more likely to experience revision surgery, with no significant differences based on time to reoperation, failure, or complication percentages. PROMs similarly improved following MAT in both subjects aged ≥40 years and those <40 years at final follow-up with no significant differences in minimal clinically important difference accomplishment percentage, adverse events rate, reoperation percentage, time to reoperation, or failure rate between groups. Women may be more likely to experience revision surgery after MAT [12].

2.7   Immediate MAT or Conventional Delayed Transplantation?

In a study with level 4 of evidence, Wang et al. compared the long-run clinical and radiological results between the immediate and delayed MAT [13]. Nine menisci were transplanted straight away following total meniscectomy (immediate group, IM), and 10 menisci were delayed transplanted in subjects with the median of 35 months (range 9–92 months) following total meniscectomy (delayed group, DE). Subject's subjective clinical results including visual analog scale (VAS), IKDC, and Lysholm and Tegner scores as well as muscle strength measures were compared. Joint degeneration was assessed by both X-rays to evaluate joint space width narrowing, Kellgren-Lawrence (K-L) grade, and MRI with T2 mapping sequences to quantitatively analyze both cartilage and meniscal allograft degeneration. The median follow-up time was 10.8 years. The IKDC (IM vs. DE, 89.8 vs 80.9) and Lysholm scores (IM vs. DE, 87.7 vs 78.0) were close in two groups, while the IM group showed slightly lower VAS (IM vs. DE, 0.2 vs. 1.5), higher Tegner score (IM vs. DE, 7 vs. 3.5), and better quadriceps muscle strength. The IM group had less joint space narrowing (IM vs. DE, 0.35 mm vs. 0.71 mm), less K-L grade progression (IM vs. DE, 0.6 vs. 1.7) on X-rays, and less chondral lesion development on magnetic resonance imaging (MRI, cartilage degeneration index, IM vs. DE, 252 vs. 2038). All meniscal grafts exhibited degeneration by showing grade 3 signal on MRI and 4 (4/9) in the IM group and 8 (8/10) cases in the DE group. The T2 value of cartilage and meniscal allograft in the IM group was close to that of the healthy control and was significantly lower than that of the DE group. Compared to the conventional delayed MAT, the immediate MAT accomplished better cartilage and meniscus protection in the long run, while its superiority in PROMs was limited [13].

2.8 Return to Sports

A systematic review (level 4 of evidence) published by Ahmed et al. assessed the RTS percentage and time after MAT with ≥12-month follow-up. The return to sports percentage ranged from 20% to 91.7%. The RTS time ranged between 7.6 and 16.9 months. The return to pre-injury level had a percentage of 7% to 100%. Return to a higher level of sports had a percentage of 28.5% to 86%. The total reoperation percentage following MAT ranged between 3.1% and 80%, while the total failure ranged between 1.1% and 30.1% [14].

2.9 Scoring Parameters to Assess MRI Appearance After MAT

MRI appearance of the meniscal allograft is frequently queried and increases concerns of its viability and function. In a study with level 3 of evidence, Damasena et al. reported and validated a new scoring system for MAT MRI appearance at 1 year (MRI appearance in Meniscal Transplant Score [MIMS]), utilizing essential changes such as extrusion, meniscal signal change, loss of shape, synovitis, and bone marrow edema. MIMS was found to be a dependable technique of assessing the meniscal MAT 1 year posttransplant [15].

2.10 Autologous Semitendinosus Tendon Graft Could Function as a Meniscal Transplant

According to Rönnblad et al., the semitendinosus tendon (ST) has the potential to remodel and revascularize in an intraarticular environment. In a pilot study, Rönnblad et al. studied whether the ST graft could function as a MAT. Although this study was primarily a technical report, the follow-up data indicated that the MAT survived and adapted in shape and capabilities to an original meniscus. There were no complications and the individuals appeared to ameliorate in terms of pain and quality of life [2].

2.11 Mismatch Between Anatomic and Clinical Failures

In a study with level 3 of evidence, Song et al. investigated the degree and pattern of mismatch between anatomic and clinical failures in MAT and preoperative factors associated with the mismatch. A remarkable number of failure cases of MAT demonstrated a mismatch between anatomic and clinical failures. Even with anatomic failure, MAT did not always cause poor clinical scores or reoperations, whereas MAT could have poor outcomes without significant allograft problems. Therefore, both anatomic and clinical aspects should be taken into account when assessing MAT. In particular, type 3 failure happened more commonly in medial than in lateral MAT [3].

2.12 Accuracy of the Arthroscopic Location of the Center of the Anterior Horn During Lateral MAT

Few studies have been reported on the exactness of the provisional location of the center of the anterior horn of the lateral meniscus (AHLM). In a descriptive laboratory study, Choi et al. hypothesized that the provisional center would not coincide with the anatomic center of the AHLM. They found that without dissection of the AHLM, the determination of the anatomic center of the anterior horn is not correct during lateral MAT [4].

2.13 Aquatic Training and Bicycling Training

Strengthening programs to promote functional recuperation are treated with caution during the intermediate rehabilitation stage after MAT. In 2022, Chen et al. analyzed the impact of aquatic training (AQT) and bicycling training (BCT) during the intermediate phase of rehabilitation in amateur athletes that experienced MAT. All measured parameters for the AQT and BCT groups improved substantially following training compared with pre-training values. The IKDC score and YBT were substantially higher for AQT than for BCT. The knee flexion range of motion (ROM) and isokinetic muscle strength were substantially ameliorated in the BCT group compared to those in the AQT group. The AQT group displayed greater amelioration in dynamic balance, while BCT provided greater improvement in isokinetic muscle strength. AQT and BCT were efficacious in diminishing discomfort and improving knee symptoms and functions during intermediate-phase rehabilitation after MAT in amateur athletes [1].

2.14 Distraction Arthroplasty Plus Lateral MAT Combined with Cartilage Repair

In a study with level 3 of evidence, Lee et al. reported RTS and return to work (RTW) results following distraction arthroplasty (DA) plus lateral MAT combined with cartilage repair in active subjects with advanced OA. All subjects who experienced DA plus lateral MAT combined with cartilage repair returned to any sports and work at the last follow-up. Substantial improvements in clinical results and the radiographic joint space width were found. However, the activity ability was somewhat diminished compared with the best preoperative level [16].

2.15 Conclusions

MAT is a treatment modality for restoring knee function in subjects with irreversible meniscal injury. Adverse events (conditions requiring at least one subsequent surgery) affect about 25% of the subjects who experience MAT. Nonetheless, MAT appears to provide subjects with appropriate pain alleviation and improved function. Compared to the conventional delayed MAT, the immediate MAT accomplishes better cartilage and meniscus protection in the long run.

After a mean follow-up of about 7 years, MAT failure occurs in 34% of subjects. The median time from MAT to meniscal allograft failure is 1.3 years. Meniscal allograft tears (88%) are the primary cause of graft failure, followed by high-grade OA (12%). Subjects experiencing meniscal allograft failure are 2.7 years older at the time of MAT than subjects without failure. Subjects with high-degree preoperative OA of the index compartment have 28 times higher odds of experiencing MAT failure than subjects with low-degree preoperative OA.

References

1. Chen Y, Kim Y, Choi M. Effects of aquatic training and bicycling training on leg function and range of motion in amateur athletes with meniscal allograft transplantation during intermediate-stage rehabilitation. Healthcare. 2022;10(6):1090.
2. Rönnblad E, Rotzius P, Eriksson K. Autologous semitendinosus tendon graft could function as a meniscal transplant. Knee Surg Sports Traumatol Arthrosc. 2022;30:1520–6.
3. Song JH, Bin SI, Kim JM, Lee BS. Meniscal allograft transplantation shows a mismatch between anatomic and clinical failures. Knee Surg Sports Traumatol Arthrosc. 2022;30:1700–5.
4. Choi NH, Hwangbo BH, Kang HK, Yang BS, Victoroff BN. Accuracy of the arthroscopic location of the center of the anterior horn during lateral meniscal allograft transplantation. Orthop J Sports Med. 2022;10(5):23259671221089250.
5. Wang DY, Zhang B, Li YZ, Meng XY, Jiang D, Yu JK. The long-term chondroprotective effect of meniscal allograft transplant: a 10- to 14-year follow-up study. Am J Sports Med. 2022;50:128–37.
6. Winkler PW, Wagala NN, Hughes JD, Musahl V. High-grade preoperative osteoarthritis of the index compartment is a major predictor of meniscal

allograft failure. Arch Orthop Trauma Surg. 2022; https://doi.org/10.1007/s00402-021-04306-z.

7. Teo SJ, Tan MWP, Koh DTS, Lee KH. Medial meniscal allograft transplantation with bone plugs using a 3-tunnel technique. Arthrosc Tech. 2022;11:e217–22.

8. Vasta S, Zampogna B, Hartog TD, El Bitar Y, Uribe-Echevarria B, Amendola A. Outcomes, complications, and reoperations after meniscal allograft transplantation. Orthop J Sports Med. 2022;10(3):23259671221075310.

9. Barlow T, Coco V, Shivji F, Grassi A, Asplin L, Thompson P, et al. Patient-reported outcome and survival following meniscal allograft transplantation: an international case series. Bone Joint J. 2022;104-B:657–62.

10. Bonanzinga T, Grassi A, Altomare D, Vitale ND, Zaffagnini S, Marcacci M. Long sports career and satisfactory clinical outcomes after meniscal allograft transplantation (MAT) in young professional athletes involved in strenuous sports. Knee Surg Sports Traumatol Arthrosc. 2022;30:2314–9.

11. Palumbo NE, Matava MJ. Editorial commentary: knee meniscal allograft transplantation results in significantly improved outcomes in the majority of patients, but there is wide variability in the rate at which athletes return to sports. Arthroscopy. 2022;38: 1362–5.

12. Frank R, Gilat R, Haunschild ED, Huddleston H, Patel S, Evuarherhe A Jr, et al. Do outcomes of meniscal allograft transplantation differ based on age and sex? A comparative group analysis. Arthroscopy. 2022;38:452–465.e3.

13. Wang DY, Lee CA, Zhang B, Li YZ, Meng XY, Jiang D, et al. The immediate meniscal allograft transplantation achieved better chondroprotection and less meniscus degeneration than the conventional delayed transplantation in the long-term. Knee Surg Sports Traumatol Arthrosc. 2022;30:3708–17.

14. Ahmed AF, Rinaldi J, Noorzad AS, Zikria BA. Return to sports following meniscal allograft transplantation is possible but remains questionable: a systematic review. Arthroscopy. 2022;38:1351–61.

15. Damasena I, Onggo JR, Asplin L, Hutchinson C, Shah R, Spalding T. Extrusion, meniscal signal change, loss of shape, synovitis and bone marrow oedema are reliable scoring parameters to assess MRI appearance post meniscal transplant. Knee Surg Sports Traumatol Arthrosc. 2022;30:1527–34.

16. Lee DW, Lee DR, Kim MA, Cho SI, Lee JK, Kim JG. Patients with advanced lateral osteoarthritis can return to sports and work after distraction arthroplasty plus lateral meniscal allograft transplantation combined with cartilage repair. Knee Surg Sports Traumatol Arthrosc. 2022;30:1990–2002.

Anterior Cruciate Ligament Reconstruction

3

E. Carlos Rodríguez-Merchán,
Carlos A. Encinas-Ullán, Juan S. Ruiz-Pérez,
and Primitivo Gómez-Cardero

3.1 Introduction

According to Musahl et al., a tendency within the orthopedic community is refusal of the mental conviction that "one size fits all." Therefore, it is important to individualize the management of anterior cruciate ligament (ACL) injuries based on the subject's anatomy. During the last 20 years, greater accentuation has been placed on improving the results of ACL reconstruction (ACLR) (Figs. 3.1 and 3.2). Consequently, anatomic tunnel placement is essential in precluding graft impingement and reestablishing knee kinematics. Besides, recognition and treatment of concurrent knee injuries help to restore knee kinematics and preclude lower results and registry studies keep going to define which graft produces the best results. The use of registry studies has given various large-scale epidemiologic studies that have supported result data, such as averting allografts in children and incorporating extra-articular stabilizing techniques in younger athletes to preclude re-rupture [1]. The purpose of this chapter is to review recent developments on ACLR.

3.2 Postoperative Infection: Prevention and Treatment

According to Rodriguez-Merchan and Ribbans, around 1% of ACLR procedures develop septic arthritis in spite of intravenous antibiotic prophylaxis and other deterrent actions. Infection is most usually due to contamination in the course of autograft harvest and preparation by introducing bacteria into the knee during graft insertion. Presoaking ACL grafts in 5 mg/mL vancomycin ("vancomycin wrap") has been used to eliminate such bacterial contamination. Numerous level 3 studies have published a considerable reduction in infection percentages with no increase in graft failure percentages. However, the absence of prospective randomized control trials and these studies' heterogeneity do not permit a worldwide recommendation for vancomycin presoaking of all grafts during ACLR. Randomized controlled trials are required to prove effectiveness in diminishing sepsis percentages [2].

Because septic arthritis following ACLR is an unusual adverse event, data on preclusion approaches has not been considerably analyzed. According to Figueroa and Figueroa, recommendations that can be made from the attainable data are as follows: prophylactic intravenous antibiotics should be used preoperatively; patellar tendon autograft utilization diminishes the likelihood of a postoperative infection; and vancomycin presoaking of grafts is firmly advised, especially

E. C. Rodríguez-Merchán (✉) · C. A. Encinas-Ullán
J. S. Ruiz-Pérez · P. Gómez-Cardero
Department of Orthopedic Surgery, La Paz University Hospital, Madrid, Spain

E. C. Rodríguez-Merchán (ed.), *Advances in Orthopedic Surgery of the Knee*,
https://doi.org/10.1007/978-3-031-33061-2_3

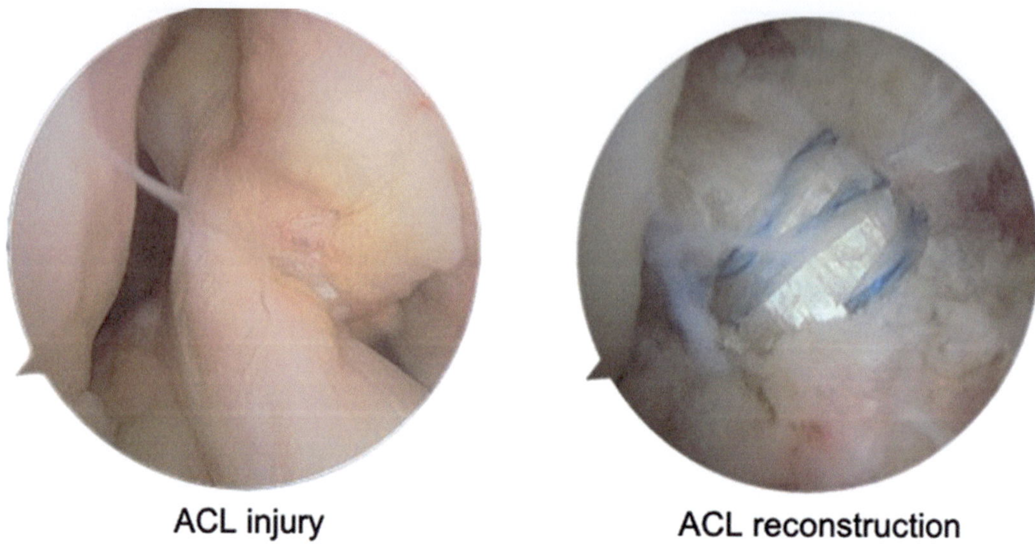

Fig. 3.1 Arthroscopic images of anterior cruciate ligament (ACL) injury (left) and ACL reconstruction (ACLR) (right)

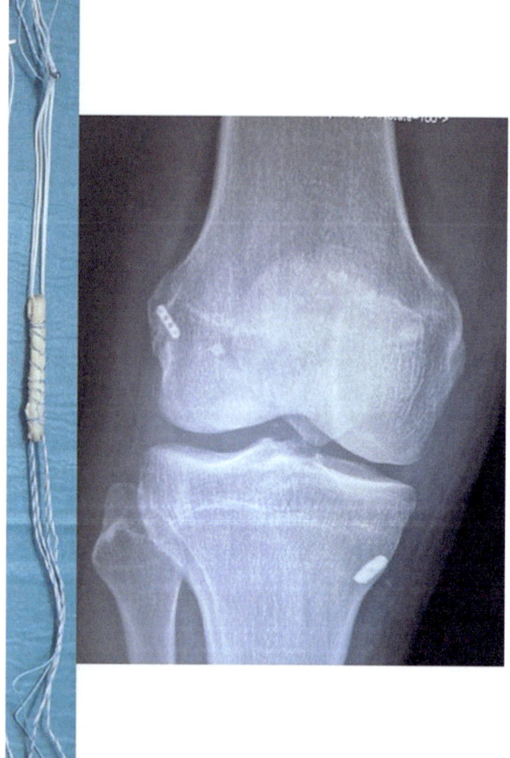

Fig. 3.2 All-inside anterior cruciate ligament reconstruction (ACLR) using only semitendinosus tendon (left) and postoperative radiographic image (right)

when carrying out hamstring autograft ACLR. When septic arthritis appears following ACLR, early treatment is essential to permit a satisfactory result. Consequently, early clinical suspicion is the most important factor to accomplish a prompt diagnosis. The management of choice is arthroscopic lavage with intravenous antibiotic treatment. Graft retention, when plausible, is relevant for attaining better functional outcomes [3].

During knee arthroscopy, irrigation fluid from the surgical field accumulates in the sterile reservoir. Whether these fluid collections and also suture material utilized during knee arthroscopy exhibit bacterial contamination over time during surgery endures unclear. Bartek et al. tried to define the contamination percentage and to analyze its potential impact on postoperative infection [4]. In a study with level 4 of evidence, 155 individuals were analyzed. Fifty-eight experienced ACLR, 63 meniscal surgery, and 34 individuals combined ACLR and meniscus repair. Bartek et al. collected pooled samples of irrigation fluid from the reservoir on the sterile drape every 15 min during the surgery. Besides, the assessed suture material of ACL graft and meniscus repair for bacterial contamination. Samples were sent for microbiological analysis; incubation time was 14 days. All individuals were seen in the outpatient department 6 weeks, 12 weeks, and 12 months postoperatively and examined for clinical signs of infection. A great statistical correlation was encountered between an advanced time span of surgery and the number of positive microbiological findings in the accumulated fluid. Suture and fixation material demonstrated a contamination rate of 28.4% (29 cases). In spite of the elevated contamination percentage, only one infection was encountered in the follow-up examinations, caused by *Staphylococcus lugdunensis*. Taking into account that bacterial contamination of accumulated fluid increases over time, the contact with the fluid reservoirs should be averted [4].

3.3   Return to Play (RTP) Testing

Hurley et al. systematically reviewed the evidence regarding return to sport assessment after ACLR and assessed the relationship between testing and secondary ACL injury (study with level 3 of evidence). Overall, 34.3% (420/1224) individuals passed the RTP testing. Those who passed the RTP testing had a statistically significant 47% lower rate of ACL graft re-rupture compared to those who did not pass the RTP testing. However, there was a barely higher, although not statistically significant, percentage of contralateral ACL rupture in those who passed the RTP testing compared to those who did not. There was a great positive correlation between a high percentage of individuals passing the ACL RTP testing in studies and ACL graft rupture percentage in those who failed. Passing RTP testing after ACLR causes an inferior percentage of ACL graft rupture, but not contralateral ACL injury. Further assessment and standardization of RTP testing is required in order to increase dependability in recognizing individuals at risk for reinjury following ACLR [5].

3.4   Factors That Affect the Incidence of Articular Cartilage Injury

Nakamae et al. studied factors that impact the incidence of articular cartilage injury in individuals with ACL injury (study with level 3 of evidence). A total of 811 individuals were enrolled. The factors that substantially impacted the incidence of cartilage injury are shown in Fig. 3.3. An older age, a longer duration between injury and surgery, and a positive pivot shift test result were positively associated with the incidence of cartilage injury in three compartments in subjects with ACL injuries. Early ACLR is advised to avert cartilage injury [6].

Zampeli et al. studied the association between the development of articular cartilage pathology and knee rotation following single-bundle ACLR (study with level 4 of evidence) [7]. Seventeen individuals that experienced single-bundle ACLR and did not have any cartilage lesions at the time of surgery based on the Outerbridge classification or meniscal injury that needed meniscectomy; >20% were studied by magnetic resonance imaging (MRI) and in the biomechanics laboratory at a 6-year minimum follow-up. Cartilage lesions that happened following ACLR were graded on MRI according to a modified Noyes scale. For cartilage assessment, the lateral and medial femoral condyles (LFC, MFC) were divided into nine segments each (lateral, central, and medial third and each third was divided into anterior, central, and posterior segment). Tibial rotation during a pivoting task was measured with optoelectronic motion analysis system and side-to-side dissimilarities of tibial rotation between the reconstructed and contralateral intact knees were estimated. The association between the total modified Noyes scale score (outcome variable) and side-to-side differences of tibial rotation after controlling for meniscectomy and meniscal repair was examined with hierarchical regression models. Side-to-side difference of tibial rotation was associated with total modified Noyes scale score. All individuals developed new

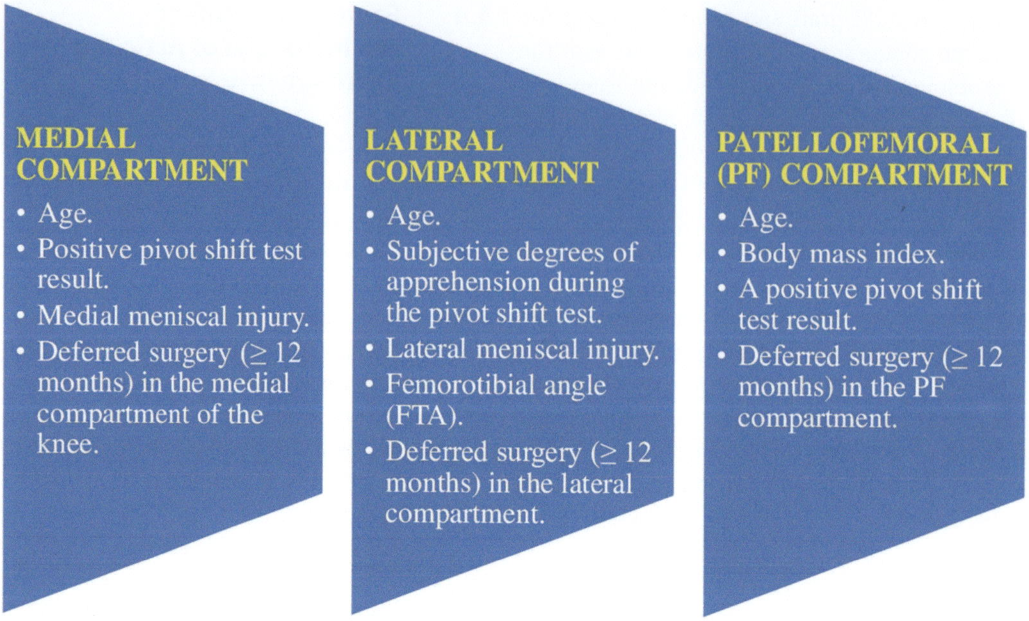

MEDIAL COMPARTMENT

- Age.
- Positive pivot shift test result.
- Medial meniscal injury.
- Deferred surgery (≥ 12 months) in the medial compartment of the knee.

LATERAL COMPARTMENT

- Age.
- Subjective degrees of apprehension during the pivot shift test.
- Lateral meniscal injury.
- Femorotibial angle (FTA).
- Deferred surgery (≥ 12 months) in the lateral compartment.

PATELLOFEMORAL (PF) COMPARTMENT

- Age.
- Body mass index.
- A positive pivot shift test result.
- Deferred surgery (≥ 12 months) in the PF compartment.

Fig. 3.3 Factors that substantially impact the incidence of cartilage injury after anterior cruciate ligament reconstruction (ACLR) [6]

cartilage lesions in MRI located principally at the central region of the lateral femoral condyle and less commonly in the central and anterior regions of the medial femoral condyle. Abnormally increased tibial rotation that persisted after ACLR was significantly associated with the development of new articular cartilage lesions at mean 8.4 years following ACLR which were located principally at the central region of the LFC and secondarily in the central and anterior regions of the MFC (more superficial lesions). The findings of this study suggested that there was emerging evidence that abnormal rotational kinematics is a potential risk factor for the pathogenesis and onset of posttraumatic articular cartilage degeneration following ACLR [7].

3.5 Quadriceps Tendon Autograft

In a study with level 3 of evidence, Winkler et al. assessed tendencies in revision ACLR, with accent on intra-articular findings, grafts, and concurrent procedures [8]. It was hypothesized that revision ACLRs over time show a tendency toward increased complexity with increased utilization of autografts over allografts. This was a two-center retrospective study including subjects experiencing revision ACLR between 2010 and 2020. Demographic and surgical information including intra-articular findings and concurrent procedures were collected and compared for the time periods 2010–2014 and 2015–2020. All collected parameters were compared between three predefined age groups (<20 years, 20–30 years, >30 years), right and left knees, and men and women. A time series analysis was carried out to evaluate tendencies in revision ACLR. This study analyzed 260 subjects with a mean age of 26.2 years at the time of the most recent revision ACLR, representing the first, second, third, and fourth revision ACLR for 214 (82%), 35 (14%), 10 (4%), and 1 (< 1%) subjects, respectively. Subjects age >30 years demonstrated a significantly longer mean time from primary ACLR to most recent revision ACLR (11.1 years), compared to subjects age <20 years (2.2 years) and age 20–30 years (5.5 years). Quadriceps tendon autograft was utilized significantly more frequently in 2015–2020 compared to 2010–2014 (49% vs. 18%) (Fig. 3.4, top). An elevated per-

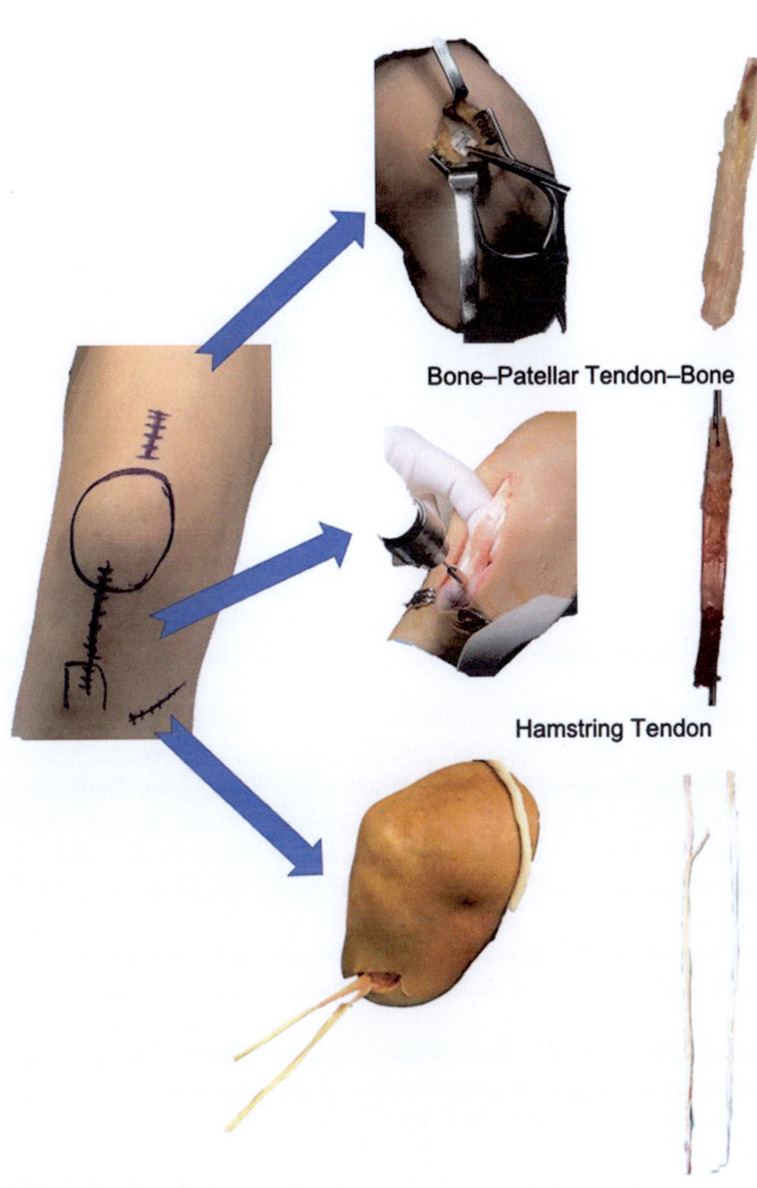

Fig. 3.4 Types of autografts used in anterior cruciate ligament reconstruction (ACLR): quadriceps tendon (top), bone-patellar tendon-bone (center), hamstring tendon (bottom)

centage of concurrently carried out procedures including meniscal repairs (45%), lateral extra-articular tenodesis (LET; 31%), osteotomies (13%), and meniscal allograft transplantations (11%) was demonstrated. Concurrent LET was associated with intact cartilage and severely abnormal preoperative knee laxity and demonstrated a statistically significant and linear increase over time. Intact cartilage (41%), concurrent medial meniscal repairs (39%), and LET (35%) were most commonly found in individuals aged <20 years. Winkler et al. stated that quadriceps tendon autograft and concurrent LET were becoming more and more popular in revision ACLR. Intact cartilage and severely abnormal preoperative knee laxity represent indications for LET in revision ACLR (Fig. 3.5). The elevated percentage of concurrent surgical techniques found demonstrated the high surgical demands of revision ACLR [8].

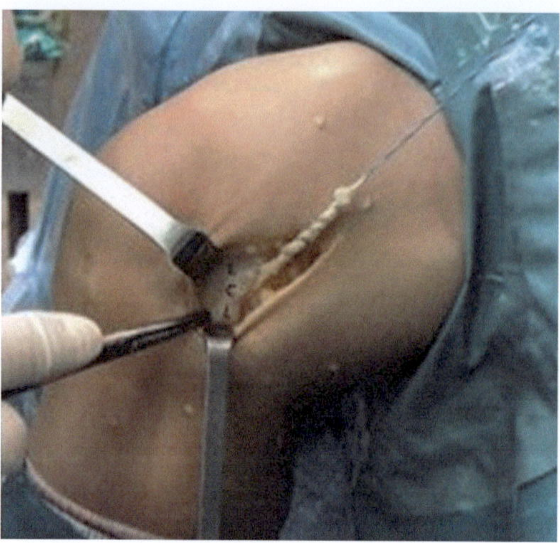

Fig. 3.5 Lemaire's lateral extra-articular tenodesis (LET) combined with anterior cruciate ligament reconstruction (ACLR). LCL = lateral collateral ligament

3.6 Biologic Agents to Optimize Outcomes

According to Kon et al., management alternatives for ACL injuries have notably developed over the past decades. Even though ACLR is a concrete fact, stimulation of ACL healing through biological methods could represent a novel conservative technique. The utilization of biologic products, such as platelet-rich plasma (PRP) or mesenchymal stem cells (MSCs), to manage partial ruptures or to improve ligamentization following ACLR, could thoroughly improve clinical results. The systematic review reported by Kon et al. concluded that no clinical superiority has been described when utilizing PRP in ACLR. Concerning ACL healing in partial tears, the application of PRP has led to encouraging results, but these findings should be validated by properly designed randomized control trials (RCTs) [9].

3.7 Quadriceps Versus Hamstring Tendon Autografts

According to Horstmann et al., comparable information of functional results of ACLR utilizing either hamstring or quadriceps tendon grafts is debatable (Fig. 3.4, bottom and top). Hortsmann et al. carried out a prospective RCT to provide information comparing both grafts regarding the functional result [10]. A two-center trial involving symptomatic subjects 18 years of age or older with an ACL tear was performed. They randomly assigned 27 subjects to quadruple hamstring tendon reconstruction and 24 to quadriceps tendon reconstruction. The subjects were assessed preoperatively, at 3, 6, 12, and 24 months postsurgery. The main outcome parameter was the side-to-side knee laxity determined with an arthrometer. Secondary outcomes included results in the International Knee Documentation Committee (IKDC) and Lysholm scores and isokinetic testing of strength in knee extension and flexion. Forty-four subjects (86%) completed the 2-year follow-up. There was substantially improved knee stability at all time intervals with no dissimilarity between the two study groups. The manual side-to-side displacement improved by 4.7 mm in subjects with hamstring tendon reconstruction and 5.5 mm in subjects with quadriceps tendon reconstruction. Besides, muscle strength and outcome scores (IKDC and Lysholm score) did not demonstrate any dissimilarities between the hamstring tendon group and the quadriceps tendon group. Subjects in the hamstring tendon group returned to their preinjury activity level after 95.2 days, while subjects in the quadriceps tendon group needed 82.1 days. Quadriceps and hamstring tendon autografts gave comparably good outcomes in primary ACLR [10].

3.8 ACLR Combined with LET

According to Viglietta et al., interest in the role of LET in averting rotatory instability and the pivot shift phenomenon after ACLR has been lately renewed (Fig. 3.5). Nonetheless, the aforementioned authors affirmed that there was still concern about overconstraint of the lateral compartment of the knee and the risk of subsequent osteoarthritis (OA) [11]. In a study with level 3 of evidence, Viglietta et al. compared long-run subjective and objective results and the percentage of OA development between subjects experiencing isolated ACLR (iACLR) with a hamstring tendon autograft and those with a combined Arnold-Coker modification of the McIntosh extra-articular procedure. Risk factors for long-run OA were evaluated. The study included 165 consecutive subjects treated at a single center by ACLR. A total of 86 subjects experienced iACLR (iACLR group) and 79 received combined intra- and extra-articular reconstruction (ACLR+LET). The IKDC, Lysholm, and Tegner activity scores were administered. Knee stability was tested through the Lachman test, the pivot shift test, and the KT-1000 knee arthrometer test. A positive pivot shift test (++/+++), laxity on the KT-1000, and referred giving-way episodes or revision ACLR were considered failures. Radiographic results were evaluated according to the Fairbank, IKDC, and Kellgren-Lawrence (K-L) scales. Radiographic assessment included both the overall tibiofemoral joint and the medial and lateral compartment separately. The mean follow-up was 15.7 years. There were no statistically significant differences in subjective scores between the two groups. A side-to-side difference > 5 mm on the KT-1000 arthrometer assessment was encountered in eight subjects in the iACLR group and in one subject in the ACLR+LET group. Nine cases of failure were encountered in the iACLR group and only one case was encountered in the ACLR+LET group. Subjects in the iACLR group had a significantly higher OA degrees than those in the ACLR+LET group for the overall tibiofemoral joint and the lateral compartment of the knee. No differences were encountered in the medial compartment. A higher level of lateral compartment OA was encountered in subjects who experienced partial lateral meniscectomy in the iACLR group compared with those in the ACLR+LET group. It was shown that meniscectomy was the most significant factor for long-run OA development. A significantly higher risk of long-run OA was encountered with iACLR than with ACLR combined with the Arnold-Coker modification of the McIntosh extra-articular technique. Knees with combined ACLR also had a significantly lower OA degree after partial lateral meniscectomy. Besides, those experiencing combined ACLR had better knee stability and lower graft rupture

percentages at the long-run follow-up. Partial meniscectomy was the principal risk factor negatively associated with OA changes [11].

Williams affirmed that LET diminishes ACL graft re-rupture percentages in high-risk subjects [12]. Moreover, he believed in iliotibial band (ITB)-related LET to restrain anterolateral rotatory instability (ALRI) in ACL that is injured and reconstructed and not in the "anterolateral ligament" or related procedures. However, Williams also expressed that the potential for conflict of a modified Lemaire LET femoral tunnel with an ACL femoral tunnel was higher than appreciated, and it risks iatrogenic ACL graft damage or compromised fixation. For MacIntosh LET, Williams uses a staple to fix a strip of ITB (left attached distally to Gerdy's tubercle) at the lateral femoral metaphysis. The tines of the staple are proximal to the ACL femoral tunnel and fixation, so conflict cannot happen. For modified Lemaire LET, the ITB graft is taken deep to the lateral collateral ligament (LCL) and attached at "Lemaire's point" on the lateral femur (proximal and posterior to the LCL femoral attachment). For fixation, Williams uses a 15-mm length suture anchor, sufficiently short to avert conflict. He presumes fixation is less strong with sutures, so the 2–3 cm of ITB graft proximal to the suture is turned distally back over the LCL and sutured to itself. This does create a thickened contour to the lateral knee, but excellent clinical results. Finally, Williams recommended the anteromedial bundle (AMB) position for the femoral tunnel, as in his experience in professional soccer players, utilizing the central "anatomic" position increases percentages of ACL graft re-rupture. Moreover, "anatomic" femoral tunnel position results in a flatter trajectory increasing the risk of conflict with a LET tunnel (or lateral physical damage in subjects with open growth plates) [12].

3.9 Tear Rates of the Ipsilateral ACL Graft Versus the Contralateral Native ACL

In a retrospective cohort study with level 3 of evidence, Ifran et al. compared the tear percentages of ipsilateral ACL grafts and the contralateral native ACL and studied the correlation of gender, age at time of surgery, and body mass index (BMI) with the occurrence of these injuries [13]. The medical records of 751 subjects who experienced ACLR with follow-up periods of 2 to 7 years were retrospectively analyzed. Survival analyses of ipsilateral ACL grafts and contralateral native ACL were carried out. The tear percentages of the ipsilateral ACL graft and contralateral ACL were 5.86% and 6.66%, respectively, with no significant difference between groups. The mean time of tears of the ipsilateral ACL and contralateral ACL was also similar at 2.64 and 2.78 years, respectively, after surgery. Both the odds of sustaining an ipsilateral ACL graft and contralateral ACL tear were also significantly reduced by 0.10 and 0.14, respectively, for every 1-year increase in age at which the reconstruction was carried out. However, graft type, gender, and BMI were not associated with an increased risk of these injuries. There was no difference between tear percentages of ipsilateral ACL graft and contralateral ACL after ACLR. Subjects who experienced ACLR at a young age were at an increased risk of both ipsilateral graft and contralateral ACL rupture following an ACLR. Subjects who are young and more likely to return to competitive sports should be counselled of the risks and advised to not disregard the rehabilitation of the contralateral knee during the immediate and back to sports period of recovery [13].

3.10 Suspensory Versus Interference Tibial Fixation of Hamstring Tendon Autografts

According to Rahardja et al., the hamstring tendon is commonly utilized to reconstruct the ACL, but there is an absence of agreement on the optimal technique of fixation [14]. Registry studies have demonstrated that the type of femoral fixation device can affect the risk of revision ACLR, but it is not clear whether the type of tibial fixation has an impact. Rahardja et al. stated that in New Zealand, over 95% of hamstring tendon grafts are fixed with an adjustable loop suspensory device on the femoral side, with variable usage between suspensory and interference devices, with or without a sheath, on the tibial side. In a cohort study with level 2 of evidence, they studied the association between the type of tibial fixation device and the risk of revision ACLR. Prospective information recorded in the New Zealand ACL Registry was analyzed. Only primary ACLRs carried out with a hamstring tendon autograft fixed with a suspensory device on the femoral side were included. A total of 6145 primary ACLRs carried out between 2014 and 2019 were studied. A total of 59.6% of hamstring tendon autografts were fixed with a suspensory device on the tibial side ($n = 3662$), 17.6% with an interference screw with a sheath ($n = 1079$), and 22.8% with an interference screw without a sheath ($n = 1404$). When compared with suspensory devices, a higher revision risk was found when utilizing an interference screw with a sheath and without a sheath. The number of graft strands and a graft diameter of ≥ 8 mm were associated with the percentage of revision; however, after adjusting for confounding parameters on the multivariate analysis, they did not significantly impact the risk of revision. In this study of hamstring tendon autografts fixed with an adjustable loop suspensory device on the femoral side during primary ACLR, the utilization of an interference screw, with or without a sheath, on the tibial side resulted in a higher revision percentage when compared with a suspensory device [14].

3.11 Combined Meniscus Repair and ACLR

In 2022 Rodriguez et al. stated that meniscal tear configurations associated with ACL tears, such as root tears and ramp lesions, were usual but less easily detected on MRI compared with a complete radial tear or a locked bucket-handle tear [15]. They also stated that timely management of these tears improves results in the setting of ACLR. Besides, they mentioned that while physical examination does not enable a definitive diagnosis of meniscal root tears and ramp lesions, high-grade laxity, including a 3+ Lachman and 3+ pivot shift, should raise suspicions for these tear configurations. MRI permits visualization of both root tears and ramp lesions, even though the gold standard for diagnosis is probing at the time of arthroscopy due to a high false-negative percentage on MRI. Up to 17% of subjects with an ACL tear have a lateral meniscal root tear; a contact mechanism and augmented posterior slope are both associated with a greater prevalence of lateral meniscal root tears and these are repaired with a tunnel technique. Rodriguez et al. mentioned that meniscal ramp lesions happened in up to 41% of subjects with ACL tears due to a contact mechanism, and they preferred repair with an inside-out technique. More than 60% of complete radial meniscal tears happened in the setting of ACL tears and were preferentially repaired with a hashtag technique for minimally separated tears and a two-tunnel technique combined with an inside-out repair for more severe tears. Buckethandle tears were more frequent in the setting of chronic ACL deficiency; concurrent with ACLR urgent meniscal repair with an inside-out technique is the gold standard, which permits for precise approximation of the tear with multiple points of fixation for improved biomechanical performance. It is critical to detect and manage these tears during ACLR because of their role as secondary stabilizers and for long-run chondral protection [15].

3.12 Early ACLR Versus Initial Non-Reconstructive Treatment with Late Crossover to Surgery

Although comparable clinical and functional results have been published after nonsurgical and surgical ACL treatment, few studies have studied the effects of early versus late ACLR with initial rehabilitation. In a cohort study with level 2 of evidence, Bergerson et al. analyzed patient-reported knee function in subjects who initially experienced non-reconstructive management after an ACL injury but who later chose to experience ACLR as compared with subjects experiencing ACLR close to the index injury and subjects managed non-reconstructively at 1 to 10 years of follow-up [16]. Outcomes from the Knee Injury and Osteoarthritis Outcome Score (KOOS) were extracted from the Swedish National Knee Ligament Registry for subjects managed with non-reconstruction, early ACLR, and initial non-reconstruction but subsequent ACL reconstruction (crossover group). The $KOOS_4$ (a mean of 4 KOOS subscales) was analyzed cross-sectionally at baseline and at the 1-, 2-, 5-, and 10-year follow-ups. Besides, the Patient Acceptable Symptom State (PASS) was applied to all KOOS subscales from baseline to the 10-year follow-up. A total of 1074 crossover, 484 non-reconstruction, and 20,352 early ACLR cases were included. The crossover group reported lower $KOOS_4$ values than the group experiencing early ACLR at baseline and at all follow-ups: baseline, −6.5; 1 year, −9.3; 2 years, −4.8; 5 years, −6.1; and 10 years, −10.9. Besides, a smaller proportion of the crossover cohort accomplished a PASS on KOOS subscales at baseline and through the 1-, 2-, 5-, and 10-year follow-ups as compared with the early ACLR group. No differences were found between crossover and non-reconstruction cases on either the $KOOS_4$ or the PASS at any follow-up. A greater proportion of subjects managed with early ACLR reported acceptable knee function and superior overall knee function as compared with individuals who chose to cross over from non-reconstructive management to ACLR [16].

3.13 ACL Injury and Knee OA

In 2022 Webster et al. published a systematic review and meta-analysis to summarize the risk for the development and incidence of knee OA after ACL injury and surgical management and compare incidence percentages between surgical and nonsurgical treatment of ACL injury. There was a near sevenfold and eightfold increase in the odds for the development of knee OA post ACL injury and ACLR. Data were too heterogenous to specify a point estimate incidence for OA after ACL injury, but OA incidence was estimated at

36% at near 10 years after reconstruction surgery. A significantly higher incidence of OA was encountered for those who experience surgical treatment at a minimum 10-year follow-up. This study showed that ACL injury notably increases the risk for development of knee OA, which is likely to be present in the long-run in about a third of subjects who have reconstruction surgery. Surgical management did not diminish OA incidence in the longer run compared with non-surgical management [17].

3.14 Concomitant Anterolateral Ligament Reconstruction

Gillet et al. affirmed that to diminish the percentage of ACL graft rupture, recent surgeries have involved anterolateral ligament reconstruction (ALLR) [18] (Fig. 3.6). This reconstruction technique harvests more knee flexor muscle tendons than isolated ACLR, but its impact on knee muscle strength recovery endures unknown. In a retrospective cohort study with level 2 of evidence, Gillet et al. evaluated the impact of ALLR with a gracilis graft on the strength of the knee extensor and flexor muscles at 6 months postoperatively. Their hypothesis was that the additional amount of knee flexor harvest for ALLR would result in impairment in knee flexor muscle strength at 6 months postoperatively. A total of 186 subjects were assigned to two cohorts according to the type of surgery: ACL + ALLR (graft: semitendinosus + gracilis, $n = 119$) or isolated ACLR (graft: semitendinosus, $n = 67$). The strength of the knee extensor and flexor muscles was evaluated utilizing an isokinetic dynamometer at 90, 180, and 240 deg./s for concentric and 30 deg./s for eccentric contractions and compared between groups utilizing analysis of variance statistical parametric mapping. Regardless of the surgery and the muscle, the injured leg produced significantly less strength than the uninjured leg throughout knee flexion and extension from 30° to 90° for each angular velocity (30, 90, 180, and 240 deg./s). However, the knee muscle strength was similar between the ACL + ALLR and ACLR groups. The addition of ALLR utilizing the gracilis tendon during ACLR did not alter the muscle recovery found at 6 months postoperatively. Although more knee flexor muscle tendons were harvested in ACL + ALLR, the postoperative strength recovery was similar to that of isolated ACLR [18].

3.15 Double-Bundle Versus Single-Bundle ACLR

In a meta-analysis with level 2 of evidence, Seppänen et al. compared arthroscopic single-bundle (SB) and double-bundle (DB) ACLRs in

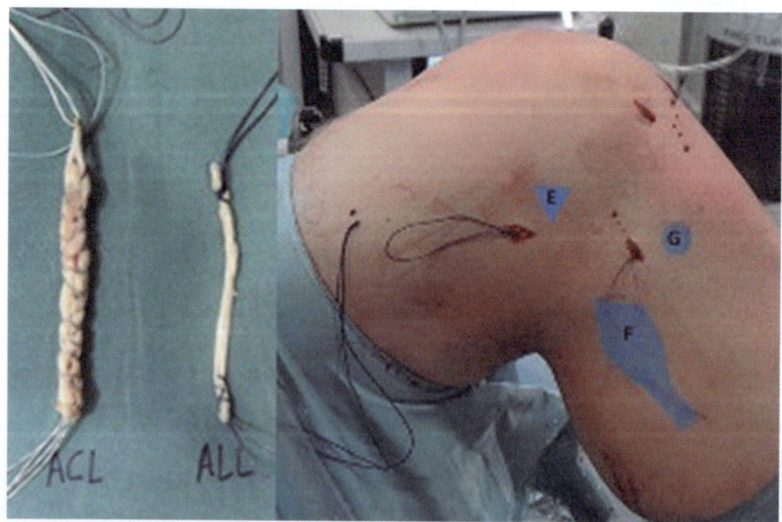

Fig. 3.6 Anterolateral ligament reconstruction (ALLR) combined with anterior cruciate ligament reconstruction (ACLR). ACL = anterior cruciate ligament; ALL = anterolateral ligament; E = lateral epicondyle; F = fibula; G = Gerdy's tubercle

the light of all accessible RCTs. A meta-analysis of this well-researched topic was carried out and subgroup analyses of the medial portal technique and the transtibial technique were added as a new idea. The hypothesis was that the DB technique was superior to the SB technique also in subgroup analyses of the medial portal and transtibial techniques. When analyzing all the included studies, the DB technique was superior to the SB technique in KT-1000/2000 assessment, IKDC subjective assessment, Lysholm scores, pivot shift, and IKDC objective assessment. Similar outcomes were also encountered in the subgroup analyses of minimum 2-years' follow-up and the transtibial technique. However, there were no dissimilarities between the two techniques in a subgroup analysis of the medial portal technique. Generally, DB ACLR led to better restoration of knee laxity and subjective results than SB ACLR. The subgroup analysis of the medial portal technique showed that orthopedic surgeons can accomplish equally as good outcomes with both techniques when femoral tunnels are drilled through the medial portal [19].

3.16 Graft Isometry During Anatomical ACLR

Moon et al. studied the surgical results of anatomical ACL according to the graft isometry measured during surgery (study with level 4 of evidence) [20]. Electrical medical records of subjects who experienced an arthroscopic ACLR through the transportal technique utilizing hamstring tendon autograft between 2012 and 2016 were retrospectively reviewed. The subjects were classified into two groups based on the graft length change throughout the knee range of motion (ROM) measured just prior to graft fixation (Group 1, graft length change ≤2 mm; Group 2, graft length change >2 mm). Comparative analyses, including a non-inferiority trial, were carried out regarding the clinical scores, knee laxity, and radiographic parameters between the groups. A total of 67 individuals were included in the study. The total change in the length of ACL graft throughout the knee ROM was 1.4 mm in Group 1 and 3 mm in Group 2. Group 1 demonstrated a relatively high (proximal) femoral tunnel and shallow (anterior) tibial tunnel compared to Group 2, but there were no apparent differences in the macroscopic view. There were no statistically significant differences in the clinical results between groups at 2 years after surgery, which satisfied the non-inferiority criterion of Group 1 in terms of clinical scores and knee laxity compared to Group 2. The surgical results of anatomical ACLR in subjects with non-isometric ACL graft were not inferior in terms of clinical scores and knee laxity, compared to those with nearly isometric ACL graft. The graft tunnel placement in the isometric position during anatomical ACLR, which is technically challenging in the clinical setting, was not an essential factor in terms of clinical results [20].

3.17 Remnant Preservation in ACLR

According to van Keulen et al., selective anteromedial or posterolateral bundle reconstruction is acknowledged as a treatment modality in partial ACLR with a biomechanically sufficient ACL remnant [21]. However, there is scarcity in literature studying clinical results of standard ACLR with preservation of residual continuous but biomechanically insufficient ACL tissue. In a study with level 3 of evidence, van Keulen et al. analyzed the impact of preservation of residual continuous but biomechanically insufficient ACL tissue in standard ACLR on complication and repeat surgery percentage and patient-reported and clinical result. The retrospective study included 134 subjects (age 23 years; Tegner 6) with an isolated acute ACL tear. In 67 individuals, residual continuous but biomechanically insufficient ACL tissue was present and preserved based on visual inspection, probing of the ACL tissue and Lachman test under arthroscopic view (standard reconstruction with tissue preservation; SRTP). These subjects were matched to 67 subjects that experienced ACLR where no residual ACL tissue could be preserved (standard reconstruction; SR) based on gender, age, and chondral and/or meniscal status. Clinical failure (recurrent instability, pathological ACL graft laxity, and/or ACL graft discontinuity), other adverse events and repeat-surgery percentage within index surgery and 1-year and within index surgery and 2-year follow-up, and patient-reported and clinical results at 1-year and at 2-year follow-up were compared. A statistically significant lower clinical failure percentage within index surgery and 1-year (SRTP, 3%; SR, 13%) and within index surgery and 2-year follow-up (SRTP, 3%; SR, 23%) and revision ACL surgery percentage within index surgery and 1-year (SRTP, 2%; ST, 10%) and within index surgery and 2-year follow-up (SRTP, 2%; SR, 18%) was encountered in the SRTP group. No statistically significant differences were observed for other studied results in subjects that were without clinical failure. This study demonstrated that in ACLR surgery, preservation of residual continuous but biomechanical insufficient ACL tissue may result in lower clinical failure percentage and ACL revision surgery percentage within index surgery and 1-year and within index surgery and 2-year follow-up compared to standard ACLR where no residual continuous ACL tissue could be preserved [21] (Fig. 3.7).

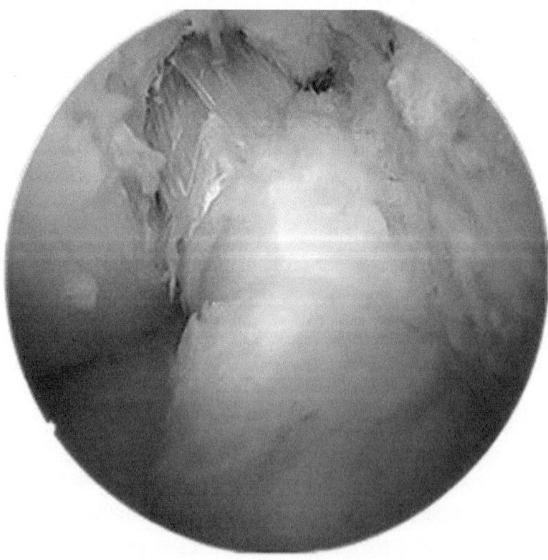

Fig. 3.7 Remnant preservation in an anterior cruciate ligament reconstruction (ACLR)

In 2022 Franciosi et al. claimed that the ACL remnant had been pointed out as a ligamentization enhancer. Nevertheless, the remaining tissue can be functional if it still provides some stability or nonfunctional. In a study with level 2 of evidence, Franciozi et al. compared the clinical outcomes and knee stability of functional vs. nonfunctional remnant preservation ACLR [22]. One hundred and seventy-five subjects with ACL injuries were included and experienced remnant preservation ACLR. They were divided into two groups accordingly to remnant tissue functionality: functional (Group F) and nonfunctional (Group NF). Primary result was defined as PROMs measured with Lysholm, IKDC, and Tegner continuous scales and improvements. Secondary results comprised of Lachman test, anterior drawer test, pivot shift test, extension and flexion deficit, graft coverage by remnant preserved tissue, and failure percentage (persistent instability or new ACL lesion). Menisci lesions, cartilage lesions, and time to surgery were also recorded for each group. One hundred and forty-four subjects were accessible at a mean of 30.2 months: 69 functional and 75 nonfunctional. Lysholm, IKDC, and Tegner functional results showed no difference between the groups, functional compared to nonfunctional: 88.4 vs. 92.2, and 83.2 vs. 87 and 6 vs. 6, respectively. Lysholm and IKDC functional result improvements showed differences between the groups: functional compared to nonfunctional (39.3 vs. 42.3 and 37.7 vs. 41.0). However, they were not clinically significant. The functional group demonstrated more stability on physical examination pre- and postoperatively. There was no difference regarding extension deficit; however, the functional group had more flexion deficit. The nonfunctional group had better graft coverage. There was no difference regarding failure rate: 4% vs. 9%. Both remnant preservation ACLR techniques were able to accomplish satisfactory functional results. A functional remnant was not related to improved functional results in comparison to a nonfunctional remnant; however, it was related to less laxity pre- and postoperatively and inferior graft coverage [22].

3.18 ACL Autograft Reconstruction Revisions with Tendon Allografts

In 2022 Vincelot-Chainard et al. reported that the number of ACLRs was steadily rising in France and also that re-tear percentages of up to 25% had been published and graft selection endured a remarkable challenge. They also stated that allografts, although rarely used in France, could be a viable alternative [23]. In a retrospective cohort study with level 4 of evidence, Vincelot-Chainard et al. analyzed the benefits of ACL revision with allografts, by determining subjective scores (IKDC score and KOOS), measuring laxity, and assessing the percentage of return to sports (RTS). Their hypothesis was that tendon allografts were dependable and could be utilized in France for ACLR revision. They performed a retrospective study including 39 subjects managed in two centers between 2004 and 2016 and followed up for at least a year. Subjects were eligible if they had experienced tendon allograft reconstruction for ACL revision with or without rupture of a peripheral plane. They excluded underage subjects and subjects with a history of ligament injury in the contralateral knee. The mean age was 32 years. The allografts were extensor mechanisms, anterior or posterior tibial tendons, fascia lata tendons, hamstring tendons, and a short fibular tendon. They were attained from French and Belgian tissue banks. They were utilized for the reconstruction of 39 ACLs and 11 collateral ligaments. The IKDC score and KOOS were determined in all individuals. Laximetry was carried out in 31 subjects by an independent examiner. The mean follow-up was 3.5 years. Arthroscopic release was needed in one subject, and two subjects experienced re-tears. No deep surgical site infections were found. The subjective IKDC score and the KOOS improved significantly, from 53.6 to 80.7 and from 60.4 to 83.2, respectively. The mean postoperative differential laxity was 1.4 mm (KT 1000) and 1.6 mm (GNRB®). Of the three individuals who were professional athletes, two had returned to sports at the same level one year later, and among the recreational athletes, 54% had resumed their prior sporting activities. The conclusion of this study was that in the setting of complex ligament reconstruction revision, tendon allografts were dependable and could be utilized [23].

3.19 Return to Work After ACLR

In 2022 Arimaa et al. affirmed that among people of working age, the return to work (RTW) after ACLR is an important marker of success of surgery. They determined when subjects were able to RTW after ACLR and recognized factors that were associated with the timing of RTW. They utilized logistic regression analyses to study patient-related factors that may be associated with the length of RTW (above vs. below the median 59 days) after arthroscopic ACLR in a large group of subjects working in the public sector in Finland ($n = 803$; $n = 334$ men, $n = 469$ women; mean age 41 years). The mean length of RTW was 65 days. Higher odds ratios were found for age groups 40–49 and ≥ 50 years compared with ≤ 30 years old, for lower-level nonmanual and manual work compared with higher-level nonmanual work, and for those who had been on sick leave >30 days in the previous year. Sex, comorbid conditions, preceding antidepressant management, and concomitant surgical procedures were not associated with the length of RTW. Factors associated with prolonged sick leave beyond the median time of 59 days were higher age, lower occupational status, and preoperative sick leaves [24].

3.20 Factors Affecting Graft Healing After ACLR

In a study with level 4 of evidence, Okutan et al. analyzed the anatomic, operative, and biological factors that impacted graft healing after single-bundle ACLR [25]. One hundred fourteen subjects who experienced anatomic single-bundle

ACLR with quadrupled hamstring tendon autografts between 2016 and 2019 were retrospectively studied. Ninety-four subjects met the inclusion criteria with minimum follow-up of 12 months. Subjects were assessed with multiple clinical measurements, including International Knee Documentation Committee Subjective Knee Form (IKDC-SKF), Lyshom Scores, and Marx Activity Scale. To assess graft healing, the signal-to-noise quotient (SNQ) was measured at intra-articular graft and intra-tunnel integration were assessed on MRI at one year after surgery. Potential factors impacting graft healing, including age, sex, BMI, time from injury to surgery, posterior tibial slope, lateral femoral condyle ratio, notch width index, meniscal injury, remnant preservation, tunnel aperture locations, graft size, graft bending angle, and graft/remaining notch volume ratio were assessed for their association with graft SNQ value by stepwise regression analysis. A total of 94 subjects were assessed with a mean follow-up of 28.5 months. The results are shown in Fig. 3.8. There was no correlation between graft SNQ values and IKDC-SKF and Lysholm scores. There was no correlation between graft SNQ values and International Knee Documentation Committee (IKDC) and Lysholm scores. Tibial slope, remnant preservation, and graft/remaining notch volume ratio were significant independent associated factors of graft SNQ value at one year. The graft SNQ values were also weakly correlated with femoral tunnel integration and the Marx Activity Scale. Okutan et al. concluded that these factors should be taken into account for ensuring the ideal graft healing and for the return to sport (RTS) decision-making [25].

3.21 Anteromedial Versus Central Femoral Tunnel Placement After Single-Bundle ACLR

In a study with level 2 of evidence, Zhang et al. compared clinical results and graft healing after ACLR with anteromedial and central femoral tunnel placement [26]. During 2016 and 2018, 110 consecutive subjects experienced single-bundle ACLR; 85 subjects met the inclusion criteria, and each subject experienced 3D-CT (3D computed tomography) within 1 week and MRI 1.5 years after the operation. The central point of the femoral tunnel and signal-to-noise quotient (SNQ) of three regions of interest (ROIs) in the intra-articular graft were estimated to study the tunnel position and graft healing extent. Clinical evaluations, including functional scores, KT-2000 arthrometer measurements, and pivot shift tests, were assessed at the 2-year follow-up. Subjects were divided into two groups depending on the femoral tunnel position: the anteromedial position group (Group A) and the center position group (Group B). Seventy-one subjects were accessible for the 2-year follow-up and MRI

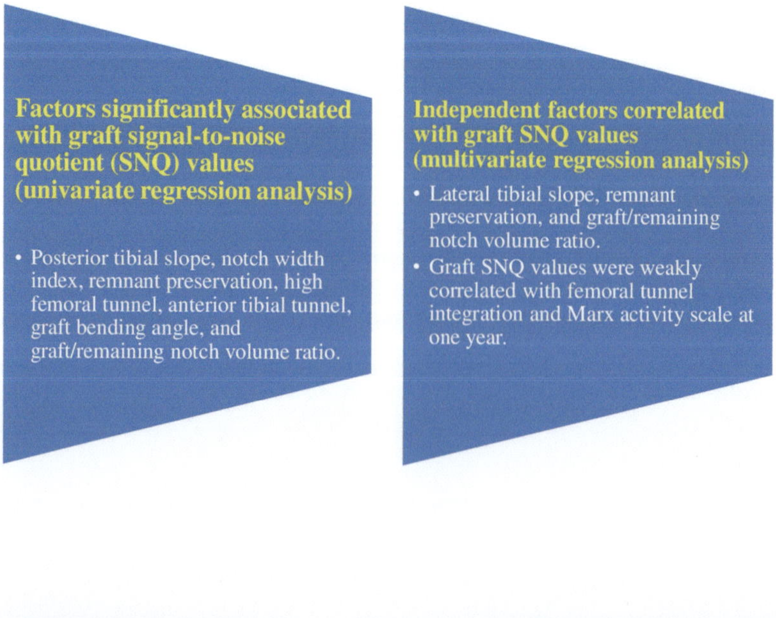

Fig. 3.8 Factors that impact graft healing after single-bundle anterior cruciate ligament reconstruction (ACLR) [25]

examination – 34 subjects in Group A and 35 subjects in Group B – and 2 subjects were excluded for an eccentric tunnel position. No graft failure happened and compared with the preoperative evaluation outcomes, the results of both groups improved at the final follow-up. Group A was significantly better than Group B regarding the KT-2000 arthrometer measurements. No significant differences were found in terms of functional scores, pivot shift test results, or the SNQ between groups. No differences in clinical results or graft healing were encountered between anteromedial and central femoral tunnel placements in single-bundle ACLR. The conclusion of Zhang et al. was that satisfactory clinical results, knee stability, and graft healing can be attained for both femoral tunnel placements [26].

3.22   ACLR in Small-Statured Female Individuals

According to Goto et al., the choice of graft for ACLR remains debatable, and the quadriceps tendon (QT) autograft is a good option for ACLR. However, concerns regarding its utilization in short-statured individuals, related to donor site morbidity, anterior knee pain, or loss of muscle strength, remain. In a study with level 4 of evidence, Goto et al. compared muscle strength and morbidity between individuals with short and normal statures following ACLR with a QT autograft. A total of 73 women (mean age, 33.8 years) who experienced primary ACLR between 2016 and 2019 were included. Subjects were categorized into two groups: group S, with a height $\leq$ 163 cm, and group L, with a height > 163 cm. Muscle strength, harvesting site morbidity, and ACL return to sport after injury scale (ACL-RSI) were assessed, with a mean timing of the follow-up of 9 months. The mean quadriceps strength for the isokinetic measurements at 60° and 240° were 65.0% and 74.0% in group S, respectively, and 70.0% and 75.7% in group L, respectively. There was no significant difference in the postoperative muscle strength or mean ACL-RSI (group S, 70.0; group L, 65.9) between the groups. No donor site morbidity was

found in either group. Muscle strength recovery, morbidity, and readiness to return to sports were similar in both groups, which supported the possibility of QT autografts for women with a small stature [27].

3.23   Factors Affecting Graft Failure and Return to Play After ACLR

In 2022 Liu et al. expressed that the posterior tibial slope (PTS) was considered a risk factor for ACL injury. However, the impact of PTS on graft failure following ACLR remained relatively unknown [28]. In a systematic review with level 4 of evidence, Liu et al. investigated whether PTS could be a potential risk factor for graft failure after ACLR. Observational studies reporting the associations of medial tibial plateau slope (MTPS) or lateral tibial plateau slope (LTPS) with graft failure after ACLR were assessed. Twenty studies implicating 12 case-control studies, 4 retrospective studies, and 4 cross-sectional studies including 5326 subjects met the final inclusion criteria. The elevated heterogeneity and the characteristics of nonrandomized controlled trials limited data synthesis. Fifteen of the 20 included studies found a significant association between increased PTS and ACL graft failure, while 5 studies concluded that increased PTS was not associated with ACL graft failure. Ten studies suggested that MTPS was associated with ACL graft failure, and six studies suggested that LTPS was associated with ACL graft failure. The mean MTPS values for the nonfailure group ranged from 3.5° to 14.4°. For the graft failure group, MTPS ranged from 4.71° to 17.2°. The mean LTPS values for the nonfailure group ranged from 2.9° to 11.9°. For the graft failure group, LTPS ranged from 5.5° to 13.3°. The reported PTS values that caused ACL graft failure was greater than 7.4° to 17°. Increased PTS was associated with a higher risk of ACL graft failure after ACLR. In spite of various methods of measuring PTS have elevated dependability, there is still vast disagreement in the actual value of PTS [28].

In 2022 Balendra et al. stated that modern ACLR techniques have led to improved results in professional footballers [29]. In a study with level 4 of evidence, Balendra et al. evaluated patient, surgical, and postoperative factors that impacted percentages and time to RTP as well as ACL re-rupture percentages. They performed a retrospective review of consecutive ACLR undertaken in professional footballers between 2005 and 2018. Two hundred and thirty-two knees in 215 professional footballers (17 bilateral) were included. Two hundred five (88.9%) were male and average age at surgery was 23.3 years. Two hundred and twenty-two (96.1%) returned to professional football, with 209 (90.1%) returning to the same or higher Tegner level. Subgroup analysis showed three factors that independently impacted RTP percentage: Players under 25 years had a higher percentage of RTP (99.3% vs 90.2%); a subsequent operation before RTP reduced RTP percentage from 98.2% to 89.7%; experiencing meniscal surgery at ACLR reduced RTP percentage. The mean time to RTP from surgery was 10.5 months. Factors encountered to increase RTP time included age under 25 (11.0 vs. 9.7 months), recurrent effusions (11.4 vs. 10.2 months), and medial meniscal repair at ACLR compared to meniscectomy (12.5 vs. 9.6 months). The surgical technique varied over the study period in relation to graft type, femoral tunnel position, and addition of LET. Overall, the re-rupture rate was 8.2% at 2 years. Patella tendon autograft in an anteromedial bundle femoral tunnel position with addition of LET had the lowest re-rupture percentage (2%). Primary ACLR in professional footballers yielded high percentages of RTP (96.1%), with 90.1% at the same level or higher, at a mean 10.5 months. Subjects under 25 years not only had a significantly higher RTP percentage, but also had a lengthier period of rehabilitation [29].

3.24 ACLR with Hamstring Tendon Graft and Femoral Cortical Button Fixation

According to Hagemans et al., the short-run results of ACLR with bone-patellar tendon-bone or hamstring tendon (HT) graft are excellent with good clinical stability and PROMs [30] (Fig. 3.3, center and bottom). They stated that although some studies had reported the long-run results of bone-patellar tendon-bone graft ACLR, few had reported the results of HT graft ACLR. In a case series with a level 4 of evidence, Hagemans et al. assessed clinical and radiographic results of HT graft ACLR with femoral cortical button fixation at a minimum 20-year follow-up. A prospective study was carried out in which all individuals experiencing isolated transtibial primary ACLR between 1994 and 1996 with HT graft and femoral cortical button fixation were evaluated clinically and radiographically. Follow-up was attained in 48 of 94 subjects (51%). Median age at operation was 31 years; median follow-up was 21 years; 65% were men; and 48% had meniscal injury at surgery and experienced partial meniscectomy. Graft rupture, reoperation, and contralateral injury percentages were evaluated; clinical stability was measured utilizing the KT-1000 arthrometer; PROMs were evaluated (IKDC, Lysholm, Forgotten Joint Score, Tegner activity, KOOS, ACL Quality of Life [ACL-QOL], EuroQol 5-Dimension 5-Level [EQ-5D-5L]); and radiographic OA (defined as K-L grade $\geq$ 2) was evaluated for the ipsilateral and the contralateral knee. Graft rupture happened in 4 subjects (8%), contralateral injury in 4 subjects (8%), and reoperation in 15 subjects (31%), which consisted principally of meniscal tears or hardware removal. In subjects with an intact graft, excellent PROMs were found, with a median Lysholm of 90, subjective IKDC of 86, and KOOS-Sports of 86. There was low awareness of the operated knee (Forgotten Joint Score, 81) and good quality of life (ACL-QOL, 85; EQ-5D-5L, 0.87). Median side-to-side difference, as measured with the KT-1000 arthrometer, was 1 mm. Radiographic OA was evident in 49% of ipsilateral and 10% of contralateral knees and was associated with meniscectomy at index surgery and decreased PROMs at follow-up. Long-run results of transtibial HT graft ACLR with femoral cortical button fixation were generally good with a low failure percentage, low awareness of the operated knee, and good clinical stability. Radiographic OA was evident in about half of the subjects at 20-year follow-up and was associated with meniscectomy at index surgery and diminished PROMs at follow-up [30].

3.25 Revision ACLR

In 2022 Marx et al. stated that although there had been substantial improvement in ACL reconstructive surgery, graft failure remained a devastating adverse event for some subjects. Besides, revision procedures were inherently more complex and technically challenging [31]. In a study with level 3 of evidence, Marx et al. analyzed prevalence of short-run adverse events after these procedures and compared tendencies in operative length, relative valuation, and reimbursement after primary versus revision ACLR. Primary and revision arthroscopic ACLR cases were identified on the American College of Surgeons' NSQIP database utilizing Current Procedural Terminology (CPT) and International Classification of Diseases (ICD) codes between January 1, 2012, and December 31, 2017. Demographics, subject variables, and surgical variables were compared between primary and revision groups. Logistic regression was utilized to recognize independent risk factors for revision ACLR. Diverse 30-day outcome measures were compared between the primary and revision ACL reconstruction groups. Diverse measures of valuation – including total relative value units (RVUs) and reimbursement per minute – were estimated and compared between the two groups. A total of 8292 individuals – 8135 primary and 157 revision procedures – were included in the final cohort. Higher ASA (American Society of Anesthesiology) scores were associated with revision ACLRs. Subjects experiencing revision procedures were less likely to have an ASA score of 1 and more likely to have an ASA score of 2 or 3. Revision ACLR was associated with higher percentages of poor 30-day outcome measures, including unplanned readmission, reoperation, return to the operating room, and surgical adverse events. The total RVUs and reimbursement for revision procedures were significantly greater than those for primary procedures. However, when accounting for operative time, the RVU/minute and reimbursement/minute were similar between the two groups. Relative to primary ACLR, revision ACL procedures were associated with worse short-run results – including unplanned readmission, reoperation, return to the operating room, and surgical adverse events. A greater ASA score was independently predictive of revision ACL surgery [31].

In 2022 Kanakamedala et al. stated that **revision ACLR** procedures were frequently technically and intellectually challenging. Also, that with careful preoperative assessment and planning, the likelihood of success could be maximized. They also affirmed that comprehending the diverse etiologies of and contributors to primary ACLR failure could guide the surgical plan in terms of whether concomitant procedures were required. Also, although successful results had been published with both one-stage and two-stage revision ACLRs, adequate patient selection was essential. Overall, clinical results including PROMs, graft failure percentages, and RTS were worse after revision ACLR compared with primary ACLR [32].

3.26 ACLR in Children and Adolescents

Taking into account that there are limited epidemiologic data examining the incidence of pediatric ACLR over the past decade, Brodeur et al. performed a descriptive epidemiology study to examine statewide population tendencies in the prevalence of ACLR in a pediatric population [33]. Inpatient and outpatient claims for pediatric patients who experienced ACLR between 2009 and 2017 were recognized in the New York Statewide Planning and Research Cooperative System database via ICD, Revision 9, Clinical Modification; ICD, Revision 10, Clinical Modification and Procedural Classification System; or Current Procedural Terminology codes. New York population data for each year between 2009 and 2017 were utilized from the New York State Department of Health to estimate the percentages of ACLR per 100,000 people aged 3 to 19 years and establish the 95% confidence limits. The percentages were then stratified by age, sex, and insurance. Two-year percentages of revision and contralateral ACLR were also analyzed by sex. Between 2009 and 2017, 20,170 pediatric ACLRs were recognized. The percentages of pediatric ACLR increased steadily from 49.3 per

100,000 in 2009 to a peak of 61 in 2014 and diminished to 51.8 by 2017. The age group 15 to 17 years had the highest percentages of ACLR of all age groups, peaking at 198.5 per 100,000. Analysis by sex demonstrated that ACLR percentages between men and women were not different. Males had a 2-year ipsilateral revision percentage of 4.3%, while females had a percentage of 3.3%. Females had a contralateral ACLR percentage of 4%, while males had a percentage of 2.6%. Pediatric ACLR percentages continued to rise until 2014, but there was a demonstrable reduction in percentages after 2014. This decline in pediatric ACLR may point to the effectiveness of injury prevention programs or changes in practice management. The elevated revision percentage in men and high contralateral surgery percentage in women can help guide patient counseling for RTP and adverse events risk [33].

Malige et al. presented a current concept review of revision ACLR in pediatric patients, discussing risk factors for re-rupture, physical examination and imaging, treatment principles and surgical techniques, postoperative rehabilitation, and clinical results. They stated that surgical treatment should be individualized, and the graft type, fixation devices, tunnel placement, and complementary procedures (e.g., LET) should be tailored to the patient's needs and previous surgeries. Rehabilitation programs should also be centered around eccentric strengthening, isometric quadriceps strengthening, active flexion ROM of the knee, and an emphasis on closed-chain exercises. In spite of adherence to strict surgical and postoperative rehabilitation principles, graft re-failure percentage is elevated, and return to sports percentage is low. Re-rupture of the ACL in the pediatric population is a challenging adverse event that needs special attention. Diagnostic assessment of repeat ACL ruptures must be similar to primary injuries. Although results after revision ACLR are expectedly worse than after primary reconstruction, athletes do return to sport after adequate rehabilitation. Further research is required to continue to improve results in this high-risk population, aimed at continued knee stability, graft survivorship, and improved quality of life [34].

According to Kew et al., sports injuries have increased in the pediatric and adolescent population [35]. RTS testing and criteria have been increasingly utilized; however, the recommendations for RTP in adolescents are not clear. In a retrospective cohort study with level 4 of evidence, Kew et al. compared strength and function at the time of the return-to-sport progression to those with and without a failed ACLR. A total of 105 adolescent patients with primary ACLR were evaluated at the time of return to sport. Kew et al. identified graft failures/contralateral injury through medical records, clinic visits, or phone interviews at minimum 2 years of postsurgical follow-up. All individuals completed bilateral isokinetic strength tests of the knee extensor/flexor groups and hop tests. Strength was expressed as torque normalized to mass (Nm/kg), and limb symmetry index was expressed as a percentage of the uninvolved limb's strength. All subjects completed result surveys. A total of 100 of 105 subjects (95.2%) were included with 4 years of follow-up, with 28 (28%) sustaining subsequent injury (12% graft, 16% contralateral). Subjects with graft failure showed stronger quadriceps strength (2.00 Nm/kg) compared with those with contralateral ACL injury (1.58 Nm/kg) and subjects that did not have a secondary injury (1.58 Nm/kg), greater quadriceps strength symmetry (85.7%) compared with subjects without secondary injury ACL (72.9%), and a greater proportion of hamstring grafts compared with those without reinjury. Adolescent subjects who sustained ACLR graft failure had greater and more symmetric quadriceps strength at the time of return to sport compared with subjects with no secondary injury [35].

In a therapeutic study with level 3 of evidence, Toker et al. assessed the SB and DB ACLR in terms of graft survival, adverse events, and PROMs in adolescent athletes [36]. In a retrospective study, 89 elite adolescent athletes who experienced either SB or DB ACLR were included. All individuals were then divided into two groups: group 1 including 51 subjects with SB ACLR (31 male, 20 female; mean age = 15.4 years) and group 2 including 38 subjects with DB ACL (30 male, 8 female; mean age = 15.7 years). Clinical data were attained, comprising skeletal maturity, sports type, ACLR technique, Lachman scores, KT-1000™ arthrometer measurement, and additional meniscal procedures as well as IKDC score, Cincinnati score, and graft size. The mean follow-up period was 53.1 months in group 1 and 46.4 months in group 2. The type of ACLR technique (SB or DB), gender, skeletal maturity, sports type, additional meniscal procedures, and Lachman scores were not associated with the re-rupture of the ACL. Moreover, the ACLR technique did not impact the percentage of re-rupture of an ACL. There were 21 re-ruptures (23.5%) and 11 (12.3%) contralateral ACL ruptures in total. Among 21 re-ruptures, 12 of them were in the DB group, while nine of them in the SB group. The groups did not differ with respect to age, the injured side, the time from injury to surgery, the postoperative follow-up time, or the preoperative physical examination results from the KT-1000 device, Cincinnati score, IKDC objective and subjective score, Lachman test, and pivot shift test. There were no differences in the re-rupture of an ACL, PROMs, and adverse events in adolescent elite players, when either an SB or DB technique was carried out [36].

3.27 Rates of Infection After ACLR Among Pediatric Patients and Adolescent Patients (Compared with Young Adult Patients)

In 2022 Elsenberg et al. stated that numerous publications had shown an increase in the number of ACLR procedures carried out in children. Also, in spite of this, most knowledge of surgical site infection percentages after these procedures were based on adult publications and information was currently limited in children [37]. In a retrospective comparative study with level 3 of evidence, Eisenberg et al. studied the percentages of infection after ACLR among pediatric patients and adolescent patients (compared with young adult patients) using the MarketScan Commercial Claims and Encounters Database. The Truven Health Analytics MarketScan Commercial Claims and Encounters database was evaluated to access health care utilization information for privately insured subjects aged 5 to 30 years old. ACLR records carried out between 2006 and 2018 were recognized utilizing Current Procedural Terminology (CPT) codes. ICD Ninth Revision (ICD-9) codes, Tenth (ICD-10) codes, and CPT codes were utilized to recognize subjects needing treatment for infection. All individuals had at least 180 days of insurance coverage after intervention. A total of 44,501 subjects aged below 18 years old and 63,495 subjects aged 18 to 30 years old that experienced arthroscopic ACLR were recognized. There were no dissimilarities in infection percentages between those below 18 years old (0.52%) and those above 18 years old (0.46%). However, among subjects below 18 years old, subjects below 15 years old had a significantly lower percentage of infection at 0.37% compared with adolescents (15 to 17 years old) at 0.55%. Among young adults, males had higher percentages of infection than females (0.52% vs. 0.37%), while no dissimilarity was found in the pediatric and adolescent population (0.58% vs. 0.47%). This study showed that percentages of infection after ACLR in a pediatric/adolescent population are low (0.52%) and similar to percentages in young adults. Infection percentages following ACLR seemed to be slightly lower in subjects under 15 years of age (0.37%) [37].

3.28 Conclusions

In anterior cruciate ligament (ACL) reconstruction (ACLR), anatomic tunnel placement is essential in precluding graft impingement and reestablishing knee kinematics. Besides, recognition and treatment of concurrent knee injuries help to restore knee kinematics and preclude lower results. Allografts must be avoided in children. In younger athletes extra-articular stabilizing techniques must be incorporated to preclude re-rupture. An older age, a longer duration between injury and surgery, and a positive pivot shift test result are positively associated with the incidence of cartilage injury in three compartments in subjects with ACL injuries. Early ACLR is advised to avert cartilage injury. Abnormal rotational kinematics is a potential risk factor for the pathogenesis and onset of posttraumatic articular cartilage degeneration following ACLR. Quadriceps tendon autograft and concurrent LET are becoming more and more popular in revision ACLR. Intact cartilage and severely abnormal preoperative knee laxity represent indications for LET in revision ACLR. Quadriceps and hamstring tendon autografts give comparably good outcomes in primary ACLR. Subjects who experienced ACLR at a young age are at an increased risk of both ipsilateral graft and contralateral ACL rupture following an ACLR. It is critical to detect and manage meniscal tears during ACLR because of their role as secondary stabilizers and for long-run chondral protection. Relative to primary ACLR, revision ACL procedures are associated with worse short-run results – including unplanned readmission, reoperation, return to the operating room, and surgical adverse events. A greater ASA score is independently predictive of revision ACL surgery.

References

1. Musahl V, Nazzal EM, Lucidi GA, Serrano R, Hughes JD, Margheritini F, et al. Current trends in the anterior cruciate ligament part 1: biology and biomechanics. Knee Surg Sports Traumatol Arthrosc. 2022;30:20–33.
2. Rodriguez-Merchan EC, Ribbans WJ. The role of vancomycin-soaking of the graft in anterior cruciate ligament reconstruction. J ISAKOS. 2022;7:94–8.
3. Figueroa D, Figueroa F. Postoperative infection after anterior cruciate ligament reconstruction: prevention and management. Instr Course Lect. 2022;71:489–95.
4. Bartek B, Winkler T, Garbe A, Schelberger T, Perka C, Jung T. Bacterial contamination of irrigation fluid and suture material during ACL reconstruction and meniscus surgery: low infection rate despite increasing contamination over surgery time. Knee Surg Sports Traumatol Arthrosc. 2022;30:246–52.
5. Hurley ET, Mojica ES, Haskel JD, Mannino BJ, Alaia M, Strauss EJ, Jazrawi LM, et al. Return to play testing following anterior cruciate reconstruction - a systematic review & meta-analysis. Knee. 2022;34:134–40.
6. Nakamae A, Miyamoto A, Kamei G, Eguchi A, Shimizu R, Akao M, et al. An older age, a longer duration between injury and surgery, and positive pivot shift test results increase the prevalence of articular cartilage injury during ACL reconstruction in all three compartments of the knee in patients with ACL injuries. Knee Surg Sports Traumatol Arthrosc. 2022;30:219–30.
7. Zampeli F, Pappas E, Velonakis G, Roumpelakis IM, Poulou LS, Papagiannis GI, et al. Development of new cartilage lesions after ACL reconstruction is associated with abnormal knee rotation. Knee Surg Sports Traumatol Arthrosc. 2022;30:842–51.
8. Winkler PW, Vivacqua T, Thomassen S, Lovse L, Lesniak BP, Getgood AMJ, et al. Quadriceps tendon autograft is becoming increasingly popular in revision ACL reconstruction. Knee Surg Sports Traumatol Arthrosc. 2022;30:149–60.
9. Kon E, Di Matteo B, Altomare D, Iacono F, Kurpyakov A, Lychagin A, et al. Biologic agents to optimize outcomes following ACL repair and reconstruction: a systematic review of clinical evidence. J Orthop Res. 2022;40:10–28.
10. Horstmann H, Petri M, Tegtbur U, Felmet G, Krettek C, Jagodzinski M. Quadriceps and hamstring tendon autografts in ACL reconstruction yield comparably good results in a prospective, randomized controlled trial. Arch Orthop Trauma Surg. 2022;142:281–9.
11. Viglietta E, Ponzo A, Monaco E, Iorio R, Drogo P, Andreozzi V, et al. ACL reconstruction combined with the Arnold-Coker modification of the MacIntosh lateral extra-articular tenodesis: long-term clinical and radiological outcomes. Am J Sports Med. 2022;50:404–14.
12. Williams A. Editorial commentary: Lateral extra-articular tenodesis reduces anterior cruciate ligament graft rerupture rates: proper anterior cruciate ligament and lateral extra-articular tenodesis technique is vital to prevent complications. Arthroscopy. 2022;38:870–2.
13. Ifran NN, Mok YR, Krishna L. Tear rates of the ipsilateral ACL graft and the contralateral native ACL are similar following ACL reconstruction. J Knee Surg. 2022;35:308–11.
14. Rahardja R, Love H, Clatworthy MG, Monk AP, Young SW. Suspensory versus interference tibial fixation of hamstring tendon autografts in anterior cruciate ligament reconstruction: results from the New Zealand ACL registry. Am J Sports Med. 2022;50:904–11.
15. Rodriguez AN, LaPrade RF, Geeslin AG. Combined meniscus repair and anterior cruciate ligament reconstruction. Arthroscopy. 2022;38:670–2.
16. Bergerson E, Persson K, Svantesson E, Horvath A, Olsson Wållgren J, et al. Superior outcome of early ACL reconstruction versus initial non-reconstructive treatment with late crossover to surgery: a study from the Swedish National Knee Ligament Registry. Am J Sports Med. 2022;50:896–903.
17. Webster KE, Hewett TE. Anterior cruciate ligament injury and knee osteoarthritis: an umbrella system-

atic review and meta-analysis. Clin J Sport Med. 2022;32:145–52.

18. Gillet B, Blache Y, Rogowski I, Vigne G, Capel O, Sonnery-Cottet B, et al. Isokinetic strength after ACL reconstruction: influence of concomitant anterolateral ligament reconstruction. Sports Health. 2022;14:176–82.

19. Seppänen A, Suomalainen P, Huhtala H, Mäenpää H, Kiekara T, Järvelä T. Double bundle ACL reconstruction leads to better restoration of knee laxity and subjective outcomes than single bundle ACL reconstruction. Knee Surg Sports Traumatol Arthrosc. 2022;30:1795–808.

20. Moon HS, Choi CH, Yoo JH, Jung M, Lee TH, Hong KB, et al. Graft isometry during anatomical ACL reconstruction has little effect on surgical outcomes. Knee Surg Sports Traumatol Arthrosc. 2022;30:1594–604.

21. van Keulen LZ, Hoogeslag RAG, Brouwer RW, Huis IN, 't Veld R, Verdonschot N. The importance of continuous remnant preservation in anterior cruciate ligament reconstruction. Knee Surg Sports Traumatol Arthrosc. 2022;30:1818–27.

22. Franciozi CE, Minami FK, Ambra LF, Galvão PHSAF, Schumacher FC, Kubota MS. Remnant preserving ACL reconstruction with a functional remnant is related to improved laxity but not to improved clinical outcomes in comparison to a nonfunctional remnant. Knee Surg Sports Traumatol Arthrosc. 2022;30:1543–51.

23. Vincelot-Chainard C, Buisson X, Taburet JF, Djian P, Robert H. ACL autograft reconstruction revisions with tendon allografts: Possibilities and outcomes. A one-year follow-up of 39 patients. Orthop Traumatol Surg Res. 2022;108(3):102832.

24. Arimaa A, Knifsund J, Keskinen H, Kivimäki M, Aalto V, Oksanen T, et al. Return to work following anterior cruciate ligament reconstruction. Acta Orthop. 2022;93:554–9.

25. Okutan AE, Kalkışım M, Gürün E, Ayas MS, Aynacı O. Tibial slope, remnant preservation, and graft size are the most important factors affecting graft healing after ACL reconstruction. Knee Surg Sports Traumatol Arthrosc. 2022;30:1584–93.

26. Zhang J, Ma Y, Pang C, Wang H, Jiang Y, Ao Y. No differences in clinical outcomes and graft healing between anteromedial and central femoral tunnel placement after single bundle ACL reconstruction. Knee Surg Sports Traumatol Arthrosc. 2021;29:1734–41.

27. Goto K, Duthon VB, Menetrey J. Anterior cruciate ligament reconstruction using quadriceps tendon autograft is a viable option for small-statured female patients. Knee Surg Sports Traumatol Arthrosc. 2022;30:2358–63.

28. Liu Z, Jiang J, Yi Q, Teng Y, Liu X, He J, Zhang K, et al. An increased posterior tibial slope is associated with a higher risk of graft failure following ACL reconstruction: a systematic review. Knee Surg Sports Traumatol Arthrosc. 2022;30:2377–87.

29. Balendra G, Jones M, Borque KA, Willinger L, Pinheiro VH, Williams A. Factors affecting return to play and graft re-rupture after primary ACL reconstruction in professional footballers. Knee Surg Sports Traumatol Arthrosc. 2022;30:2200–8.

30. Hagemans FJA, Jonkers FJ, van Dam MJJ, von Gerhardt AL, van der List JP. Clinical and radiographic outcomes of anterior cruciate ligament reconstruction with hamstring tendon graft and femoral cortical button fixation at minimum 20-year follow-up. Am J Sports Med. 2020;48:2962–9.

31. Marx JS, Plantz MA, Gerlach EB, Carney J, Swiatek PR, Cantrell CK, et al. Revision ACL reconstruction has higher incidence of 30-day hospital readmission, reoperation, and surgical complications relative to primary procedures. Knee Surg Sports Traumatol Arthrosc. 2022;30:1605–10.

32. Kanakamedala AC, Edgar CM, Fanelli GC, Musahl V, Alaia MJ. Surgical considerations in revision anterior cruciate ligament reconstruction. Instr Course Lect. 2022;71:475–87.

33. Brodeur PG, Licht AH, Modest JM, Testa EJ, Gil JA, Cruz AI Jr. Epidemiology and revision rates of pediatric ACL reconstruction in New York State. Am J Sports Med. 2022;50:1222–8.

34. Malige A, Leska T, Baghdadi S, Ganley T. Pediatric revision anterior cruciate ligament reconstruction: current concepts review. Clin J Sport Med. 2022;32:139–44.

35. Kew ME, Bodkin S, Diduch DR, Brockmeier SF, Lesevic M, Hart JM, et al. Reinjury rates in adolescent patients 2 years following ACL reconstruction. J Pediatr Orthop. 2022;42:90–5.

36. Toker B, Erden T, Dikmen G, Özden VE, Fıratlı G, Taşer Ö. Clinical outcomes of single-bundle versus double-bundle ACL reconstruction in adolescent elite athletes: a retrospective comparative study. Acta Orthop Traumatol Turc. 2022;56:20–5.

37. Eisenberg MT, Block AM, Vopat ML, Olsen MA, Nepple JJ. Rates of infection after ACL reconstruction in pediatric and adolescent patients: a MarketScan Database study of 44,501 patients. J Pediatr Orthop. 2022;42:e362–6.

Patellofemoral Osteoarthritis: Treatment Other than Patellofemoral Arthroplasty

E. Carlos Rodríguez-Merchán, Hortensia De la Corte-Rodríguez, Carlos A. Encinas-Ullán, Juan S. Ruiz-Pérez, and Primitivo Gómez-Cardero

4.1 Introduction

According to Kamat et al., the patellofemoral (PF) component of the knee joint is influenced by a wide range of degenerative causes without implicating the other parts of the knee. Besides, PF joint degeneration is frequently the presenting pathology in early knee osteoarthritis (OA) and missed due to a variable presentation (Fig. 4.1).

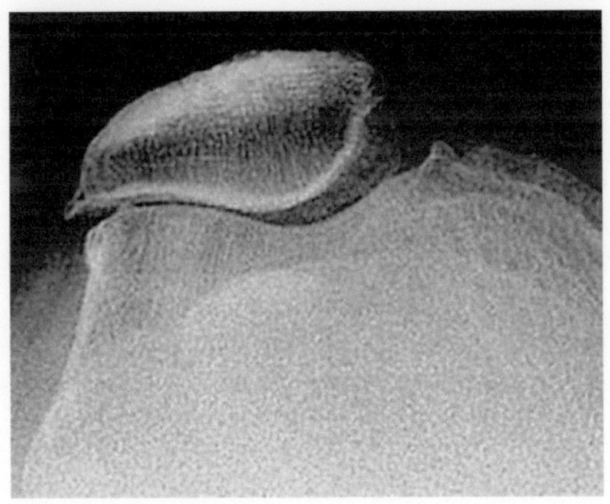

Fig. 4.1 Patellofemoral osteoarthritis

tAccurate examination and focused investigation can help with early diagnosis and guide management. Diverse aspects to management need to be addressed after thorough assessment [1]. The purpose of this chapter is to review recent developments on the treatment of PF OA other than PF arthroplasty.

4.2 Risk Factors of PF Joint OA

In 2022 Kuwabara et al. presented a synthesis of recent literature regarding the management of PF OA. Risk factors of PF joint OA include patella malalignment or maltracking, injury to supportive structures including the medial patellofemoral ligament (MPFL), dysfunction of hamstring and quadriceps coordination, lower extremity alignment, trochlear dysplasia, patellar trauma, or anterior cruciate ligament (ACL) surgery [2].

4.3 Diagnosis

According to Kuwabara et al., special physical examination maneuvers include patellar grind test, apprehension test, and lateral patellar tilt angle. Radiographs that should be attained first line include weight-bearing bilateral anteroposterior (AP), lateral, and Merchant views. Computed tomography (CT) and magnetic resonance imaging (MRI) are utilized to evaluate

E. C. Rodríguez-Merchán (✉) · C. A. Encinas-Ullán
J. S. Ruiz-Pérez · P. Gómez-Cardero
Department of Orthopedic Surgery, La Paz University Hospital, Madrid, Spain

H. De la Corte-Rodríguez
Department of Physical and Rehabilitation Medicine, La Paz University Hospital, Madrid, Spain

E. C. Rodríguez-Merchán (ed.), *Advances in Orthopedic Surgery of the Knee*,
https://doi.org/10.1007/978-3-031-33061-2_4

trochlear dysplasia, excessive patellar height, and tibial tubercle-trochlear groove (TT-TG) distance [2].

4.4 Nonoperative Treatment

4.4.1 General Concepts

Nonoperative treatment alternatives include nonpharmacologic management (patient education, self-management, physical therapy, weight loss), extracorporeal shockwave therapy (ESWT), cold therapy, taping, bracing, and orthotics. Pharmacologic management options discussed include NSAIDs (nonsteroidal anti-inflammatory drugs), acetaminophen, oral narcotics, and duloxetine. Injection therapies include glucocorticoids, hyaluronic acid, platelet-rich plasma (PRP), and other regenerative therapies (bone marrow aspirate concentrate [BMAC], adipose, or mesenchymal stem cells [MSCs]). Other treatment alternatives include radiofrequency ablation and botulinum toxin [2].

4.4.2 Knee Taping in Addition to a Supervised Exercise Protocol

Shah et al. studied the impact of knee taping in addition to a supervised exercise protocol on the pain intensity and functional status of subjects with PF OA. Their study was based on a randomized, controlled pretest-posttest experimental group design. Following an initial screening, 40 subjects with PF OA (mean age 55) were randomly assigned to one of two groups, group A or group B ($n = 20$ each). Group A experienced knee taping and participated in a supervised exercise program, while group B only participated in a supervised exercise program. For 4 weeks, both groups received their prescribed treatment 5 consecutive days each week. At baseline (day 1 pre-intervention) and 4 weeks post-intervention, the visual analog scale (VAS) and the Western Ontario and McMaster Universities Osteoarthritis Index (WOMAC) scores were attained. When comparing the outcome scores at 4 weeks post-intervention with baseline scores, the within-group analysis showed significant mean differences for the results within groups A and B, but a nonsignificant mean difference for the results of VAS within group B. Similarly, when the scores of VAS and WOMAC were compared at 4 weeks post-intervention, there was a significant mean difference between groups A and B. In subjects with PF OA, combining knee taping with a supervised exercise protocol was more efficacious than the supervised exercise protocol alone in alleviating pain and improving functional status [3].

4.5 Surgical Treatment

4.5.1 General Concepts

The algorithm for the surgical management of PF joint OA can begin with the arthroscopic evaluation of the PF articular cartilage to address mechanical symptoms and to assess/treat lateral soft tissue with or without overhanging lateral osteophytes. If individuals fail to have symptomatic improvement, a tibial tubercle osteotomy (TTO) can be considered in those individuals less than 50 years of age or active patients >50 years old. In individuals with severe PF joint OA, refractory to the above managements, PF arthroplasty (PFA) should be contemplated. While early PFA designs and techniques were less than encouraging, more recent implant designs and surgical techniques have shown robust outcomes in the literature. PF OA is a challenging orthopedic problem to manage, in that it can frequently affect younger individuals, with otherwise well-functioning knees. It is a unique entity compared to tibiofemoral OA with different epidemiology, biomechanics and risk factors, and management alternatives [2].

4.5.2 Arthroscopic Debridement Plus Intra-Articular Injection of Microfragmented Adipose Tissue

In a retrospective case series with level 4 of evidence, Vasso et al. reported the clinical and functional results of a series of subjects with isolated primary PF OA managed with intra-articular injection of microfragmented autologous adipose tissue plus knee arthroscopy [4]. The outcomes were also analyzed in relation to the age and body mass index (BMI) of subjects and to the stage of PF OA. Twenty-three individuals with early-to-moderate (stages 1–3 according to the Iwano classification system) PF OA who received this treatment were retrospectively analyzed, with a mean follow-up of 22.1 months. Individuals were evaluated utilizing the International Knee Society (IKS) knee and function and VAS scores and relative to their capacity for climbing stairs. Differences in improvements of IKS and VAS scores in relation to age (<60 vs. ≥60 years), BMI (<30 vs. ≥30 kg/m^2), and stage of PF OA (stages 1–2 vs. stage 3) were eventually studied. The mean IKS knee score substantially improved from 35.6 points preoperatively to 61.9 points at the latest follow-up, while the mean IKS function score substantially improved from 52 points preoperatively to 82.3 points at the latest follow-up. The mean VAS score significantly diminished from 8.7 preoperatively to 5.2 at the latest follow-up. A significant improvement in the capacity to climb stairs was observed. No significant differences in improvements of IKS knee and function and VAS scores were encountered in relation to age, body mass index (BMI), or stage of PF OA. Intra-articular injection of microfragmented autologous adipose tissue following arthroscopic debridement significantly improved overall clinical and functional scores in individuals with early or moderate isolated primary PF OA at a mean follow-up of almost 2 years. Improvements were not significantly impacted by age, BMI, or stage of PF OA [4].

4.5.3 Patellar Thinning Osteotomy

According to Vaquero et al., isolated PF OA can be a disabling illness. When conservative management fails, surgical alternatives can be unforeseeable and might be considered too aggressive for middle-aged and active individuals [5]. In 2010 Vaquero et al. analyzed the clinical and radiological outcomes of a coronal osteotomy implicating thinning of the patella in a selected group of subjects with isolated PF OA. Since 1991, 31 patients (35 knees) have been treated, of whom 34 were accessible for follow-up at a mean of 9.1 years. The Knee Society Score (KSS), the Patellar score, and the Short Form-36 questionnaire (SF-36) were utilized for clinical assessment. They also studied the radiological features to confirm bone healing and evaluate the progression of OA. A substantial improvement in the functional scores and radiological parameters was found. All individuals except one were satisfied with the procedure. Radiological progression of the PF OA was slowed but radiological tibiofemoral OA progressed in 23 (65%) cases, with a total knee arthroplasty (TKA) becoming necessary in four cases without technical problems in resurfacing the patella. They compared the outcomes with other forms of surgical management published in the literature. Patellar thinning osteotomy offered good clinical and radiological results, presenting an alternative technique of managing PF OA [5].

4.5.4 Open Partial Lateral Facetectomy

PF OA is a frequent illness which might happen alone or in association with tibiofemoral OA. In cases of isolated symptomatic PF OA with typical lateral malalignment and formation of osteophytes at the lateral border of the PF joint, Martens et al. carried out a lateral facetectomy of the patella and associated lateral retinaculum release (Fig. 4.2). The outcomes of a prospective

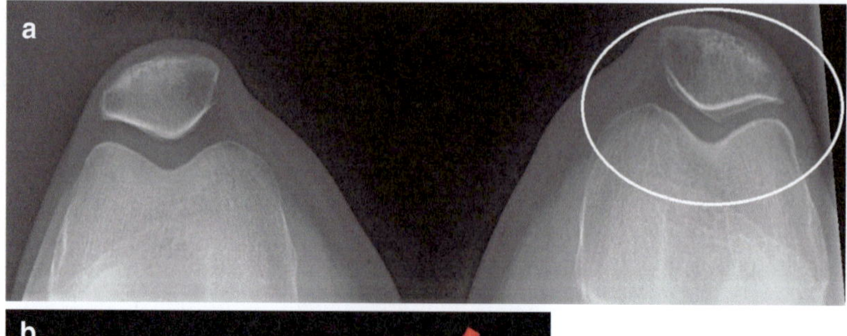

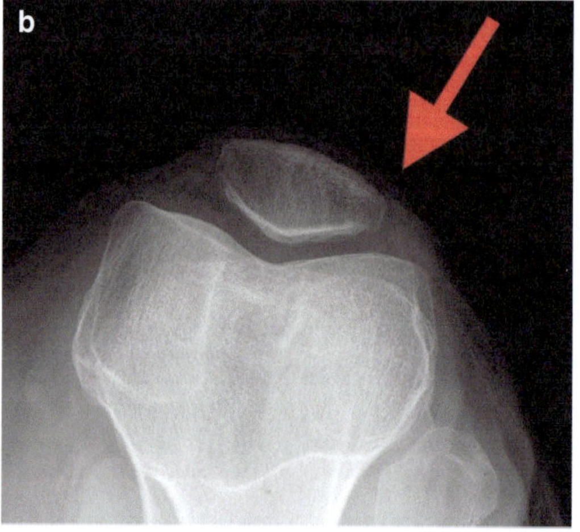

Fig. 4.2 (**a, b**) Open partial lateral facetectomy for patellofemoral osteoarthritis: (**a**) preoperative radiograph of the patellofemoral joint on axial view (circle). (**b**) Postoperative view (arrow)

study of 20 cases with a mean follow-up of 2 years were reported. A good-to-moderate outcome was attained in 90%. The average age was 60 years. Martens et al. had two failures with a subjective rating of poor. The main reason was tibiofemoral OA too far advanced at the time of the operation, which then progressed in the postoperative course. Besides, the technique resulted in noticeable improvement for many cases and carried only a small risk. Further reconstructive surgery of the knee was not excluded. Because of the minor surgery and quick recovery, this technique presented a valid option to more involved operations such as patellectomy, Bandi or Maquet reconstructive procedures, or PF arthroplasty (PFA) [6].

In a therapeutic study with level 4 of evidence, Yercan et al. investigated the effect of the partial lateral facetectomy of the patella on middle-aged to elderly subjects with isolated lateral PF OA. Between 1991 and 2000, they carried out partial lateral facetectomy on 11 knees in 11 individuals with an average age of 62 years. The mean follow-up was 8 years. The average KSS improved from a preoperative score of 150 to a score of 176 at latest follow-up. Follow-up radiographs demonstrated slow progression of OA in the PF and tibiofemoral compartments, but radiographic appearance did not always correlate with clinical symptoms. The success of this surgical procedure depended largely on alleviation of pain. Partial lateral facetectomy was relatively simple and efficacious surgical management for middle-aged to elderly active subjects with isolated lateral PF OA who want to maintain activity level [7].

The main aim of an article with a level 4 of evidence published in Wang et al. in 2021 was to examine the therapeutic impact of a modified partial lateral facetectomy of the patella for stage III lateral PF OA, which included partial lateral patella articular facet that was resected, coronal Z-shaped incision to lengthen lateral retinaculum, and patellar perimeter electrocoagulation to denervate [8]. Between December 2008 and January 2013, 36 knees of 32 individuals with severe PF OA were treated with the aforementioned modified partial patellar lateral facetectomy. All subjects were stage III according to the Iwano scale, and their patellas were all Wiberg type III or Baumgartl type IV in shape. The study group included 6 men and 26 women with an average age of 54.03 years and an average illness course of 8.67 years. The modified Kujala scores were utilized to assess PF function, and the congruence angle was utilized to assess the patellar position. KSS was utilized to assess overall knee function. Six knees of five cases were lost to follow-up. Thirty knees of 27 cases were followed up for 5 years, with an average follow-up time of 60 months. The average preoperative modified Kujala score was 15.93, and the average score at last follow-up was 32.03. The satisfactory PF function was accomplished in 28 knees (93.33%). The congruence angle improved from preoperative +23.07 degrees to 11.91 degrees at the last follow-up. The average preoperative KSS were 110.40 points, which increased to 156.77 points at the last postoperative follow-up. Pain was significantly alleviated, and the ability to climb stairs was substantially improved. All scores demonstrated statistically significant improvements after surgery. No adverse events were found. This modified partial lateral facetectomy of the patella for stage III lateral PF OA alleviated pain and partially improved function. This modified procedure was relatively simple, safe, and an efficacious management method for middle-aged and elderly subjects with PF OA. Moreover, this surgical technique can be utilized as an alternative or prephase to TKA [8].

In 2012 Wetzels et al. stated that excision of the eroded lateral patellar facet had been suggested as an acceptable treatment for short-run pain reduction in individuals with isolated PF OA and that the outcome of this procedure in the long run was not known. Therefore, they reviewed the outcomes of 155 subjects (168 knees) treated with lateral facetectomy at an average follow-up of 10.9 years. During follow-up, 62 knees (36.9%) had failed and were revised to either TKA (60 knees), PFA (one case), or total patellectomy (one case). The average time to reoperation in the failure group was 8 years. The Kaplan-Meier survival percentages with reoperation as endpoint were 85% at 5 years, 67.2% at 10 years, and 46.7% at 20 years. At final follow-up, 79 (74.5%) of the knees that had not been reoperated were rated as either good or fair, which corresponded to 47% of the original group. This study showed that a satisfactory result after lateral patellar facetectomy for isolated PF OA could be expected in about half of the cases at 10-year follow-up [9].

According to Lopez-Franco et al., knee OA mainly affecting the lateral facet of the patella, especially in young individuals, was a definite challenge to the surgeon. In 2013 Lopez-Franco et al. studied the long-run result of a simple operation such as the partial lateral facetectomy on middle-aged to elderly individuals with predominant lateral PF OA. A retrospective, long-term study of 39 knees (28 females, mean age at surgery 61 years old) with a minimum follow-up of 10 years was carried out. Assessments included preoperative and postoperative questionnaires, physical examinations, and radiographs. The main parameters included the initial anterior pain alleviation, with higher scores utilizing the KSS (which improved in 84% of the knees), and the eventual failure of the technique, including percentage of subjects that needed secondary TKA (30% of the knees). Partial lateral facetectomy aiming to decrease the high pressure in the lateral facet of the patella confirmed frequent pain alleviation. This surgical procedure being minimally invasive, relatively simple, and efficacious in selected subjects was a valid early option to more complex procedures and did not prevent further reconstructive surgery in case of illness progression [10].

4.5.5 Arthroscopic Patellar Lateral Facetectomy

According to Ferrari et al., isolated PF OA is relatively frequent, with the lateral facet of the patella being the most commonly affected part. This problem can be a result of a patellar maltracking syndrome, patella instability, or idiopathic degenerative changes. A thorough diagnostic workup with a physical examination and imaging tests are compulsory for an adequate diagnosis and to rule out other causes of PF knee pain. These individuals are frequently treated nonoperatively with exercises for patella mobility, intra-articular injections, braces, patellar tracking, quadriceps balance and strength, and activity modification. Subjects with lateral patellar pain that is refractory to nonoperative management, and who have a clear bony deformity on the patella overriding the lateral aspect of the trochlea, can benefit from surgical treatment. Ferrari et al. advised an arthroscopic lateral patellar facetectomy because the joint can be dynamically evaluated, treated, and reassessed intraoperatively to ensure that normal bony contact has been reestablished [11].

4.5.6 Lateral Facetectomy Plus Insall's Realignment Procedure

In 2013 Montserrat et al. assessed the long-term results of lateral facetectomy plus Insall's realignment procedure to treat isolated PF OA [12]. All consecutive subjects experiencing this procedure with a follow-up between 10 and 14 years were included in this study. Subjects were excluded if they had previous patellar dislocation, patellar fracture, tibiofemoral OA (except mild cases), or follow-up <10 or >14 years. Failure cases (need for TKA) of this surgical procedure before 10 years of follow-up were considered in the overall failure percentage. Clinical, functional, and radiographic results were attained at baseline and compared to postoperative values. Forty-three subjects (mean age 59.7 years) had a follow-up between 10 and 14 years and were finally included in this study. The failure percentage in the whole series and included subjects was 26.4 and 16.3% for a mean follow-up of 9.2 years and 11.7 years, respectively. PF pain, need for NSAIDs, longitudinal and transversal patellar glide tests, Zholen's sign, and knee effusion substantially improved in the follow-up. Postoperative KSS anatomical, functional, and total scores and Kujala's score were significantly higher compared to preoperative values. The patellar tilt and shift substantially improved postoperatively, whereas the PF OA was not modified

with respect to preoperative evaluation. The lateral facetectomy plus Insall's realignment procedure was a successful treatment for isolated PF OA from a clinical, functional, and radiographic point of view in the long-run follow-up [12].

In 2014 Montserrat et al. reported the survival analysis of partial lateral facetectomy and Insall's procedure in subjects with isolated PF OA and evaluated the risk and protective factors for failure of the procedure [13]. From 1992 to 2004, all subjects with isolated PF OA who met the inclusion criteria and experienced this procedure were enrolled. Risk and protective factors for failure (failure considered as the need for TKA) were evaluated by comparing attained baseline information between failed and non-failed cases. Eighty-seven cases (mean age 61.8 years, mean follow-up 9.6 years) were included. Twenty-three failed cases were encountered. Mean survival time was 13.6 years. At 13 years (last failure case), the cumulative survival was 59.3%. Baseline medial tibiofemoral pain, genu flexum, and worst grade of tibiofemoral OA were significant risk factors for failure. In contrast, higher anatomical and total KSS scores, absence of knee effusion, higher value of the Caton-Deschamps index, and lateral position of the patella were all protective factors against failure. The treatment for isolated PF OA through partial lateral facetectomy and Insall's procedure showed good long-run survival. The presence of preoperative medial tibiofemoral pain, genu flexum, and incipient tibiofemoral OA increased the risk of failure of this procedure. In contrast, higher anatomical and total KSS scores, lack of knee effusion, higher value of the Caton-Deschamps index, and lateral position of the patella were encountered to protect against failure [13].

4.5.7 Arthroscopic Debridement, Facetectomy, and Synovectomy

In 2021 Zhao stated that isolated PF OA affects climbing, squatting, and standing up movements in daily life and sports. Also, various surgical procedures have been developed to address the various causes, different degrees of cartilage degeneration, and combined lesions. Zhao et al. reported an arthroscopic PF arthroplasty technique (arthroscopic debridement, facetectomy, and synovectomy), with the main purpose to reduce the pain originating from the PF joint and related structures. The critical points of this technique were PF denervation and partial patellar facetectomy. This clinical experience showed that this technique was efficacious to address all kinds of PF OA [14].

4.5.8 Arthroscopic Lateral Patellar Facetectomy and Lateral Release

In a case series with level 4 of evidence, Douiri et al. analyzed the clinical outcomes and survival curve of arthroscopic lateral patellar facetectomy and lateral release for isolated PF OA [15]. All subjects experiencing arthroscopic lateral patellar facetectomy and lateral release between January 2008 and January 2018 were assessed retrospectively. The inclusion criteria were diagnosis of isolated symptomatic lateral PF OA; PF OA with kissing lesions (defined as a lesion on both the patella and trochlea, which were in direct contact); arthroscopic lateral patellar facetectomy and lateral release; and two-year minimum follow-up. Assessment included preoperative and postoperative subjective International Knee Documentation Committee (IKDC), Knee Injury and Osteoarthritis Outcome Score (KOOS) scores, and visual analogue pain scale (VAS) score. The primary endpoint determining the survival curve was revision of lateral facetectomy. A retrospective analysis was performed on 61 consecutive arthroscopic lateral patellar facetectomy and lateral release procedures, carried out in 55 subjects for a diagnosis of isolated PF OA. Five individuals were lost to follow-up, leaving 56 knees (50 individuals) accessible at a mean follow-up of 7.5 years. The cohort included 37 women and 13 men with a mean age of 59 years. Nine subjects (18%) experienced revision surgery: six TKAs, two high tibial osteotomies, and one revision arthroscopic lateral patellar facetectomy. The mean time from arthroscopic

facetectomy to TKA was 51 months. The survival curve rate was 86% at 7.5 years. Both KOOS and IKDC scores improved significantly. The mean VAS diminished from 6.98 preoperatively to 2.06 at the last follow-up. Arthroscopic lateral patellar facetectomy and lateral release for isolated PF OA showed sustained significant improvement in knee clinical outcome scores and pain with a low percentage of adverse events and revision surgery at mid-run follow-up. This operation can be advised in cases of symptomatic isolated PF OA [15].

According to Lopez-Franco, isolated PF OA is not uncommon, and treatment remains debatable. Several surgical procedures have been carried out to manage this disease. The success of surgery highly depends on the technique and the patient selection. The surgeon can choose between a relatively extreme TKA, with predictable outcomes, or operations demanding less surgical dissection and resection, but offering less certainty. Partial lateral facetectomy is a minimally invasive procedure that is simple and efficacious enough in selected subjects with up to 10 years of follow-up. An even less aggressive technique, the arthroscopic partial lateral facetectomy in combination with lateral retinacular release, has been demonstrated to be safe, practical, reproducible, and with a low percentage of adverse events and revision surgery at mid-run follow-up [16].

4.6 Conclusions

In subjects with patellofemoral (PF) osteoarthritis (OA), combining knee taping with a supervised exercise protocol is more efficacious than the supervised exercise protocol alone in alleviating pain and improving functional status. Intra-articular injection of microfragmented autologous adipose tissue following arthroscopic debridement significantly improves overall clinical and functional scores in subjects with early or moderate isolated primary PF OA. Partial lateral facetectomy (open or arthroscopic), lateral facetectomy plus Insall's realignment, arthroscopic lateral patellar facetectomy and lateral release, and arthroscopic PF arthroplasty technique

(PF denervation, partial patellar facetectomy, arthroscopic debridement, facetectomy, and synovectomy) are valid options for the treatment of isolated PF OA.

References

1. Kamat Y, Prabhakar A, Shetty V, Naik A. Patellofemoral joint degeneration: a review of current management. J Clin Orthop Trauma. 2021;24:101690.
2. Kuwabara A, Cinque M, Ray T, Sherman SL. Treatment options for patellofemoral arthritis. Curr Rev Musculoskelet Med. 2022;15:90–106.
3. Shah MN, Shaphe MA, Qasheesh M, Reza MK, Alghadir AH, Iqbal A, et al. Efficacy of knee taping in addition to a supervised exercise protocol to manage pain and functional status in individuals with patellofemoral osteoarthritis: a randomized, controlled clinical trial. Pain Res Manag. 2022;2022:2856457.
4. Vasso M, Corona K, Capasso L, Toro G, Schiavone PA. Intraarticular injection of microfragmented adipose tissue plus arthroscopy in isolated primary patellofemoral osteoarthritis is clinically effective and not affected by age, BMI, or stage of osteoarthritis. J Orthop Traumatol. 2022;23(1):7.
5. Vaquero J, Calvo JA, Chana F, Perez-Mañanes R. The patellar thinning osteotomy in patellofemoral arthritis: four to 18 years' follow-up. J Bone Joint Surg Br. 2010;92:1385–91.
6. Martens M, De Rycke J. Facetectomy of the patella in patellofemoral osteoarthritis. Acta Orthop Belg. 1990;56:563–7.
7. Yercan HS, Ait Si Selmi T, Neyret P. The treatment of patellofemoral osteoarthritis with partial lateral facetectomy. Clin Orthop Relat Res. 2005;436:14–9.
8. Wang M, Li X, Li P, Wang H, Gao W. Modified partial lateral facetectomy of the patella for stage III patellofemoral osteoarthritis with 5-year follow-up. J Knee Surg. 2021;34:1142–8.
9. Wetzels T, Bellemans J. Patellofemoral osteoarthritis treated by partial lateral facetectomy: results at long-term follow up. Knee. 2012;19:411–5.
10. Lopez-Franco M, Murciano-Anton MA, Fernandez-Aceñero MJ, De Lucas-Villarrubia JC, Lopez-Martín N, Gomez-Barrena E. Evaluation of a minimally aggressive method of patellofemoral osteoarthritis treatment at 10 years minimum follow-up. Knee. 2013;20:476–81.
11. Ferrari MB, Sanchez G, Chahla J, Moatshe G, LaPrade RF. Arthroscopic patellar lateral facetectomy. Arthrosc Tech. 2017;6:e357–62.
12. Montserrat F, Alentorn-Geli E, Leon V, Gines-Cespedosa A, Rigol P. Treatment of isolated patellofemoral osteoarthritis with lateral facetectomy plus Insall's realignment procedure: long-term follow-up. Knee Surg Sports Traumatol Arthrosc. 2013;21:2572–7.
13. Montserrat F, Alentorn-Geli E, Leon V, Gines-Cespedosa A, Rigol P. Partial lateral facetectomy plus Insall's procedure for the treatment of isolated patellofemoral osteoarthritis: survival analysis. Knee Surg Sports Traumatol Arthrosc. 2014;22:88–96.
14. Zhao J. Arthroscopic debridement, facetectomy, and synovectomy for isolated patellofemoral osteoarthritis. Arthrosc Tech. 2021;10:e2741–5.
15. Douiri A, Lavoué V, Galvin J, Boileau P, Trojani C. Arthroscopic lateral patellar facetectomy and lateral release can be recommended for isolated patellofemoral osteoarthritis. Arthroscopy. 2022;38:892–9.
16. Lopez-Franco M. Editorial commentary: isolated patellofemoral osteoarthritis may be treated arthroscopically: arthroscopic partial lateral facetectomy is a good alternative to more aggressive techniques. Arthroscopy. 2022;38:900–1.

Patellofemoral Arthroplasty

E. Carlos Rodríguez-Merchán,
Carlos A. Encinas-Ullán, Juan S. Ruiz-Pérez,
and Primitivo Gómez-Cardero

5.1 Introduction

In a narrative review of the literature published in 2020, Rodriguez-Merchan summarized the situation of patellofemoral (PF) arthroplasty (PFA) in the management of isolated PF osteoarthritis (OA) and gave an account of the clinical outcomes of PFA for the management of isolated PF degenerative OA of the knee. He stated that PF OA affects up to 24% of women and 11% of men over the age of 55 years who suffer from symptomatic knee OA. The article described fairly good results of PFA survivorship and functional results at short- and mid-run follow-up in the setting of isolated PF OA. Success of PFA depended on accurate subject selection rather than prosthetic failure or wear. The main cause of PFA failure was advancement of tibiofemoral OA. In contemporary times, encouraging outcomes have been achieved by the association of PFA and unicompartmental knee arthroplasty (UKA). Therefore, subjects with isolated PF OA with severe anterior knee pain may be candidates for PFA (Fig. 5.1). The success of the surgical procedure and the long-run survivorship of PFA were related to a good surgical technique and observation to meticulous indications and contraindications in subject selection. Newer prostheses have also played a role to improved outcomes. Thus, PFA is an option for younger subjects with isolated PF OA [1].

In a report with level 5 of evidence published in 2022, Hoogervorst and Arendt claimed that isolated PF OA was a frequent source of anterior knee pain in subjects over the age of 40 years. Also, PFA was an alternative to address PF AO when the nonoperative or joint-preserving treatment has failed. For the aforementioned authors, the objectives of PFA were to diminish pain and increase function of the knee in a bone and ligament-preserving fashion while maintaining or optimizing its kinematics. They also mentioned that over the last decades, advances have been made in optimizing implant designs, addressing adverse events, and improving functional and patient-reported outcomes (PROMs). Adequate subject selection had demonstrated to be imperative [2]. The purpose of this chapter is to review recent developments on PFA.

E. C. Rodríguez-Merchán (✉) · C. A. Encinas-Ullán
J. S. Ruiz-Pérez · P. Gómez-Cardero
Department of Orthopedic Surgery, La Paz University
Hospital, Madrid, Spain

© The Author(s), under exclusive license to Springer Nature Switzerland AG 2023
E. C. Rodríguez-Merchán (ed.), *Advances in Orthopedic Surgery of the Knee*,
https://doi.org/10.1007/978-3-031-33061-2_5

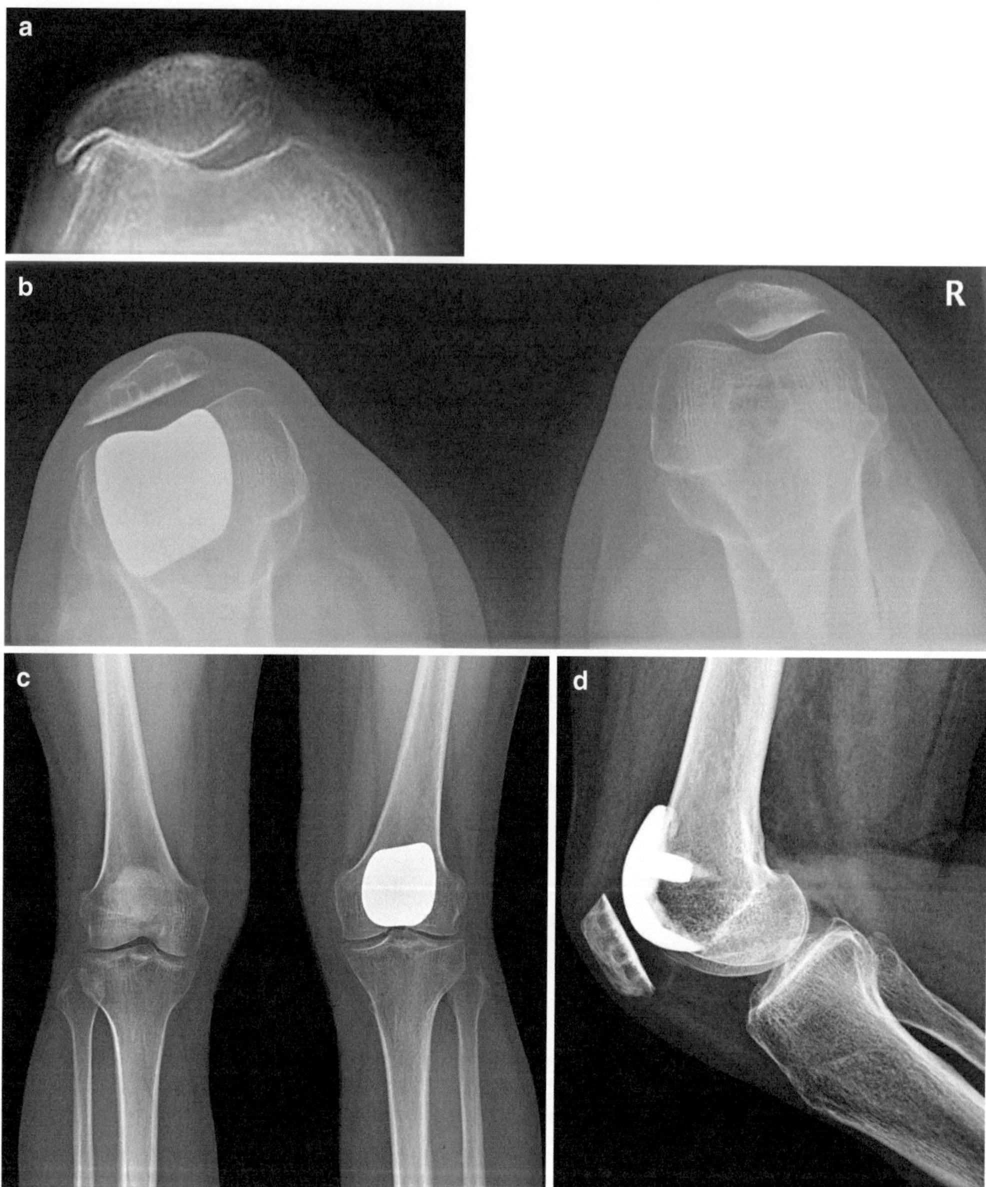

Fig. 5.1 (**a–d**) Patellofemoral (PF) arthroplasty in isolated PF osteoarthritis: (**a**) preoperative axial radiograph. (**b**) Postoperative axial view. (**c**) Postoperative anteroposterior (AP) radiograph of the knee. (**d**) Postoperative lateral view of the knee

5.2 PFA in Isolated PF OA

5.2.1 Survivorship and Functional Outcomes

In 2017 van der List et al. performed a systematic review (level 4 of evidence) to assess overall PFA survivorship and functional results. A search was carried out utilizing PubMed, Embase, and Cochrane systems, and the registries were searched. Twenty-three cohort studies and one registry reported survivorship utilizing Kaplan-Meier curve, while 51 cohort studies reported functional results of PFA. Twelve studies were level 2 studies, while 45 studies were level 3 or 4 studies. Heterogeneity was principally observed in the type of prosthesis and year the cohort started. Nine hundred revisions in 9619 PFAs were published yielding 5-, 10-, 15-, and 20-year PFA survivorships of 91.7%, 83.3%, 74.9%, and 66.6%, respectively, and an annual revision rate of 2.18. Functional results were published in 2587 PFAs with an overall score of 82.2% of the maximum score. Knee Society Score (KSS) and Knee Function Score were 87.5% and 81.6%, respectively. This systematic review demonstrated that fairly good outcomes of PFA survivorship and functional results had been reported at short- and midterm follow-up in the setting of isolated PF OA. Heterogeneity existed principally in prosthesis design and year the cohort began [3].

5.2.2 Preoperative Bone Scans Can Predict Survivorship

In 2020 Baker et al. stated that isolated PF joint OA had been identified in 10% of the population presenting with symptomatic knee OA. Also, patient selection was important in order to improve survivorship following PFA [4]. Baker et al. compared the utilization of a preoperative bone scan versus a magnetic resonance imaging (MRI) to identify the patient with isolated PF OA. This was a retrospective review of 32 individuals experiencing isolated PFA for PF OA utilizing the same implant design. Sixteen subjects received a preoperative bone scan to confirm isolated PF OA. These subjects were matched by age and gender to subjects where an MRI was utilized to determine isolated PF OA. The bone scan cohort contained 13 women and three men with an average age of 48 years and average follow-up of 52 months. There was no significant difference in age, body mass index (BMI), follow-up, or pre-operative range of motion (ROM) between the groups. The MRI and bone scan results were reported by a radiologist specializing in orthopedic radiology. Survivorship was 100% in the PFA group selected utilizing a preoperative bone scan. Revision surgery with conversion to total knee arthroplasty (TKA) was needed in 5 of 16 subjects (31%) when an MRI was utilized to recognize isolated PF OA. Revision in all subjects in the MRI group was due to progression of knee OA in the tibiofemoral joint. There were no cases of implant-related failures. PFA utilizing a modern design implant showed 100% survivorship when a preoperative bone scan was utilized for patient selection to confirm isolated PF OA. In the group where only an MRI was utilized, there was a 31% failure due to progression of the illness. Based on this study, Baker et al. advised the utilization of a bone scan as a tool in the selection criteria for subjects experiencing PFA [4].

5.2.3 Patient-Reported Outcomes

In 2021 Abeysekera et al. presented the experience of a single center on PFA, in terms of PROMs. From January 2005 to January 2016, 42 subjects with isolated PF OA were treated. The subjects were evaluated utilizing the OKS preoperatively and one, five, and eight year(s) after surgery. Among 42 subjects who experienced PFA, only 25 individuals (31 limbs implicated) had records up to 5 years. There was a substantial clinical improvement of OKS postoperatively, diminishing the score on average by 10.4 one year after surgery and 8.9 five years after surgery. This improvement was independent of the types of implants, gender, age, and BMI. The conclusion of Abeysekera et al. was that PFA can significantly improve the knee function, and this improvement is independent of the type of implant, gender, age, and BMI. However, they also mentioned that further studies were required to evaluate the long-run results of PFA [5].

According to Dai et al., PFA was acknowledged in 2021 as the method for the treatment of isolated PF OA. However, few previous studies had evaluated the PROMs and risk factors of less improvement of PROMs in subjects experiencing PFA. They performed a retrospective analysis, including all subjects who had experienced PFA. A total of 46 PFAs were studied with a mean follow-up of 37 months. The mean age at surgery was 61.1 years. Subjects demonstrated significant improvement in all PROMs. Subjects with trochlear dysplasia (TD) preoperatively have greater improvement in OKS and Kujala score postoperatively (19.2 vs. 23.1). Longer duration of symptoms (DOSs, ≥1 year) had a greater mean improvement in OKS and Kujala score. According to the measurement of patella height, subjects with patella alta (Caton-Deschamps index [CDI] ≥1.3) demonstrated less improvement in both OKS and Kujala score. PFA was a safe and efficacious surgery with good PROMs. Patella alta with a CDI ≥1.3 and duration of preoperative symptoms ≤1 year were risk factors for diminished OKS and Kujala score improvement, while the preoperative presence of TD was a significantly predictive factor for increased OKS improvement [6].

5.2.4 Obesity Does Not Affect Patient-Reported Outcomes

In 2022 Tishelman et al. stated that PFA had collected attention in recent years as an efficacious option to TKA for subjects with symptomatic, isolated PF joint OA. Also, obesity had previously been recognized as a risk factor for revision surgery, but its effect on PROMs had not been assessed. A retrospective review of a consecutive series of PFA surgeries was performed. Subjects were dichotomized by BMI as obese (O, BMI >30) or nonobese (NO, BMI: 18.5–25). Demographic, surgical data, and PROMs were collected and studied accordingly. Seventy-six subjects (41 nonobese, 35 obese) were recognized. Subjects who were obese presented with significantly worse preoperative PROMs regarding knee-specific quality of life, physical function, and mental health. No significant difference was found in improvement in knee function scores between subjects who were obese or nonobese. Besides, no difference in the percentage of PFA revision was found and there were no postoperative adverse events reported. Obese subjects with isolated PFA can expect the same improvement in function as nonobese subjects after PFA. This chapter emphasized the priority of subject selection in PFA and challenged the notion that surgeons should exclude subjects from experiencing a PFA on the basis of obesity [7].

5.2.5 Obesity Linked to High Risk of Revision and Progression of Medial Tibiofemoral OA

Marullo et al. studied the effect of obesity on patient result, procedure failure percentage, and OA progression in the tibiofemoral compartments in a series of isolated PFAs carried out with a third-generation implant [8]. The study population was subjects who had experienced third-generation PFA between 2007 and 2017. Subjects were categorized by BMI as obese (O, BMI > 30 kg/m^2) or nonobese (NO, BMI < 30 kg/m^2). Preoperative and postoperative clinical and functional evaluation included knee ROM, KSS, University of California Los Angeles (UCLA) Activity Score, Tegner Activity Level Scale, and VAS for pain. Preoperative and postoperative radiographs were assessed for progression of tibiofemoral compartment OA, changes in patellar height, and knee coronal alignment. A total of 120 PFAs with a mean follow-up of 6.9 years were included: 25 in the O group and 95 in the NO group. Significant improvement was found in knee ROM, clinical and functional KSS, UCLA Activity Score, Tegner score, and VAS for pain without intergroup differences. Worsening of the medial Kellgren-Lawrence (K-L) grade (but not the lateral K-L grade) was more common in the O than the NO group during the follow-up period. Failure happened in 4.2% of NO and in 20% of O group subjects; the difference was solely due to failure because of OA progression in the tibiofemoral compartment (16% in the O group). There were no between-group differences in the failure percentage for any cause other than OA progression (4.2% in the NO group, 4% in the O group). An equal improvement in function after PFA was found in both obese and nonobese subjects; however, the elevated failure percentage due to OA progression in the medial tibiofemoral compartment warrants caution when considering PFA in obese subjects [8].

5.2.6 PFA in Patients with PF OA with Trochlear Dysplasia

In 2022 Yang et al. stated that the influence of trochlear dysplasia on PFA had almost never been published in the literature [9]. They studied the efficacy of PFA in subjects with PF OA associated with trochlear dysplasia. From January 2014 to March 2018, 35 subjects with PF OA and trochlear dysplasia (29 women and 6 men), who experienced PFA, were included in the retrospective study. Radiological measurements including the patellar tilt (PT), congruence angle (CA), Blackburne-Peel ratio (BPR), TT-TG distance, and lateral trochlear inclination (LTI) were evaluated pre- and postoperatively to assess the changes in PF alignment. The PROMs were evaluated utilizing the OKS. The mean follow-up time was 2 years. The intraclass correlation coefficients were excellent for all measurements. The PF alignment and knee function were significantly improved postoperatively. The PT diminished from 23.3° preoperatively to 6.4° postoperatively. The CA diminished from 32.3° preoperatively to 10.2° postoperatively. The lateral trochlear inclination increased from 8.3° preoperatively to 16.0° postoperatively. The TT-TG distance diminished from 18.2 mm preoperatively to 11.5 mm postoperatively. The BPR did not significantly change postoperatively. The average OKS improved from 19.5 preoperatively to 29.2 at 6 months postoperatively, 37.9 at 1 year postoperatively, and 39.1 at final follow-up. No individual developed PF malalignment or prosthesis loosening during short-run follow-up. PFA yielded favorable therapeutic outcomes in subjects with PF OA associated with trochlear dysplasia [9].

5.2.7 Conversion of PFA to a TKA: Patellar Button Compatibility

In a review of contemporary literature, McDonald and Kurmis compared TKA to PFA. The findings of this study suggested that surgeons can reliably retain well-fixed, undamaged, dome-shaped all-polyethylene patellar buttons in the conversion of a PFA to TKA with the anticipation of adequate mid-run performance and survivorship, as long as congruent tracking with the new tibiofemoral components is accomplished. The aforementioned authors stated that this outcome is likely translatable to the majority of contemporary, all-polyethylene, dome-shaped patellar buttons, even with manufacturer mismatch [10].

5.3 PFA in Posttraumatic PF Osteoarthritis

According to Konan and Haddad, PFAs have been successfully utilized in the treatment of isolated PF joint OA. In 2016 they hypothesized that in posttraumatic PF OA, isolated unicompartmental arthroplasty should be associated with dependable pain alleviation, subject satisfaction, and functional result at mid-run follow-up. Fifty-one Avon PFJ (Stryker, Mahwah, NJ) isolated unicompartmental arthroplasties (47 individuals; 29 men, 18 women) were recognized at a mean follow-up of 7.1 years. The average age at surgery was 57 years. All subjects reported excellent pain alleviation, satisfaction, and functional results. Median Oxford Knee Score (OKS) was 38 at latest follow-up with a significant improvement from preoperative scores. There were two revisions: one for pain and one for progression of OA. The probability of survival (Kaplan-Meyer analysis) with revision as end point was 96.1%. The study demonstrated good mid-run outcomes for the Avon PFJ (Stryker, Mahwah, NJ) system in posttraumatic PF OA, at mid-run follow-up in a relatively young subject group [11].

5.4 Inlay PF Arthroplasty

In a retrospective study of prospectively collected information with level 3 of evidence, Feucht et al. analyzed whether preoperative PF anatomy was associated with clinical improvement and failure percentage after isolated PFA utilizing a modern inlay-type trochlear implant [12]. Prospectively collected 2-year information of subjects treated with isolated inlay PFA (HemiCAP® Wave, Arthrosurface, Franklin, MA, USA) between 2009 and 2016 and accessible digitalized preoperative imaging (plain radiographs in three planes and MRI) were retrospectively studied. All subjects were assessed utilizing the WOMAC (Western Ontario and McMaster Universities Osteoarthrtis Index) score, Lysholm score, and visual analog scale (VAS) for pain. Subjects revised to TKA or not accomplishing the minimal clinically important difference (MCID) for the total WOMAC score or VAS pain were considered failures. Preoperative imaging was studied regarding the following aspects: tibiofemoral OA, PF OA, trochlear dysplasia (Dejour classification), patellar height (Insall-Salvati index [ISI]; patellotrochlear index [PTI]), and position of the tibial tuberosity (tibial tubercle-trochlear groove [TT-TG] and TT-PCL [posterior cruciate ligament] distance). A total of 41 subjects (61% women) with a mean age of 48 years could be included. Fifteen subjects (37%) were considered failures, with 5 subjects (12%) revised to TKA and 10 subjects (24%) not accomplishing MCID for WOMAC total or VAS for pain. Failures had a significantly higher ISI and a significantly lower PTI. Moreover, the proportion of individuals with a pathologic ISI (>1.2), a pathologic PTI (<0.28), and without trochlear dysplasia were significantly higher in failures. Significantly greater improvements in clinical result scores were found in individuals with a higher preoperative degree of PF OA, ISI $\leq$ 1.2, PTI $\geq$ 0.28, TT-PCL distance $\leq$21 mm, and a dysplastic trochlea. Preoperative PF anatomy was significantly associated with clinical improvement and failure percentage following isolated inlay PFA. Less improvement and a higher failure percentage must be expected in subjects with patella alta (ISI > 1.2 and PTI < 0.28), absence of trochlear dysplasia, and a lateralized position of the tibial tuberosity (TT-PCL distance >21 mm). Concomitant procedures such as tibial tuberosity transfer might be considered in such subjects [12].

In a retrospective case series with level 4 of evidence, Imhoff et al. assessed the clinical results of subjects with a minimum 2-year follow-up after contemporary PF inlay arthroplasty (PFIA) and tried to identify potential risk factors for failure in a multicenter study [13]. All subjects who experienced implantation of PFIA between 09/2009 and 11/2016 at 11 specialized orthopedic referral centers were enrolled in the study and were assessed retrospectively at a minimum 2-year follow-up. Clinical results included the WOMAC score, Knee Injury and Osteoarthritis Outcome Score (KOOS), Tegner Scale, VAS for pain, and subjective subject satisfaction. Pre- and perioperative risk factors were compared among failures and non-failures to establish potential risk factors. A total of 263 subjects (85% follow-up rate) could be enrolled. The mean age at the time of index surgery was 49 years with a mean postoperative follow-up of 45 months. The overall failure rate was 11% (28 subjects), of which 18% (5 subjects) were subjects with patella resurfacing at index surgery and 82% (23 individuals) were subjects without initial patella resurfacing. At final follow-up, 93% of the subjects who did not fail were satisfied with the procedure with a mean transformed WOMAC Score of 84.5 points, a mean KOOS of 73.3 points, a mean Tegner score of 3.4 points, and a mean VAS score for pain of 2.4 points. An increased BMI was significantly correlated with a worse postoperative result. Concomitant procedures addressing PF instability or malalignment, the lack of PF resurfacing at the index surgery, and a high BMI were significantly correlated with failure in this subject group. PFIA demonstrated elevated subject satisfaction with good functional results at short-run follow-up and thus can be considered a viable treatment alternative in young subjects suffering from isolated PF OA. Imhoff et al. advised patellar resurfacing at index surgery to diminish the risk of failure [13].

5.5   Onlay PF Arthroplasty

In 2021 Villa et al. stated that PFA for isolated PF OA remained debatable due to variable postoperative results and high failure percentages. Also, second-generation (2G) onlay prostheses had been associated with improved postoperative outcomes. Villa et al. performed a systematic review to assess the overall survivorship and functional results of 2G PFA. The mean age of the subjects was 59.7. When analyzing all studies, weighted survival at mean follow-up of 5.52 was 87.72%. Subanalysis of studies with minimum 5 years of follow-up demonstrated a survival of 94.24%. The most frequent operative adverse event was OA progression for all implants. The percentage of revisions and conversions reported after analyzing all studies was 1.37% and 7.82%, respectively. Villa et al. concluded that safe and acceptable results of functional outcomes and PFA survivorship can result from 2G PFAs at both short- and mid-run follow-up for subjects with isolated PF OA [14].

5.6   Conclusions

PFA utilizing a modern design implant shows 100% survivorship when a preoperative bone scan is utilized for subject selection to confirm isolated PF OA. If only MRI is utilized, there is a 31% failure due to progression of the illness. PFA can significantly improve the knee function, and this improvement is independent of the type of implant, gender, age, and BMI. Obese subjects with isolated PF OA can expect the same improvement in function as nonobese subjects after PFA. An equal improvement in function after PFA has been found in both obese and nonobese subjects; however, the elevated failure percentage due to OA progression in the medial tibiofemoral compartment warrants caution when considering PFA in obese subjects. PFA yields favorable therapeutic outcomes in subjects with PF OA associated with trochlear dys-

plasia. Good mid-run outcomes for the Avon PFJ system have been demonstrated in posttraumatic PF OA, at mid-run follow-up in a relatively young subject group. The probability of survival (Kaplan-Meyer analysis) of the Avon PFJ system with revision as end point is 96.1%. In inlay PFA, less improvement and a higher failure percentage must be expected in subjects with patella alta, absence of trochlear dysplasia, and a lateralized position of the tibial tuberosity. Concomitant procedures such as tibial tuberosity transfer might be considered in such subjects. In onlay PFA, studies with minimum 5 years of follow-up have demonstrated a survival of 94.24%. The most frequent operative adverse event is OA progression. The percentage of revisions and conversions is 1.37% and 7.82%, respectively.

References

1. Rodriguez-Merchan EC. The Present situation of patellofemoral arthroplasty in the management of solitary patellofemoral osteoarthritis. Arch Bone Jt Surg. 2020;8:325–31.
2. Hoogervorst P, Arendt EA. Patellofemoral arthroplasty: expert opinion. J Exp Orthop. 2022;9(1):24.
3. van der List JP, Chawla H, Zuiderbaan HA, Pearle AD. Survivorship and functional outcomes of patellofemoral arthroplasty: a systematic review. Knee Surg Sports Traumatol Arthrosc. 2017;25:2622–31.
4. Baker JF, Caborn DN, Schlief TJ, Fain TB, Smith LS, Malkani AL. Isolated patellofemoral joint arthroplasty: can preoperative bone scans predict survivorship? J Arthroplast. 2020;35:57–60.
5. Abeysekera WYM, Schenk W. Patient-related outcomes of patellofemoral arthroplasty: experience of a single center. Arthroplasty. 2021;3(1):19.
6. Dai Y, Diao N, Lin W, Yang G, Kang H, Wang F. Patient-reported outcomes and risk factors for decreased improvement after patellofemoral arthroplasty. J Knee Surg. 2021; https://doi.org/10.1055/s-0041-1735159.
7. Tishelman JC, Pyne A, Kahlenberg CA, Gruskay JA, Strickland SM. Obesity does not affect patient-reported outcomes following patellofemoral arthroplasty. J Knee Surg. 2022;35:312–6.
8. Marullo M, Bargagliotti M, Vigano M, Lacagnina C, Romagnoli S. Patellofemoral arthroplasty: obesity linked to high risk of revision and progression of

medial tibiofemoral osteoarthritis. Knee Surg Sports Traumatol Arthrosc. 2022;30:4115–22.

9. Yang G, Wang J, Dai Y, Lin W, Niu J, et al. Patellofemoral arthroplasty improves patellofemoral alignment in patients with patellofemoral osteoarthritis with trochlear dysplasia. J Knee Surg. 2022;35:331–6.

10. McDonald LK, Kurmis AP. Patellar button compatibility in the conversion of patellofemoral arthroplasty to a total knee arthroplasty: a review of the contemporary literature. J Orthop Surg (Hong Kong). 2022;30(1):10225536221084147.

11. Konan S, Haddad FS. Midterm outcome of Avon patellofemoral arthroplasty for posttraumatic unicompartmental osteoarthritis. J Arthroplast. 2016;31:2657–9.

12. Feucht MJ, Lutz PM, Ketzer C, Rupp MC, Cotic M, Imhoff AB, et al. Preoperative patellofemoral anatomy affects failure rate after isolated patellofemoral inlay arthroplasty. Arch Orthop Trauma Surg. 2020;140:2029–39.

13. Imhoff AB, Bartsch E, Becher C, Behrens P, Bode G, Cotic M, et al. The lack of retropatellar resurfacing at index surgery is significantly associated with failure in patients following patellofemoral inlay arthroplasty: a multi-center study of more than 260 patients. Knee Surg Sports Traumatol Arthrosc. 2022;30:1212–9.

14. Villa JC, Paoli AR, Nelson-Williams HW, Badr RN, Harper KD. Onlay patellofemoral arthroplasty in patients with isolated patellofemoral arthritis: a systematic review. J Arthroplast. 2021;36:2642–9.

Patellofemoral Arthroplasty Versus Total Knee Arthroplasty for Isolated Patellofemoral Osteoarthritis

6

E. Carlos Rodríguez-Merchán,
Carlos A. Encinas-Ullán, Juan S. Ruiz-Pérez,
and Primitivo Gómez-Cardero

6.1 Introduction

It has been reported that both patellofemoral arthroplasty (PFA) and total knee arthroplasty (TKA) are successful in treating isolated patellofemoral (PF) osteoarthritis (OA), but the complication percentages following PFA are concerning [1]. In 2019 Bunyoz et al. claimed that due to inconsistent outcomes and high failure percentages, TKA was more frequently utilized to manage isolated PF OA in spite of the theoretical advantage of PFA. Also, it was perceived that second-generation (2G) PFA might have improved the results of surgery [2].

In 2019 Woon et al. stated that PFA and TKA were accepted treatments for end-stage isolated PF OA. However, adverse events and reoperations had historically differed between the two procedures [3]. In 2021 Peng et al. affirmed that isolated PF OA was a frequent subtype of knee OA, leading to a huge economic burden on health care systems. Even though previous studies had demonstrated that PFA and TKA had good clinical effects, it remained largely unclear which treatment was more effective for individuals with isolated PF OA [4]. The purpose of this chapter is to review recent developments on PFA versus TKA for isolated PF OA.

6.2 Clinical Results

Dahm et al. identified all individuals at their institution who experienced PFA or total TKA as treatment for isolated PF OA between January 2003 and December 2005. Twenty-three PFA and 22 TKA individuals met inclusion criteria. Mean age was 60 years and 69 years, respectively. Mean follow-up was 29 months in the PFA group and 27 months in the TKA group. Mean postoperative Knee Society Clinical Rating System (KSCRS) scores were 89 and 90 in the PFA and TKA cohorts, respectively. Mean UCLA (University of California Los Angeles) scores were 6.6 and 4.2, respectively. Mean blood loss and hospital stay were significantly lower among PFA individuals. Linear regression analysis showed that blood loss, hospital stay, and functional results were not influenced by age as an independent variable. No significant adverse events happened in the PFA group. There was one deep vein thrombosis (DVT) in the TKA group. PFA yielded clinical results comparable to that of TKA as treatment for isolated PF OA and might be a less invasive alternative for this select subgroup of individuals [5].

E. C. Rodríguez-Merchán (✉) · C. A. Encinas-Ullán
J. S. Ruiz-Pérez · P. Gómez-Cardero
Department of Orthopedic Surgery, La Paz University
Hospital, Madrid, Spain

6.3   Cost-Effectiveness Analysis

Fredborg et al. evaluated the cost-effectiveness of PFA in comparison with TKA for the treatment of isolated PF OA based on prospectively collected information on health results and resource utilization from a blinded, randomized clinical trial (RCT). A total of 100 individuals with isolated PF OA were randomized to receive either PFA or TKA by experienced knee surgeons trained in using both implants. Individuals completed patient-reported outcomes (PROMs) including EuroQol five-dimension questionnaire (EQ-5D) and 6-Item Short-Form Health Survey questionnaire (SF-6D) prior to the procedure. The scores were completed again after six weeks; after three, six, and nine months; and again after one and two years post-surgery and yearly henceforth. Time-weighted outcome measures were constructed. Cost data were obtained from clinical registrations and patient-reported questionnaires. This study provided robust evidence that PFA from a one-year hospital management perspective is cheaper and provides better results than TKA when applied to individuals with isolated PF OA and carried out by experienced knee surgeons [6].

6.4   Systematic Reviews and Meta-Analyses

Peng et al. compared postoperative function, adverse events, revision percentages, level of physical activity, and satisfaction rate between PFA and TKA. The pooled outcomes demonstrated that both the PFA group and the TKA group had improved postoperative indicators, suggesting that the two operation modes could improve the knee function and quality of life of individuals. Throughout the first 2 years postoperatively, higher activity level and better functional recovery were found for PFA compared with TKA in this study; furthermore, the differences between the two operation modes were statistically significant. Peng et al. encountered no significant difference in adverse events, revision percentages, and satisfaction rate between the two procedures. Although there was no found difference in the adverse events, revision percentages, and satisfaction percentage between PFA and TKA, PFA was superior to TKA in terms of knee function and physical activity in the first 2 years postoperatively. Consequently, PFA was a safe, efficacious, and less invasive treatment for individuals with isolated PF OA. The findings of this study suggested that PFA might be more appropriate for younger patients with high activity needs. Patient selection is, therefore, thought to be of crucial importance. Individualized surgical plan should be designed according to the individual's age, body mass index (BMI), knee OA site, and activity level and combined with the surgeon's personal experience [4].

In a systematic review and meta-analysis, Li et al. compared second-generation (2G) PFA with TKA in treating isolated PF OA by evaluating the rates of revisions, adverse events, and PROMs. For the revision rate and adverse events, there were no significant differences between 2G PFA and TKA. For isolated PF OA, 2G PFA showed similar outcomes to TKA with respect to the rates of revisions, adverse events, and PROMs [7].

In 2022 Elbardesy et al. stated that both PFA and TKA were accepted surgical alternatives for end-stage isolated PF OA. They performed a systematic review and meta-analysis to compare results of PFA and TKA by assessment of the PROMs. No significant difference was encountered between both TKA and PFA in the context of operating time. No significant difference after 5 years' follow-up was observed between the two treatment alternatives in terms of UCLA score and patient satisfaction. PFA demonstrated significant improvement in WOMAC (Western Ontario and McMaster Universities Osteoarthritis Index) score at five-year follow-up, less postoperative inpatient time, better cost-effectiveness, and significantly less blood loss. PFA appeared to be a feasible option to TKA for the management of isolated PF OA in adequately selected individuals. PFA demonstrated less postoperative inpatient time and blood loss with similar PROMs to the TKA. Furthermore, it was an economically beneficial joint-preserving procedure [8].

6.4.1 Patient-Reported Outcomes (PROMs)

In a systematic review with level 4 of evidence, Bunyoz et al. compared the results of 2G PFA and TKA by evaluation of PROMs. The postoperative weighted mean AKSS (American Knee Society Score) knee scores were 88.6 in the second-generation PFA group and 91.8 in the TKA group. The postoperative weighted mean AKSS function score was 79.5 in the 2G PFA group and 86.4 in the TKA group. There was no significant difference in the mean AKSS knee or function scores between the second-generation PFA group and the TKA group. The postoperative weighted mean Oxford Knee Score (OKS) was 36.7 and the postoperative weighted mean WOMAC (Western Ontario and McMaster Universities Osteoarthritis Index) score was 24.4. The revision percentage was higher in the 2G PFA group (113 revisions [8.4%]) than in the TKA group (3 revisions [1.3%]). Progression of OA was most frequently noted as the reason for revision of PFA, and it was noted in 60 cases (53.1%); this was followed by pain in 33 cases (29.2%). Excellent postoperative weighted mean AKSS knee scores were encountered in both the 2G PFA group and in the TKA group, suggesting that both surgical alternatives can result in satisfying PROMs. Higher revision percentages in the 2G PFA studies might in part be due to challenges related to patient selection. Based on assessment of PROMs, the use of 2G PFA appeared to be an equal alternative to TKA for the management of isolated PF OA in adequately selected individuals [2].

6.4.2 Adverse Events

In 2012 Dy et al. stated that both PFA and TKA are successful in treating isolated PF OA, but the complication percentages following PFA were concerning. In a systematic review of level 3 therapeutic studies (level 3 of evidence), Dy et al. compared the prevalence of adverse events, reoperations, and revision after PFA and TKA for PF OA. There was a higher likelihood of any reoperation and revision in PFA compared to TKA. Reoperation and revision were more likely in first-generation PFA (1G-PFA) than the 2G PFA. When comparing 2G PFA to TKA, there was no significant difference in reoperation, revision, pain, or mechanical complications. Individuals who underwent PFA rather than TKA were more likely to experience adverse events and required reoperation or revision, but subgroup analysis suggested a relation to implant design. There was no significant difference in reoperation, revision, pain, or mechanical complications between 2G PFA and TKA [1].

6.4.3 Reoperation Rates

Woon et al. carried out a systematic review to report on the reoperation percentages between TKA and modern PFA for isolated PF OA (Fig. 6.1). The weighted percentage of either conversion or revision arthroplasty in the PFA group and the TKA group was 6.34 and 0.11, respectively. The weighted rate of return to the operating room for bony and soft tissue procedures was 1.06 and 0.79, respectively. The weighted percentage of manipulation under anesthesia (MUA) was 0.32 and 1.23, respectively. Patients who experienced PFA may be more likely to return to the operating room for conversion to TKA and/or revision surgery than those who underwent TKA [3].

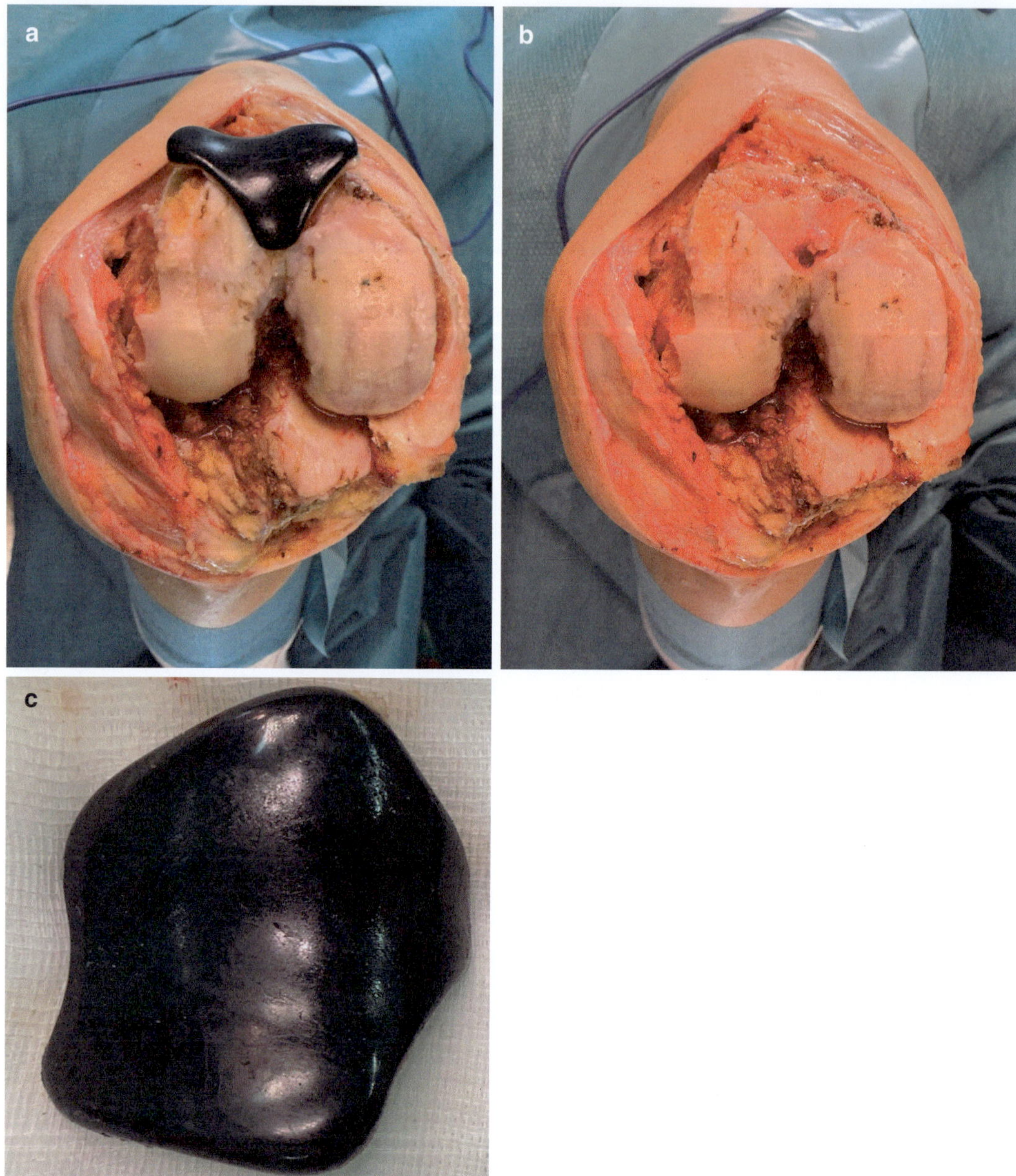

Fig. 6.1 (**a–c**) Patellofemoral arthroplasty (PFA) that required revision total knee arthroplasty (TKA) due to pain caused by progression of femorotibial osteoarthritis: (**a**) intraoperative image during revision before removal of the femoral component, (**b**) intraoperative image after removal of the femoral component of the PFA, (**c**) femoral component already removed

6.5   Conclusions

Patellofemoral arthroplasty (PFA) yields clinical results comparable to that of total knee arthroplasty (TKA) as treatment for isolated patellofemoral osteoarthritis (PF OA) and might be a less invasive alternative for a select subgroup of subjects. PFA from a one-year hospital management perspective is cheaper and provides better results than TKA when applied to subjects with isolated PF OA and carried out by experienced knee surgeons. PFA might be more appropriate for younger subjects with high activity needs. Subject selection is of crucial importance. An individualized surgical plan should be designed according to the subject's age, body mass index (BMI), knee OA site, and activity level and combined with the surgeon's personal experience. For isolated PF OA, secondgeneration (2G) PFA yields similar outcomes to TKA with respect to the rates of revisions, adverse events, and patientreported outcome measures (PROMs). PFA demonstrates less postoperative inpatient time and blood loss with similar PROMs to the TKA. Furthermore, it is an economically beneficial joint-preserving procedure. Based on assessment of PROMs, the use of 2G PFA appears to be an equal alternative to TKA for the management of isolated PF OA in adequately selected subjects. Subjects who underwent PFA rather than TKA are more likely to experience adverse events and required reoperation or revision. However, there is no significant difference in reoperation, revision, pain, or mechanical complications between 2G PFA and TKA.

References

1. Dy CJ, Franco N, Ma Y, Mazumdar M, McCarthy MM, Gonzalez Della Valle A. Complications after patello-femoral versus total knee replacement in the treatment of isolated patello-femoral osteoarthritis. A meta-analysis. Knee Surg Sports Traumatol Arthrosc. 2012;20:2174–90.
2. Bunyoz KI, Lustig S, Troelsen A. Similar postoperative patient-reported outcome in both second generation patellofemoral arthroplasty and total knee arthroplasty for treatment of isolated patellofemoral osteoarthritis: a systematic review. Knee Surg Sports Traumatol Arthrosc. 2019;27:2226–37.
3. Woon CYL, Christ AB, Goto R, Shanaghan K, Shubin Stein BE, Gonzalez Della Valle A. Return to the operating room after patellofemoral arthroplasty versus total knee arthroplasty for isolated patellofemoral arthritis—a systematic review. Int Orthop. 2019;43:1611–20.
4. Peng G, Liu M, Guan Z, Hou Y, Liu Q, Sun X, et al. Patellofemoral arthroplasty versus total knee arthroplasty for isolated patellofemoral osteoarthritis: a systematic review and meta-analysis. J Orthop Surg Res. 2021;16(1):264.
5. Dahm DL, Al-Rayashi W, Dajani K, Shah JP, Levy BA, Stuart MJ. Patellofemoral arthroplasty versus total knee arthroplasty in patients with isolated patellofemoral osteoarthritis. Am J Orthop (Belle Mead NJ). 2010;39:487–91.
6. Fredborg C, Odgaard A, Sørensen J. Patellofemoral arthroplasty is cheaper and more effective in the short term than total knee arthroplasty for isolated patellofemoral osteoarthritis: cost-effectiveness analysis based on a randomized trial. Bone Joint J. 2020;102-B:449–57.
7. Li C, Li Z, Shi L, Gao F, Sun W. The short-term effectiveness and safety of second-generation patellofemoral arthroplasty and total knee arthroplasty on isolated patellofemoral osteoarthritis: a systematic review and meta-analysis. J Orthop Surg Res. 2021;16(1):358.
8. Elbardesy H, McLeod A, Gul R, Harty J. Midterm results of modern patellofemoral arthroplasty versus total knee arthroplasty for isolated patellofemoral arthritis: systematic review and meta-analysis of comparative studies. Arch Orthop Trauma Surg. 2022;142:851–9.

Medial Unicompartmental Knee Arthroplasty

7

E. Carlos Rodríguez-Merchán,
Carlos A. Encinas-Ullán, Juan S. Ruiz-Pérez,
Primitivo Gómez-Cardero,
and Hortensia De la Corte-Rodríguez

7.1 Introduction

It has been reported that medial unicompartmental knee arthroplasty (MUKA) has advantages over total knee arthroplasty (TKA) including fewer adverse events and faster recovery; however, it has also been claimed that MUKAs have higher revision percentages (Fig. 7.1). Understanding reasons for MUKA failure might, therefore, allow for optimized clinical results [1]. According to Porteous et al., the perioperative and short-run benefits of MUKA were well supported in the literature. However, there remained concern regarding the higher revision percentage when compared with TKA [2].

In 2022 Gaudiani et al. claimed that while MUKA had shown benefits over TKA in selected individuals, component placement continued to be challenging with conventional surgical instruments, resulting in higher early failure percentages. Also, robotic-arm-assisted MUKA (RA-MUKA) had shown to be successful in component positioning through preoperative planning and intraoperative adjustability [3].

According to Roche et al., improper alignment and implant positioning following MUKA has been shown to lead to postoperative pain and increase the prevalence of revision procedures. Also, the utilization of RA-MUKA has become an area of interest to help overcome these chal-

E. C. Rodríguez-Merchán (✉) · C. A. Encinas-Ullán
J. S. Ruiz-Pérez · P. Gómez-Cardero
Department of Orthopedic Surgery, La Paz University
Hospital, Madrid, Spain

H. De la Corte-Rodríguez
Department of Physical and Rehabilitation Medicine,
La Paz University Hospital, Madrid, Spain

lenges. Besides, Roche et al. mentioned that the accuracy of intraoperative alignment compared with standing long-leg X-rays postoperatively after RA-MUKA had been in question [4]. In 2022 Wang et al. affirmed that a forgotten joint was considered the final objective of joint replacement [5].

According to Cavagnaro et al., MUKA has an infection rate of 0.1–0.8%. Besides, these authors expressed that in spite of the wide amount of lit-erature about septic TKA management, few data were accessible for MUKA infection treatment [6]. In 2022 Ly et al. stated that while good mid-run outcomes for treating spontaneous knee osteonecrosis (SPONK) with MUKA had been published, concerns remained about implant sur-vival at the long run [7]. The purpose of this chapter is to review recent developments on MUKA.

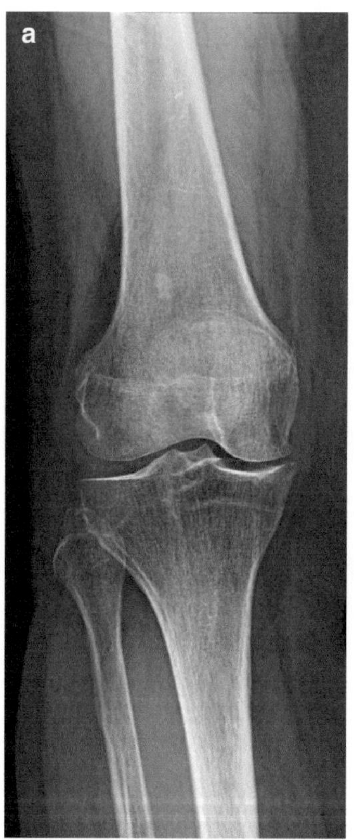

Fig. 7.1 All-poly medial unicompartmental knee arthro-plasty (MUKA): (**a**) preoperative anteroposterior (AP) radiograph. (**b**) Bone cuts made to prepare the implanta-tion of MUKA. (**c**) Intraoperative view of MUKA in knee flexion. (**d**) Intraoperative view in knee extension. (**e**) Postoperative AP view. (**f**) Postoperative lateral radiograph

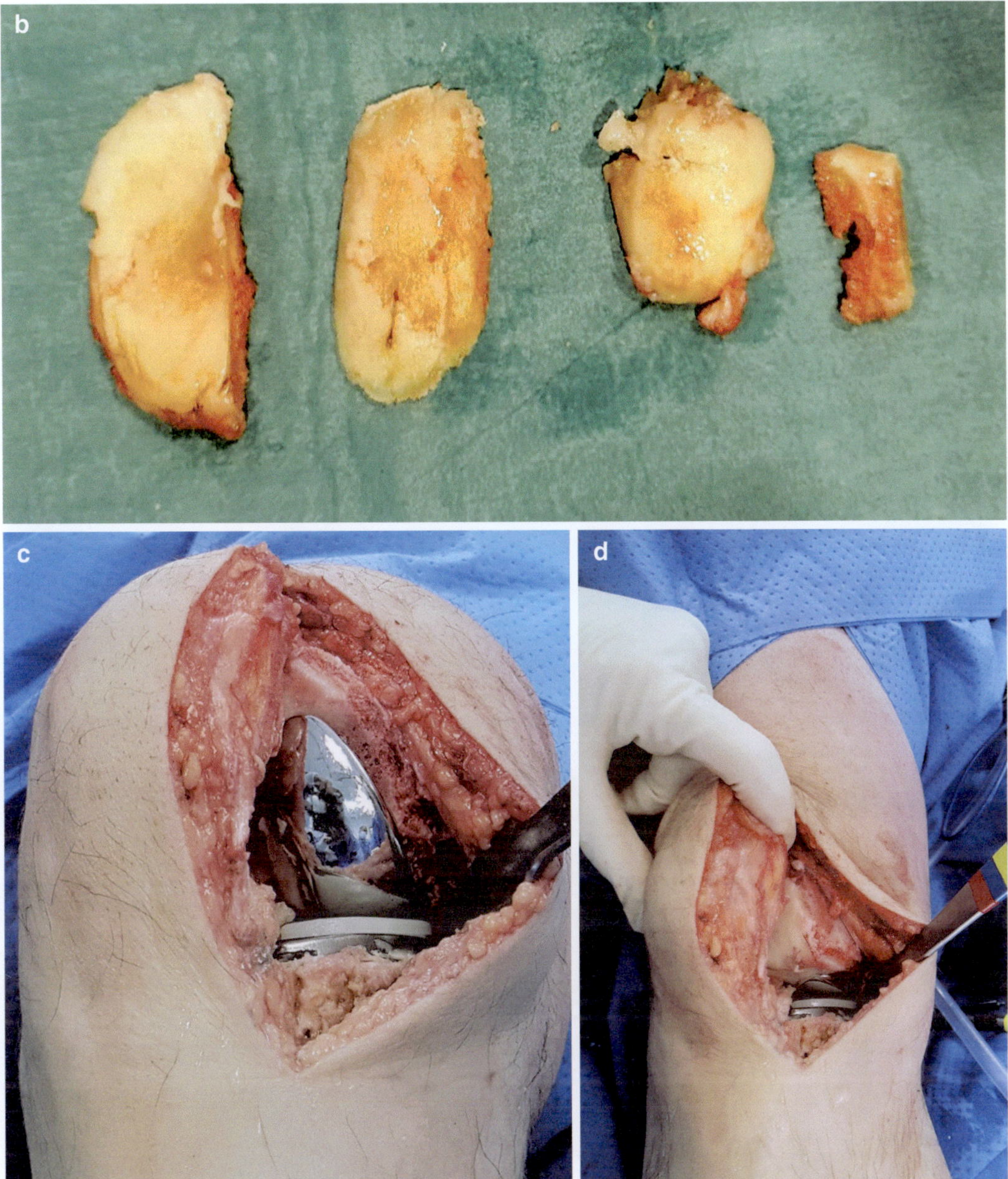

Fig. 7.1 (continued)

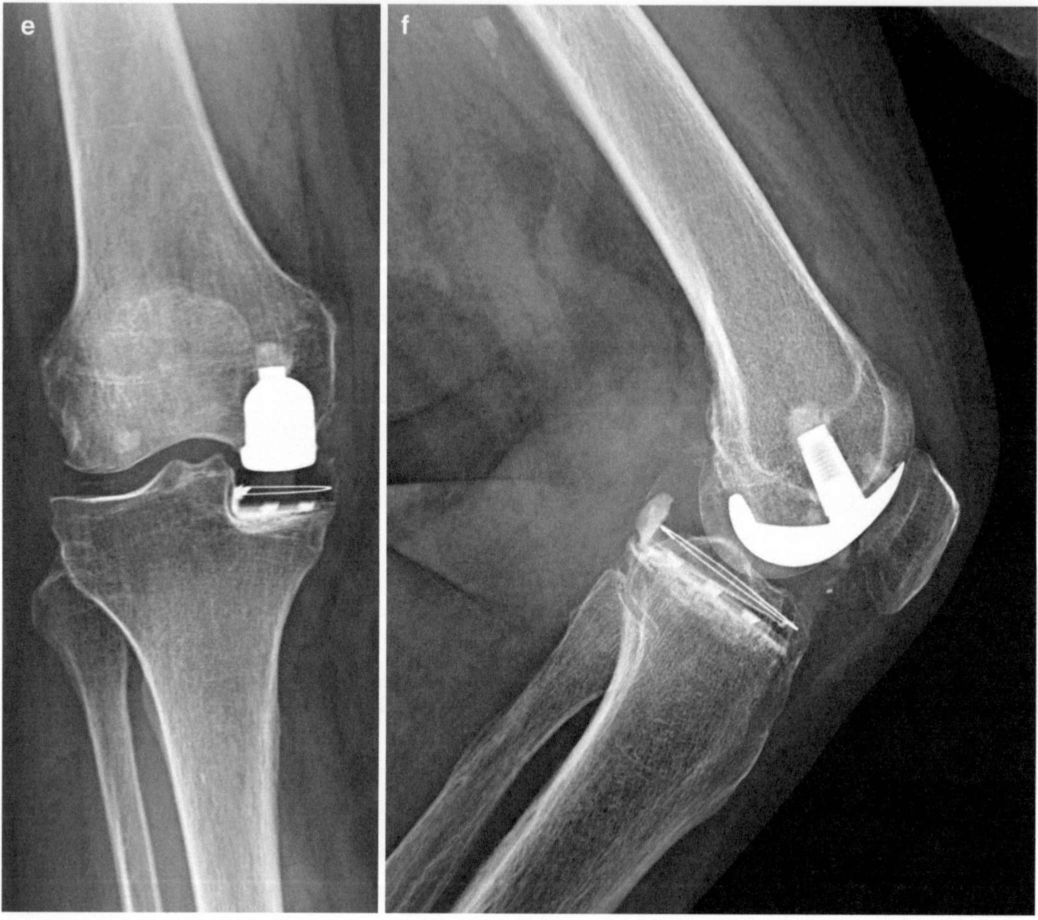

Fig. 7.1 (continued)

7.2　Predictors of a Forgotten Joint After MUKA

According to Wang et al., a forgotten joint is considered the final objective of joint replacement [5]. In a retrospective cohort study, Wang et al. analyzed the predictive factors of a forgotten joint following fixed-bearing MUKA. They utilized prospectively collected information from 302 cases of MUKA with a minimum of 2-year follow-up. The primary outcome was the accomplishment of a forgotten joint following UKA, according to the Forgotten Joint Score (FJS-12) at the last follow-up. Individuals with FJS-12 > 84 were considered to have forgotten MUKA. Of subjects, 94 (31.1%) accomplished a forgotten joint post-surgery. Multivariate logistic regression analysis showed that preoperative hip-

knee-ankle angle (HKAA), anatomic lateral distal femoral angle (ALDFA), and postoperative HKAA and HKAA changes were independent predictors of a forgotten joint. The likelihood of accomplishing a forgotten joint increased by 29% with a 1° increase in ALDFA. Preoperative HKAA, postoperative HKAA, HKAA changes (ΔHKAA), and results exhibited a nonlinear relationship. The likelihood of accomplishing a forgotten joint was the highest with preoperative HKAA >172.0°, postoperative HKAA of 176–178.5°, and ΔHKAA <5.5°. To accomplish the forgotten joint state, the ideal HKAA (hip-knee-ankle angle) range after fixed-bearing MUKA was 176–178.5° and ΔHKAA (HKAA changes) should be <5.5°. Subjects with smaller preoperative ALDFA (anatomic lateral distal femoral angle) and HKAA had a lower likelihood of accomplishing a forgotten joint following MUKA [5].

7.3   MUKA in Patients Under the Age of 60 Years

In a study with level 4 of evidence, Kyriakidis et al. systematically reviewed the clinical and functional results after MUKA in subjects under the age of 60 years old [8]. Utilizing the Preferred Reporting Items for Systematic Reviews and Meta-Analyses guidelines, studies between 2012 and April 2022, on individuals 18–60 years old who have had a MUKA assessing patient-reported outcome measures (PROMs), were included. The clinical Knee Society Score (KSS) was considered the primary outcome. Pre- and postoperative range of motion (ROM), PROMs, adverse events, and survival were recorded. Paired sample t testing was carried out to compare the preoperative with postoperative KSS. Seventeen articles comprising 2083 MUKAs were included. The follow-up range was between 1 and 15 years. In eligible studies, all reported results were improved after MUKA. The mean clinical KSS was significantly improved from 45.5 preoperatively to 89.4 postoperatively. Mean implant survival ranged 86–96.5% at 10 years' follow-up. There was no significant difference between mobile and fixed bearing in terms of ROM and clinical KSS. In total, 92 revisions and 7 reoperations with implant retention were reported. MUKA for medial OA was a safe, dependable, and efficacious treatment alternative for subjects of 60 years or younger. It provided pain alleviation, satisfactory activity level, excellent clinical results, and up to 96.5% implant survival at 10-year follow-up [8].

7.4   Medial MUKA with Patellar Denervation

Suwankomonkul et al. performed a prospective comparative study (level 3 of evidence) to evaluate the short-run outcomes of anterior knee pain and adverse events following medial UKA with patellar denervation (PD) or without PD in medial compartment osteoarthritis (OA) and severe patellofemoral (PF) OA subjects [9]. A total of 66 subjects with medial compartment and severe PF OA were allocated to MUKA with or without patella denervation. The primary outcomes were Kujala anterior knee pain scale and adverse events measured at 6 months after the surgery. Sixty-six subjects (37 subjects experiencing MUKA with PD and 27 subjects experiencing MUKA without PD) of medial compartment and severe lateral facet PF OA (62 women, 4 men; mean age 60.16 years; 17 PF grade III, 49 PF grade IV) were included in the study. The mean preoperative Kujala scores were 54.96 in the no-PD group (group I) and 47.77 in the PD group (group II). All baseline parameters were also comparable between treatment groups except the preoperative Kujala score. The mean final value of the Kujala score was 70.22 in the no-PD group (group I) and 80.10 in the PD group (group II). The mean difference of the Kujala score was statistically significantly higher by 9.88 points in the PD group when compared to the no-PD group. There were no adverse events in both groups after surgery. Patellar denervation appeared to provide short-run benefits improving the Kujala score in individuals with PF OA experiencing MUKA [9].

7.5   Pulsed Electromagnetic Fields After MUKA

In a study with level 2 of evidence, D'Ambrosi et al. evaluated pain alleviation and clinical results in subjects experiencing MUKA stimulated with pulsed electromagnetic fields (PEMFs) compared to a control group [10]. A prospective randomized controlled trial (RCT) was carried out in which 72 subjects experiencing MUKA were randomized into a control group or an experimental PEMF group. The subjects allocated to the experimental group were instructed to use PEMFs for 4 h per day for 60 days. They were assessed before a surgery and then during the time points corresponding to 1 month, 2 months, 6 months, 12 months, and 36 months after the surgery. No placebo group was included in the RCT. Clinical evaluation included the Visual Analogue Scale (VAS) for pain, Oxford Knee Score (OKS), Short Form 36 (SF-36) health survey questionnaire, and joint swelling. During each follow-up visit, the consumption of nonsteroidal anti-inflammatory drugs (NSAIDs) was recorded. The VAS diminished on follow-up visits in both groups; a statistically significant difference between the groups was found during the 6-, 12-, and 36-month follow-ups in favor of the PEMF group. One month after MUKA, the rates of subjects utilizing NSAIDs in the PEMF and control group were 71% and 92%, respectively. At the 2-month point, 15% of the subjects in the PEMF group utilized NSAIDs compared to 39% in the control group. The objective knee girth assessment demonstrated a statistically significant difference at 6, 12, and 36 months with improved values found in the PEMF group. The subjective evaluation of the swelling showed a statistically significant difference at 2, 6, 12, and 36 months with better values seen in the PEMF group. Besides, the OKS result was significantly higher in the experimental group during all the follow-ups. The utilization of PEMFs led to significant pain alleviation, better clinical improvement, and lower NSAIDs consumption after MUKA when compared to the control group [10].

7.6 St Georg Sled MUKA

According to Porteous et al., the perioperative and short-run benefits of UKA were well supported in the literature. However, there remained concern regarding the higher revision percentage when compared with TKA [2]. In a study with level 4 of evidence, Porteous et al. analyzed the functional result and survivorship of a large series of fixed bearing, MUKAs (St Georg Sled), with a minimum of 20 years' follow-up. Between 1974 and 1994, 399 individuals (496 knees) experienced a medial fixed-bearing UKA. Prospective information was collected preoperatively and at regular intervals postoperatively using the Bristol Knee Score (BKS), OKS, and WOMAC scores. Kaplan-Meier survival analysis was utilized to establish survivorship, with revision or need for revision as end point and differences evaluated utilizing the

Mantel-Cox log rank test. Functional knee scores improved postoperatively, but showed a slight reduction from 10 years of follow-up onwards. Survivorship was estimated as 86% at 10 years, 80% at 15 years, and 78% at 20 years. Sixty knees were revised, with progression of illness in another compartment the most frequent reason. Eighty-eight percent were revised using a primary prosthesis. For subjects over the age of 65 years at the time of index procedure, 93% died with a functioning prosthesis in situ. MUKA showed good long-run function and survivorship and represented an excellent surgical alternative for subjects over 65 years of age, where few individuals will need a revision procedure [2].

7.7 Infection in MUKA

In 2022 Cavagnaro et al. stated that MUKA had an infection rate of 0.1–0.8%. Also, in spite of the wide amount of literature about septic TKA management, few data were accessible for MUKA infection treatment [6]. In their article they presented the clinical and radiological results along with complication rates of a series of septic MUKA treated with two-stage exchange. They retrospectively reviewed 16 subjects treated with staged MUKA revision for infection between June 2015 and September 2019 in a single bone infection unit. Clinical scores (VAS, KSS, OKS, postoperative ROM), radiological parameters (osseointegration, loosening, and radiolucencies), and adverse events were reported. The mean follow-up was 33.5 months. Mean age at surgery was 68.5. All but two were MUKA. The mean number of previous surgeries was 2.9. The mean ROM, VAS, KSS, and OKS of the series improved significantly. Radiological analysis did not demonstrate any migration or implant loosening. Ten constrained condylar and six posterior stabilized prosthesis were finally implanted. One intraoperative pathogen isolation was recorded and managed with suppressive therapy and good final result. The implant survivorship free from infection was 100% at the final follow-up. The overall survival percentage for any reason of revision was 100%. According to the outcomes of this study, staged revision represented a dependable and efficacious alternative in delayed and late MUKA infections. This technique provided optimal clinical and radiological outcomes with acceptable complication rates [6].

7.8 Hypoallergenic MUKA

7.8.1 Return to Sports: Medial Mobile-Bearing Hypoallergenic TiNbN UKA Versus Medial Fixed-Bearing Hypoallergenic Uni Oxinium

Monti et al. have compared the percentage of return to sports (RTS) in subjects who experienced surgery for mobile-bearing MUKA with either hypoallergenic TiNbN or with oxidized zirconium alloy implants [11]. The records of two consecutive groups for a total of 90 hypoallergenic implants were prospectively studied. The first group consisted of 41 consecutive series of medial mobile-bearing hypoallergenic TiNbN MUKA, while the second group consisted of 49 consecutive medial fixed-bearing hypoallergenic Uni Oxinium. The clinical assessment involved evaluating each subject's University of California, Los Angeles (UCLA), activity scores and the High-Activity Arthroplasty Score (HAAS). Each subject was clinically assessed on the day prior to surgery (T0), then after a minimum follow-up period of 12 months (T1), and finally after 24 months (T2). The only preoperative difference between the two groups involved preoperative BMI with significantly higher BMI in the TiNbN group. Both groups reported significant improvement at each follow-up compared with the previous and also at the final follow-up with respect to UCLA activity score and HAAS, except for the UCLA activity score in TiNbN between T1 and T2. Furthermore, BMI improved significantly at the final follow-up, but only in the TiNbN group. Both TiNbN and Oxinium UKA procedures enabled individuals to return to an acceptable level of sports activity with excellent radiographic results after the final follow-up regardless of the age, gender, BMI, and bearing type [11].

7.8.2 Titanium Niobium Nitride (TiNbN) Alloy Implants Versus Fixed-Bearing Oxidized Zirconium Alloy Implants

D'Ambrosi et al. compared clinical and radiological results of subjects who had experienced a mobile-bearing MUKA with either titanium niobium nitride (TiNbN) alloy implants or with fixed-bearing oxidized zirconium alloy implants [12]. The records of two consecutive groups for a total of 86 hypoallergenic implants were prospectively studied. The first group consisted of 49 consecutive implantations of the hypoallergenic MUKA Journey Uni Oxinium (Ox group), while the second consisted of 37 consecutive series of MUKA Oxford (TiNbN group). All subjects were assessed by two independent surgeons who were not implicated in the index surgery. The clinical assessment consisted of evaluating each subject's OKS and KSS day before surgery (T_0) and with two consecutive follow-ups at T_1 (minimum follow-up 9 months) and T_2 (minimum follow-up 24 months). The two groups were homogeneous in all preoperative values, except BMI and duration of final follow-up (both statistically higher in the TiNbN group). Both groups demonstrated a clinically significant improvement for all scores at final follow-up. The only differences between the two groups implicated a higher preoperative Oxford score in the TiNbN group and different tibial and femoral angles at the final follow-up. Both TiNbN and Oxinium MUKA procedures enabled subjects from good to excellent clinical and radiographic results after the final follow-up, regardless of the age, gender, BMI, bearing type, and implant size [12].

7.9 Robotic-Assisted MUKA (RAMUKA)

7.9.1 Accuracy of Intraoperative Mechanical Axis Alignment to Long-Leg Radiographs

According to Roche et al., improper alignment and implant positioning following MUKA has been shown to lead to postoperative pain and increase the prevalence of revision procedures. Also, the utilization of RA-MUKA has become an area of interest to help overcome these challenges. Besides, Roche et al. mentioned that the accuracy of intraoperative alignment compared with standing long-leg X-rays postoperatively after medial RA-MUKA had been in question [4]. In their study Roche et al. tried to determine the final mean intraoperative coronal alignment in extension using an image-based intraoperative navigation system and compared the final intraoperative alignment to 6-week weight-bearing (WB) long-leg X-rays. Subjects who experienced RA-MUKA for medial compartmental OA were recognized from January 1, 2018, to August 31, 2019, through the aforementioned author institution's joint registry. The query yielded 136 (72 right and 64 left) subjects with a mean age of 72.02 years and mean BMI of 28.65 kg/m^2 who experienced RA-MUKA. Final intraoperative alignment was compared with WB long leg X-rays 6 weeks postoperatively by measuring the mechanical alignment. Mean intraoperative coronal alignment after resections and trialing was 4.39 varus degrees for the right knee and 4.81 varus degrees for the left knee. WB long-leg X-rays 6 weeks postoperatively showed mechanical axis alignment for the right and left knees to be 3.01 varus and 3.7 varus degrees, respectively. This resulted in a change in alignment of 1.36 and 1.12 degrees for the right and left knees, respectively. RA-MUKA showed excellent consistency when comparing postoperative WB long-leg X-rays to final intraoperative image-based non-WB alignment [4].

7.9.2 Survivorship and Outcomes

In 2022 Gaudiani et al. stated that while UKA had shown benefits over TKA in selected individuals, component placement continued to be challenging with conventional surgical instruments, resulting in higher early failure percentages. Also, RA-MUKA had shown to be successful in component positioning through preoperative planning and intraoperative adjustability [3]. Gaudiani et al. evaluated the 5-year

clinical results of medial RA-MUKA. They published a retrospective review of a single-center prospectively maintained cohort of 133 subjects (146 knees) indicated for MUKA from 2009 to 2013. Perioperative data and 2- and 5-year Knee Injury Osteoarthritis Outcome Score (KOOS), Western Ontario and McMaster Universities Osteoarthritis Score (WOMAC), and Forgotten Joint Score (FJS) outcome measures were collected. Five-year follow-up was recorded in 119 subjects (131 knees). Mean follow-up was 5.1 years. Mean age and BMI were 68 years and 29.3 kg/m^2, respectively. At 2-year follow-up, mean KOOS, WOMAC, and FJS were 71.5, 14.3, and 79.1, respectively. At 5-year follow-up, mean KOOS, WOMAC, and FJS were 71.6, 14.2, and 80.9, respectively. Mean change in KOOS and WOMAC was 34.6 and 11.0, respectively. For subject satisfaction at last follow-up, 89% of subjects were very satisfied/satisfied and 5% were dissatisfied. For subject activity expectations at last follow-up, 85% met activity expectations, 52% were more active than before, 25% have the same level of activity, 23% were less active than before, and 89% were walking without support. All subjects returned to driving after surgery at a mean of 15.2 days. Survivorship was 95% at 5 years. One knee (1%) had a PF revision, two knees (1.3%) were revised to different partial knee replacements, and five knees (3.4%) were converted to TKA. Overall, medial RA-MUKA showed improved PROMs, high subject satisfaction, met expectations, and excellent functional recovery. Mid-run survivorship was excellent. However, Gaudiani et al. also stated that longitudinal follow-up was required to assess long-run results of RA-MUKA procedures [3].

7.10 Revision Indications for MUKA

According to Tay et al., MUKA has advantages over TKA including fewer adverse events and faster recovery; however, MUKAs also have higher revision percentages. Understanding reasons for MUKA failure might, therefore, allow for optimized clinical results [1]. In a systematic review, Tay et al. tried to identify failure modes for MUKAs and examine differences by implant bearing, cement utilization, and time. The most frequent failure modes were aseptic loosening (24%) and OA progression (30%). Earliest failures (<6 months) were due to infection (40%), bearing dislocation (20%), and fracture (20%); mid-run failures (>2 years to 5 years) were due to OA progression (33%), aseptic loosening (17%), and pain (21%); and late-run (>10 years) failures were mostly due to OA progression (56%). Percentages of failure from wear were higher with fixed-bearing prostheses (5% cf. 0.3%), whereas percentages of bearing dislocations were higher with mobile-bearing prostheses (14% cf. 0%). With cemented components, there was a high percentage of failure due to aseptic loosening (27%), which was diminished with uncemented components (4%). MUKA failure modes differed depending on implant design, cement utilization, and time from surgery [1].

7.11 Long-Term Survival of MUKA in Spontaneous Knee Osteonecrosis

In 2022 Ly et al. stated that while good mid-run outcomes for treating spontaneous knee osteonecrosis (SPONK) with MUKA had been published, concerns remained about implant survival at the long run [7]. In a case-control study with level 4 of evidence published, Ly et al. compared results and survivorship of MUKA for SPONK versus OA at a minimum of 10 years. The study included MUKA for femoral SPONK operated between 1996 and 2010 with a minimum 10-year follow-up ($n = 47$). Each case was matched with a MUKA for OA based on body mass index (BMI), gender, and age. KSS, adverse events, and radiological (loosening) data were collected at the last follow-up. Kaplan-Meier survivorship analysis was carried out utilizing revision implant removal as end point. The mean follow-up was 13.2 years. Mean age and BMI were 72.9 years and 25.5 Kg/m^2 in the SPONK group. At the last follow-up, knee and function KSS were 89.5 and 79 in the SPONK group versus 90 and 81.7 in the

control group. Adverse events and radiological results demonstrated no significant differences. The survival percentage free from any revision was 85.1% at the last follow-up in the SPONK group and 93.6% in the control group. The main cause for revision was aseptic tibial loosening (57.1%) in the SPONK group. The 15-year survival estimate was 83% in the SPONK group. Satisfactory clinical results at the long run following MUKA for femoral SPONK were found, similar to those after UKA for OA, in spite of a higher risk of tibial loosening in the SPONK group. No symptomatic femoral loosening leading to a revision was encountered [7].

7.12 Optimized MUKA Outcome

In 2022 Mikkelsen et al. investigated changes to MUKA revision risk over the last 20 years compared with total TKA, examined external and patient factors for correlation to MUKA revision risk, and described the survival probability for current MUKA and TKA practice [13]. All knee arthroplasties reported to the Danish Knee Arthroplasty Register from 1997 to 2017 were linked to the National Patient Register and the Civil Registration System for comorbidity, emigration, and mortality information. All primary MUKA and TKA subjects with primary OA were included and propensity score matched 4 TKAs to 1 MUKA. Revision and mortality were analyzed utilizing competing risk Cox regression with a shared gamma frailty component. The matched group included 48,195 primary knee arthroplasties (9639 MUKAs). From 1997–2001 to 2012–2017, the 3-year hazard ratio diminished from 5.5 to 1.5 due to increased MUKA survival. Cementless fixation, an elevated percentage usage of MUKA, and augmented surgical volume diminished MUKA revision risk and augmented in occurrence parallel to the decreasing revision risks. MUKA practice utilizing cementless fixation at a high usage unit had a 3-year implant survival of 96%, 1.1% lower than TKA practice. MUKA revision risk diminished over the last 20 years, nearing that of TKA surgery. High usage percentages, surgical volume, and the utilization of cementless fixation had augmented during the study and were associated with diminished MUKA revision risks [13].

7.13 Conclusions

A forgotten joint is considered the final objective of joint replacement. To accomplish the forgotten joint state, the ideal HKAA (hip-knee-ankle angle) range after fixed-bearing MUKA was 176–178.5° and ΔHKAA (HKAA changes) should be <5.5°. Subjects with smaller preoperative ALDFA and HKAA had a lower likelihood of accomplishing a forgotten joint following MUKA. MUKA has advantages over TKA including fewer adverse events and faster recovery; however, MUKA has higher revision percentages. Patellar denervation appears to provide short-run benefits. MUKA for medial osteoarthritis (OA) is a safe, dependable, and efficacious treatment alternative for subjects of 60 years or younger. It provides pain alleviation, satisfactory activity level, excellent clinical results, and up to 96.5% implant survival at 10-year follow-up. Improper alignment and implant positioning following MUKA leads to postoperative pain and increases the prevalence of revision procedures. Roboticassisted MUKA (RA-MUKA) had shown to be successful in component positioning through preoperative planning and intraoperative adjustability. MUKA has an infection rate of 0.1–0.8%. Staged revision represents a dependable and efficacious alternative in delayed and late MUKA infections. The utilization of pulsed electromagnetic fields (PEMFs) leads to significant pain alleviation, better clinical improvement, and lower NSAIDs consumption after MUKA when compared to the control group. The most frequent failure modes of MUKA are aseptic loosening (24%) and OA progression (30%). Earliest failures (<6 months) are due to infection (40%), bearing dislocation (20%), and fracture (20%); mid-run failures (>2 years to 5 years) are due to OA progression (33%), aseptic loosening (17%), and pain (21%); and late-run (>10 years) failures are mostly due to OA progression (56%). Percentages of failure from wear are higher with fixed-bearing prostheses, whereas percentages of bearing dislocations are higher with mobile-bearing prostheses. With cemented components, there is a high percentage of failure due to aseptic loosening, which is diminished with uncemented components. Cementless fixation, an elevated percentage usage of MUKA, and augmented surgical volume diminish MUKA revision risk and augment in occurrence parallel to the decreasing revision risks. High usage percentages, surgical volume, and the utilization of cementless fixation are associated with diminished MUKA revision risks.

References

1. Tay ML, McGlashan SR, Monk AP, Young SW. Revision indications for medial unicompartmental knee arthroplasty: a systematic review. Arch Orthop Trauma Surg. 2022;142:301–14.
2. Porteous AJ, Smith JRA, Bray R, Robinson JR, White P, Murray JRD. St Georg Sled medial unicompartmental arthroplasty: survivorship analysis and function at 20 years follow up. Knee Surg Sports Traumatol Arthrosc. 2022;30:800–8.
3. Gaudiani MA, Samuel LT, Diana JN, DeBattista JL, Coon TM, Moore RE, et al. 5-year survivorship and outcomes of robotic-arm-assisted medial unicompartmental knee arthroplasty. Appl Bionics Biomech. 2022;2022:8995358.
4. Roche MW, Vakharia M, Law TY, Sabeh KG. Accuracy of intraoperative mechanical axis alignment to long-leg radiographs following robotic-arm-assisted unicompartmental knee arthroplasty. J Knee Surg. 2022; https://doi.org/10.1055/s-0042-1742647. Online ahead of print.
5. Wang Z, Deng W, Shao H, Zhou Y, Yang D, Li H. Predictors of a forgotten joint after medial fixed-bearing unicompartmental knee arthroplasty. Knee. 2022;37:103–11.
6. Cavagnaro L, Chiarlone F, Mosconi L, Zanirato A, Formica M, Burastero G. Two-stage revision for periprosthetic joint infection in unicompartmental knee arthroplasty: clinical and radiological results. Arch Orthop Trauma Surg. 2022;142:2031–8.
7. Ly L, Batailler C, Shatrov J, Servien E, Lustig S. Satisfactory outcomes of all-poly fixed bearing unicompartmental knee arthroplasty for avascular osteonecrosis versus osteoarthritis: a comparative study with 10 to 22 years of follow-up. J Arthroplast. 2022;37(9):1743–50.
8. Kyriakidis T, Asopa V, Baums M, Verdonk R, Totlis T. Unicompartmental knee arthroplasty in patients under the age of 60 years provides excellent clinical outcomes and 10-year implant survival: a systematic review: a study performed by the Early Osteoarthritis

group of ESSKA-European Knee Associates section. Knee Surg Sports Traumatol Arthrosc. 2022; https://doi.org/10.1007/s00167-022-07029-9. Online ahead of print.

9. Suwankomonkul P, Arirachakaran A, Kongtharvonskul J. Short-term improvement of patellofemoral pain in medial unicompartmental knee arthroplasty with patellar denervation: a prospective comparative study. Musculoskelet Surg. 2022;106:75–82.

10. D'Ambrosi R, Ursino C, Setti S, Scelsi M, Ursino N. Pulsed electromagnetic fields improve pain management and clinical outcomes after medial unicompartmental knee arthroplasty: a prospective randomised controlled trial. J ISAKOS. 2022;S2059-7754(22)00065-7.

11. Monti L, Franchi M, Ursino N, Mariani I, Corona K, Anghilieri FM, et al. Hypoallergenic unicompartmen-tal knee arthroplasty and return to sport: comparison between oxidized zirconium and titanium niobium nitride. Acta Biomed. 2022;93(3):e2022160.

12. D'Ambrosi R, Ursino N, Mariani I, Corona K, Anghilieri FM, Franchi E, et al. Similar clinical and radiographic outcomes after two different hypoaller-genic medial unicompartmental knee in patients with metal allergy. Eur J Orthop Surg Traumatol. 2022; https://doi.org/10.1007/s00590-022-03295-y. Online ahead of print.

13. Mikkelsen M, Price A, Pedersen AB, Gromov K, Troelsen A. Optimized medial unicompartmental knee arthroplasty outcome: learning from 20 years of propensity score matched registry data. Acta Orthop. 2022;93:390–6.

Lateral Unicompartmental Knee Arthroplasty

8

E. Carlos Rodríguez-Merchán,
Carlos A. Encinas-Ullán, Juan S. Ruiz-Pérez,
and Primitivo Gómez-Cardero

8.1 Introduction

According to Buzin et al., isolated lateral compartment osteoarthritis (OA) of the knee is an infrequent disease affecting approximately 1% of the population, which is ten times less usual than OA affecting only the medial compartment. Unicompartmental knee arthroplasty (UKA) has many possible advantages over total knee arthroplasty (TKA). The advantages of UKA include a smaller incision, preservation of more native tissue (including cruciate ligaments and bone), diminished blood loss, and better overall proprioception. When UKA was first introduced in the 1970s, the results of medial UKA (MUKA) were poor, but the few cases of lateral UKA (LUKA) showed promise. Since that time, there has been a relative scarcity of literature focused specifically on LUKA given it is an uncommon procedure [1]. The purpose of this chapter is to review the last developments on LUKA.

8.2 General Concepts on LUKA

A review of the recent literature revealed that LUKA was associated with excellent long-run clinical results and implant survivorship when carried out in properly selected individuals (Figs. 8.1 and 8.2). Implant design alternatives include fixed- versus mobile-bearing as well as metal-backed versus all-polyethylene tibial component, with improved results found with fixed-bearing designs. Three reasons cited for revision (fracture of the femoral component, fracture of the tibial component, and valgus malalignment) had been published in past literature but not lately. Presently, while uncommon, the most frequent causes of failure and need for revision are OA progression and aseptic loosening. In spite of the need for an occasional revision procedure, the survivorship of LUKA is comparable to MUKA, although it should be remarked that results of MUKA have been noticeably varied [1].

E. C. Rodríguez-Merchán (✉) · C. A. Encinas-Ullán
J. S. Ruiz-Pérez · P. Gómez-Cardero
Department of Orthopedic Surgery, La Paz University
Hospital, Madrid, Spain

© The Author(s), under exclusive license to Springer Nature Switzerland AG 2023
E. C. Rodríguez-Merchán (ed.), *Advances in Orthopedic Surgery of the Knee*,
https://doi.org/10.1007/978-3-031-33061-2_8

81

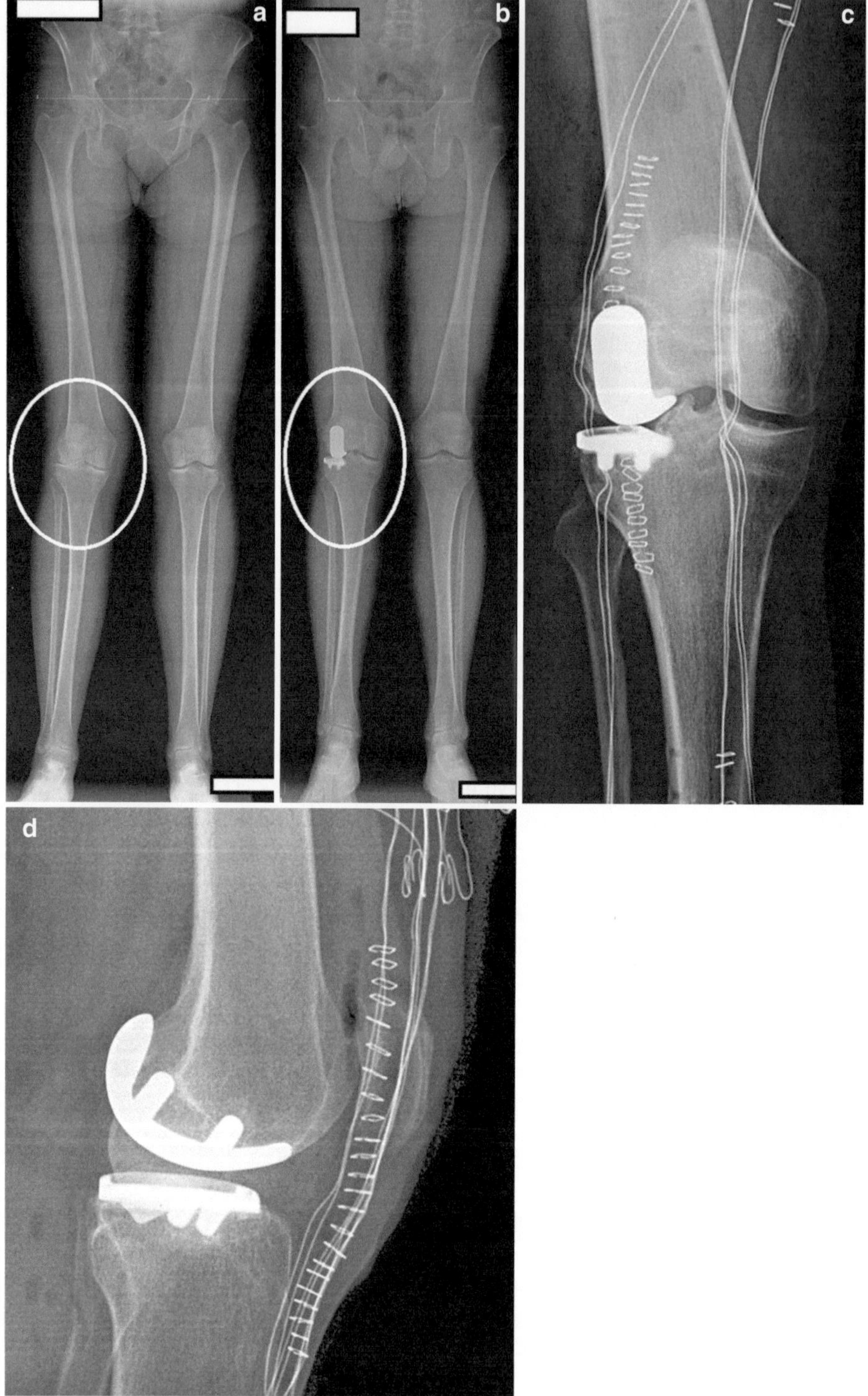

Fig. 8.1 (**a–d**) Lateral knee osteoarthritis treated with lateral unicompartmental knee arthroplasty (LUKA): (**a**) preoperative anteroposterior (AP) weight-bearing bilateral long-leg standing radiograph (circle). (**b**) Postoperative AP weight-bearing bilateral long-leg standing radiograph (circle). (**c**) Postoperative AP view. (**d**) Postoperative lateral radiograph

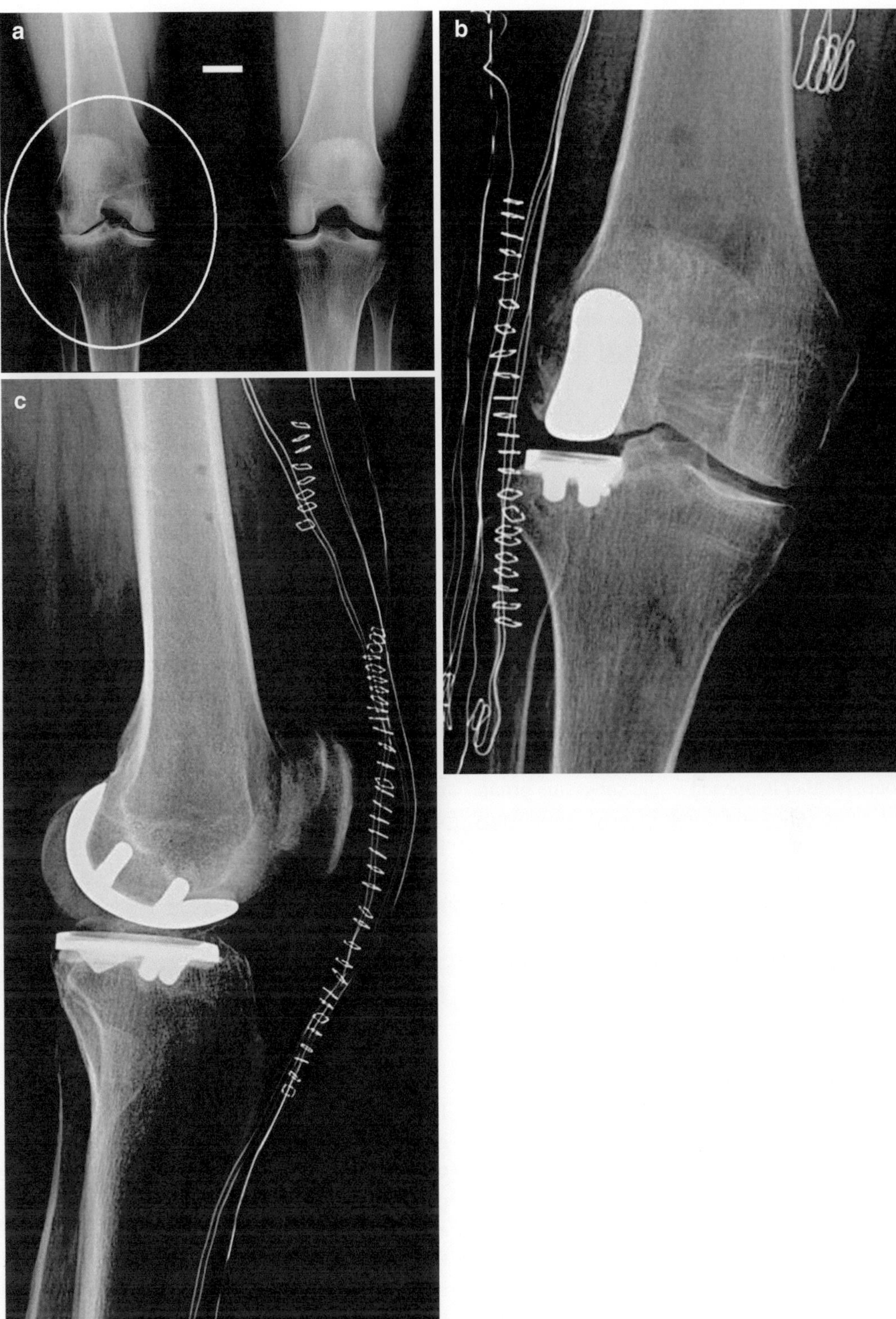

Fig. 8.2 (**a–c**) Lateral unicompartmental knee arthroplasty (LUKA) for the treatment of lateral knee osteoarthritis: (**a**) preoperative knee anteroposterior (AP) weight-bearing radiograph (circle). (**b**) Postoperative AP view. (**c**) Postoperative lateral radiograph

8.3 Medial Subvastus Approach

According to Fuller et al., UKA treats OA involving only one compartment of the knee. LUKA is principally carried out through medial parapatellar or lateral parapatellar approaches to the knee [2]. In 2022 Fuller et al. reported a medial subvastus approach to LUKA, discussed the clinical rationale behind its utilization, and offered a preliminary retrospective study on short-run results of LUKAs using the lateral versus medial subvastus approaches. A description of the medial subvastus approach was included. Besides, they reviewed 32 and 30 lateral UKAs carried out utilizing the lateral and medial subvastus approaches, respectively. Minimum follow-up duration was 1 year. KOOS-JR (Knee Injury and OA Outcome Score for Joint Replacement) knee scores were utilized for comparison. Age and body mass index (BMI) were similar between the two cohorts. Mean KOOS-JR scores for the subvastus approach group were significantly higher than those for the lateral approach group at 81.41 for medial subvastus and 74.19 for lateral. One deep infection and two revision TKAs happened in the lateral approach group. Neither happened in the subvastus group. The mean follow-up duration was significantly longer for the lateral approach group than that for the subvastus group at 749 versus 410 days. Literature on time dependence of patient-reported outcomes (PROMs) supports usage of the data, despite follow-up discrepancies. A subvastus approach for LUKA might offer improved visualization, easier conversion to TKA, and faster recovery, based on clinical observation. Preliminary outcomes suggested improved short-run knee scores compared to a lateral approach [2].

8.4 Implantation Accuracy of a LUKA

According to Keppler et al., a small proportion of patients suffer from isolated lateral OA where the sole lateral LUKA is a potential treatment alternative. There, both a medial and a lateral surgical approach can be considered [3]. In 2021 Keppler et al. investigated whether the lateral approach was superior to a modified medial approach in terms of implantation accuracy and subjective result. In a retrospective study, 175 individuals with LUKA were included between 2015 and 2020. In 82 individuals, the lateral approach was utilized, and in 93 individuals, the medial approach was utilized. To evaluate implantation accuracy, different imaging criteria on postoperative radiographs were studied. Postoperative PROMs (OKS [Oxford Knee Score], LEFS [Lower Extremity Functional Scale], and EQ-5D [EuroQol-5D]) were assessed. The tibial implant relation to the tibial plateau diameter in the lateral approach was significantly larger than in the medial approach (23.6% vs 22.2%). Significantly more deviations >15° regarding flexion position of the femoral implant and a higher number of deviations of the slope was encountered in the lateral approach. The lateral approach demonstrated a significantly higher percentage of lateral positioning of the femoral component. Post-PROMs demonstrated significant improvement in both approaches. The lateral approach was not superior regarding different radiological accuracy criteria. The Hoffa's fat pad-preserving medial approach demonstrated good outcomes in implantation accuracy and therefore was a good option to implant LUKA. Besides, significant improvement in PROMs could be shown [3].

8.5 External Rotation of the Tibial Component Should Be Avoided

In 2021 Fujita et al. stated that LUKA led to good clinical results for isolated lateral OA. However, the impact of the tibial component position on postoperative results in LUKA was yet to be established [4]. Fujita et al. studied the impact of tibial component malposition on clinical results in LUKA. This was a retrospective study of 50 knees (mean age 73.5 years) who experienced LUKA between September 2013 and January 2019. The OKS, Knee Society Score–Knee (KSSK), and Knee Society Score–Function

(KSSF) were assessed. The coronal alignment, posterior slope of tibial component, tibial component rotation relative to Akagi's line (angle α), and femoral anteroposterior axis (angle β) were measured postoperatively. The average follow-up period was 2.3 years. Clinical scores were significantly improved after LUKA. The mean coronal alignment was 0.9° varus, and the mean posterior slope was 6.8°. The mean α- and β-angles were 4.1° and 6.7° external rotation, respectively. The α-angle had significant negative correlations with postoperative OKS, KSSK, and KSSF, and β-angle had significant negative correlations with postoperative OKS and KSSK. The conclusion of this study was that excessive external rotation of the tibial component could negatively impact the postoperative results of LUKA [4].

8.6 Midterm Survivorship and Clinical Outcomes

In a systematic review of level 4 studies published in 2021, Bonanzinga et al. reviewed the accessible literature to comprehend the efficacy, the survivorship, the clinical results, and the adverse events of LUKA [5]. A review of the literature accessible about LUKA was carried out in March 2020. Mean age at surgery was 64.5 years. In 1741 individuals (65.5%), a metal back implant was utilized, and in 421 individuals (15.8%), an all-poly design was utilized. Several scores were utilized to assess clinical outcomes (OKS, AKSS [American Knee Society Score], IKS [International Knee Society], KOOS [Knee Injury and Osteoarthritis Outcome Score], WOMAC [Western Ontario and McMaster Universities Arthritis Index], VAS [visual analog scale]). Range of motion (ROM) improved with an overall mean value of 120.3°. The mean follow-up was 60.7 months, mean survivorship (absence of a revision) with a minimum 60 months of follow-up was 88.6%, and mean satisfaction of individuals was 78.5%. LUKA appeared to be an efficacious solution to manage lateral OA, based on preliminary outcomes, with survivorship and satisfaction percentage comparable to MUKA and TKA [5].

8.7 Assessment of Radiolucent Lines in Patients with LUKA

In 2021 Xue et al. assessed the radiolucent lines (RLLs) around both tibial and femoral components in individuals following LUKA [6]. They carried out a retrospective review of the records of a consecutive series of individuals who had experienced LUKA. The RLLs were evaluated with standard anteroposterior and lateral radiographs postoperatively. The patient-reported outcome measures (PROMs) included the Hospital for Special Surgery (HSS) score and OKS. The femoral component position (FCP) and femoral-tibial angle (FTA) were also recorded. A total of 198 UKAs that had adequate radiographs and outcome scores were reviewed with a median follow-up of 33 months. The outcomes suggested that 69 cases (34.8%) had RLLs on the standard radiographs. The prevalence percentages of femoral and tibial physiological RLLs were 11.6% (23/198) and 26% (52/198), respectively, of which 3% (6/198) concerned both components. All RLLs were considered "physiologic lines" that developed within 1 year after surgery. There were no significant differences among the types of RLLs in any of the result measures. No differences in FCP or FTA at the last follow-up were encountered. It was observed that one-third of UKAs had RLLs on radiographs following LUKA. All RLLs developed within 1 year after surgery. As a clinical consequence, the development of RLLs did not impact the short-run results after LUKA [6].

8.8 The Effect of Patient Age and Bearing Choice on Midterm Outcomes

According to Hartman et al., isolated lateral compartment knee OA affects between 7% and 10% of individuals with knee OA. Even though LUKA is an accepted treatment to manage this disease, it is carried out relatively seldom [7]. In a retrospective therapeutic study with level 3 of evidence, Hartman et al. assessed the mid-run survivorship, radiographic results, and PROMs.

They carried out a retrospective review of a prospectively maintained database of consecutive isolated LUKAs performed by a single surgeon at an academic institution between September 2007 and December 2015. Their primary outcome was failure defined as revision surgery to TKA. Secondary outcomes included any additional surgery for any other reason. Forty-nine consecutive individuals (27 women) with a median age of 54.7 years met the inclusion criteria. The survival percentage for the whole cohort was 86.1% at 10 years as defined by conversion to TKA. There were a total of four LUKAs (all mobile bearings) revised to TKAs. The entire cohort showed statistically significant improvements from preoperative PROMs compared with the most recent postoperative PROMs including the WOMAC, KOOS, and Tegner activity scale at a median 8.8 years of follow-up. Individuals with mobile bearing experienced higher revision to TKA and reoperation for all indications compared with fixed-bearing LUKA. In this relatively young cohort, LUKA yielded acceptable long-run survival and satisfactory improvement in functional results [7].

8.9 Survivorship and Long-Term Outcomes

In 2022 Plancher et al. stated that LUKA was an excellent alternative to alleviate disability and restore function in individuals with lateral compartment knee OA [8]. In a therapeutic study with level 3 of evidence, Plancher et al. determined the survivorship and long-run results in both younger/middle-aged and older individuals with lateral compartment OA following non-robotically assisted, fixed-bearing LUKA and to establish if an acceptable symptom state could be accomplished. All individuals were managed with fixed-bearing LUKA by a single surgeon using a lateral parapatellar approach without robotic assistance. The primary outcome variables were the KOOS, Activities of Daily Living (ADL), and Sports subscale scores. In addition, the other KOOS subscores, the Lysholm score, the achievement of the Patient Acceptable Symptom State

(PASS), and the Veterans RAND (VR-12) Physical Component Summary score (PCS) and Mental Component Summary score (MCS) were collected. Failure was defined as conversion to TKA. Individuals were divided into two groups: younger/middle-aged individuals (<60 years of age) and older individuals (≥60 years of age). A cohort of 256 individuals experienced medial ($n = 193$) or lateral ($n = 63$) UKA. Sixty-one individuals met the inclusion criteria. At mean of 10 years of follow-up, there were no significant differences between the groups in terms of any PROMs. The percentage of patients in whom PASS was achieved on the KOOS ADL and Sports subscores was 82% and 88%, respectively, in the younger group and 80% and 80%, respectively, in the older group. The mean survival estimate of the prosthesis was 15.3 years for the entire series. The estimated percentage of implant survival in the younger group was 100% at 5 and 10 years, and the estimated percentage of implant survival in the older group was 98% at 5 years and 96% at 10 years. Lateral fixed-bearing, non-robotic UKA for the management of isolated lateral compartment OA resulted in >80% of individuals reaching an acceptable symptom state in terms of both activities of daily living and sporting activities. UKA provided an excellent option that provides longevity with high PASS percentages and return to activities with a low risk of adverse events and failure [8].

8.10 Fixed-Bearing LUKA

8.10.1 Predictors of Satisfactory Outcomes

In 2021 Xue et al. stated that there was little literature accessible studying factors that may forecast functional recovery after LUKA [9]. In 2021 Xue et al. reported short- to mid-run efficacy and assessed predictors of better result following LUKA. They retrospectively reviewed 248 individuals (260 knees) who experienced LUKA from January 2013, with a mean 5-year follow-up. The primary outcome measures comprised the HSS score and patient satisfaction.

Multivariate regression analyses were performed to investigate associations between these factors with a satisfactory result. Implant survival was estimated by Kaplan-Meier analysis. Complete follow-up was accessible for 186 individuals (198 knees). At last follow-up, the HSS scores were changed from 52.1 preoperatively to 85.6. The OKS improved from 22.8 preoperatively to 42.7. The 5-year survival was 99.5%. The multivariate analysis demonstrated that the following factors tended to attain a satisfactory result: higher proportion of ASA (American Society of Anesthesiology) class I, diagnosis of primary OA, postoperative limb alignment, and higher preoperative HSS score. Individuals with valgus 9–12° reported the highest HSS scores among different subgroups. Following LUKA, postoperative results were satisfactory in individuals with lower ASA scores, diagnosis with primary OA, higher preoperative HSS scores, and those with postoperative valgus alignment. Xue et al. concluded that it was important to comprehend these correlations to help adequate patient selection to attain optimal function after LUKA [9].

8.10.2 Sports Activity and Patient-Related Outcomes

According to Zimmerer et al., unicompartmental OA increasingly affects younger individuals who have high expectations concerning their postoperative level of activity. Moreover, the aforementioned authors stated that there was no accessible information on the activity level after fixed-bearing LUKA [10]. In 2021 Zimmerer et al. reported sports activity after fixed-bearing LUKA with a minimum two-year follow up. Nineteen individuals were analyzed to establish their sporting activities at a mean follow-up of 4.6 years after fixed-bearing LUKA. The aforementioned authors also evaluated the KOOS-JR score and the University of California, Los Angeles, activity scale (UCLA scale) at baseline and latest follow-up. Prior to the onset of the first symptoms, 15 of 19 individuals were active in at least one sport compared with 13 of 19 individuals after surgery. Eighty-six percent of the individuals returned to activity. Within 6 months, 68% returned to their activities after surgery. The mean postoperative UCLA score was 6.4. Half of the individuals reached a high activity level (UCLA ≥7). Most frequent activities after surgery were long walks, biking, and hiking. High-impact activities demonstrated a significant reduction. Eighty-six percent of the individuals were able to return to regular recreational and sporting activities. In general, a shift from high-impact to low-impact activities was found. There was no difference in the number of disciplines carried out. Overall, the session length and frequency remained unchanged. However, male individuals and younger individuals participated in sports less commonly compared with preoperative levels [10].

8.10.3 Fixed-Bearing, All-Polyethylene Tibia

According to Murray et al., LUKA constitutes only 5–10% of all unicompartmental replacements carried out. The aforementioned authors stated that while the short- and medium-run benefits were well documented, there remained concern regarding the higher revision percentage when compared with TKA [11]. In 2021 Murray et al. reported the long-run clinical result and survivorship of a large series of LUKA. Between 1974 and 1994, 71 individuals (82 knees) experienced a lateral fixed-bearing St Georg Sled UKA. Prospective data was collected preoperatively and at regular intervals postoperatively using the Bristol Knee Score (BKS), with later introduction of the OKS and WOMAC scores. Kaplan-Meier survival analysis was utilized, with revision, or need for revision, as endpoint. Eighty-five percent of the individuals were female. No individuals were lost to follow-up. Functional knee scores improved postoperatively up to 10 years, at which point they showed a steady decline. Survivorship was 72% at 15 years and 68% at 20 and 25 years. Nineteen knees were revised, with progression of illness in another compartment the most frequent reason. There were two revisions due to implant fracture. In individuals aged over 70 years at the time of index procedure, 81% died with a functioning prosthesis in situ. This study represented the longest follow-up of a large series of LUKA. Outcomes of this early design of fixed-bearing UKA showed satisfactory long-run survivorship. In elderly individuals, further intervention is seldom needed. More contemporary designs or techniques may demonstrate improved long-run survivorship in time [11].

8.11 Comparison of Failure Rates of Different Prosthetic Designs

In 2022 Fratine et al. stated that LUKA is a viable solution for isolated lateral compartment OA. Several prosthetic designs are accessible such as fixed-bearing metal-backed (FB M-B), fixed-bearing all-polyethylene (FB A-P), and mobile-bearing metal-backed (MB M-B) implants [12]. In a meta-analysis, Fratini et al. compared failure percentages of different prosthetic designs. Two separate analyses were carried out among different implant designs (FB M-B vs FB A-P vs MB M-B) and different follow-ups (<5 years, between 5 and 10 years, >10 years).The failure percentage of FB M-B LUKA was significantly lower compared to other LUKA designs present in the market (0.8% vs 8.6% and 7.1% for FB M-B, FB A-P, and MB M-B, respectively). No significant difference among groups was found when comparing all implants with regard to follow-up time. Fratini et al. concluded that considering current evidence, for a surgeon approaching LUKA, the FB M-B design was preferable, given the lower failure percentages and consequently a longer implant survivorship [12].

8.12 Robotic-Assisted Lateral UKA

In 2022 Heckman et al. stated that LUKA was a popular option to TKA for individuals with isolated lateral compartment OA. Also, few studies had studied results following robotic-assisted LUKA (RA-LUKA) [13]. Heckmann et al. assessed mid-run survivorship and PROMs of RA-LUKA. A retrospective case series was performed on all RA-LUKAs carried out by a single surgeon between 2013 and 2019. Patient demographics, surgical variables, and Kozinn and Scott criteria were collected. Implant survivorship was estimated using the Kaplan-Meier method with all-cause reoperation and conversion to TKA as endpoints. Participating individuals were evaluated for patient satisfaction and the Forgotten Joint Score-12. Correlations between patient demographics and PROMs were studied. In total, 120 LUKAs were recognized, 84 of which met inclusion criteria, with a mean follow-up of 4 years. Five-year survivorship was 92.9 with all-cause reoperation as the endpoint and 100% with conversion to TKA as the endpoint. One individual was converted to TKA after the 5-year mark, resulting in a 6-year survival for conversion to TKA of 88.9%. Average Forgotten Joint Score-12 score was 82.7/100 and patient satisfaction 4.7/5. Mean coronal plane correction was 2.5° toward the mechanical axis. Neither final postoperative alignment nor failure to meet classic Kozinn and Scott criteria for UKA resulted in differences in PROMs. This study showed high mid-run survivorship and excellent PROMs with RA-LUKA. RA-LUKA was a viable treatment alternative for isolated lateral compartment OA even in individuals who do not meet classic indications [13].

In a multicenter, retrospective, observational study published in 2021, Zambiachi et al. analyzed the association between intraoperative component positioning and soft tissue balancing, as reported by robotic technology for a group of individuals who received RA-LUKA as well as short-run clinical follow-up of these individuals [14]. Between 2013 and 2016, 78 individuals (79 knees) experienced RA-LUKAs at two centers. Pre- and postoperatively, individuals were administered the KOOS and the Forgotten Joint Score-12 (FJS-12). Clinical outcomes were dichotomized based upon KOOS and FJS-12 scores into either excellent or fair outcome, considering excellent KOOS and FJS-12 to be greater than or equal to 90. Intraoperative, postimplantation robotic data relative to computed tomography-based component placement were collected and classified. Following exclusions and loss to follow-up, a total of 74 individuals (75 knees) who received RA-LUKAs were taken into account with an average follow-up of 36.3 months postoperative. Of these, 66 individuals (67 knees) were included in the clinical outcome analysis. All postoperative clinical scores demonstrated significant improvement compared with the preoperative assessment. No association was reported between three-dimensional component positioning and soft tissue balancing throughout knee ROM with overall KOOS, KOOS subscales, and FJS-12 scores. LUKA three-dimensional placement did not appear to impact short-run clinical performance. However, precise boundaries for LUKA positioning and balancing should be taken into account. Robotic assistance permitted surgeons to acquire real-time information regarding implant alignment and soft tissue balancing [14].

In 2021 Mohan et al. reported a prospective single-center clinical study of six patients (five females and one male) who experienced RA-LUKA between May 2018 and January 2020 with patient-specific 3D-CT preoperative plan. Overall satisfaction on a five-level Likert scale, clinical result based on the KOOS and MFJS (Modified Forgotten Joint Score), and radiological results based on the HKA (hip-knee-ankle) axis, femorotibial angle (FTA), and tibial posterior slope (PS) attained were compared preoperatively and postoperatively. At a mean follow-up period of 23.84 months, among six individuals 33.3% were very satisfied, 50% were satisfied, and 16.7% felt neutral. The mean KOOS changed from 63.03 to 93.95 and the mean MFJS was 75.41 postoperatively. The mean HKA axis changed from 175.81° valgus to 179.99° neutral alignment. The mean correction obtained was from 4.19° valgus deformity to 0.01°. The mean FTA and the mean PS changed from 7.34° of valgus to 1.92° of valgus and 83.44° to 85.38°, respectively. The mean preoperative and postoperative KOOS demonstrated a statistical significance, demonstrating signifi-

cant improvement with RA-LUKA. RA-LUKA was a promising surgical alternative for lateral compartment OA of the knee [15].

8.13 Revision Indications

In 2022 Tay et al. stated that LUKA was a surgical alternative for individuals with isolated lateral OA; however, the procedure had higher revision rates than MUKA. The reason for this remained unclear; therefore, a better understanding of the indications for LUKA revision were required [16]. In a systematic review, Tay et al. tried to identify revision indications for LUKA. They also investigated if revision indications were influenced by implant design and time from surgery. The main indications for LUKA revision were OA progression (35%), aseptic loosening (17%), and bearing dislocation (14%). Prevalence of revision was similar for mobile-bearing implants (7.6%) and fixed-bearing (6.4%). For mobile-bearing implants there was introduction of bearing dislocations as an additional mode of failure (24%). For fixed-bearing implants, prevalence of revision was higher for all-polyethylene (PE; 13.9%) than metal-backed (1.8%) tibial components. Early LUKA failures were associated with bearing dislocations (sequential decrease from 69% under 6 months to 0% 10+ years), while late failures were associated with OA progression (sequential increase from 0% under 6 months to 100% >10+ years). Compared with MUKA, OA progression (41%), malalignment (2.7%), instability (4%), and bearing dislocations (20%) were more frequent for LUKA. OA progression, aseptic loosening, and bearing dislocation were the three main revision indications for LUKA. Compared to MUKA, OA progression, malalignment, instability, and bearing dislocations were more frequent revision indications for LUKA. Higher survivorship of metal-backed fixed-bearing implants was observed. The findings of this article suggested that results of LUKA might be improved with more optimal alignment, gap balancing, and patient selection [16].

8.14 Conclusions

LUKA appears to be an efficacious solution to manage lateral OA, based on preliminary outcomes, with survivorship and satisfaction percentage comparable to MUKA and TKA. The estimated percentage of implant survival in the younger group (<60 years of age) is 100% at 5 and 10 years, and the estimated percentage of implant survival in the older group (>60 years of age) is 98% at 5 years and 96% at 10 years. Excessive external rotation of the tibial component negatively impacts the postoperative results of LUKA. Individuals with mobile-bearing experience higher revision to TKA and reoperation for all indications compared with fixed-bearing LUKA. Lateral fixed-bearing, non-robotic UKA for the management of isolated lateral compartment OA resulted in >80% of individuals reaching an acceptable symptom state in terms of both activities of daily living and sporting activities. The main indications for LUKA revision are OA progression (35%), aseptic loosening (17%), and bearing dislocation (14%). Prevalence of revision is similar for mobile-bearing implants (7.6%) and fixed-bearing (6.4%). For mobile-bearing implants there was introduction of bearing dislocations as an additional mode of failure (24%). For fixed-bearing implants, prevalence of revision was higher for all-polyethylene (13.9%) than metal-backed (1.8%) tibial components. Early LUKA failures are associated with bearing dislocations, while late failures are associated with OA progression. Compared with MUKA, OA progression (41%), malalignment (2.7%), instability (4%), and bearing dislocations (20%) are more frequent for LUKA. OA progression, aseptic loosening, and bearing dislocation are the three main revision indications for LUKA. Compared to MUKA, OA progression, malalignment, instability, and bearing dislocations are more frequent revision indications for LUKA.

References

1. Buzin SD, Geller JA, Yoon RS, Macaulay W. Lateral unicompartmental knee arthroplasty: a review. World J Orthop. 2021;12:197–206.
2. Fuller RM, Wicker DI, Getman GW, Christensen KS, Christensen CP. A medial subvastus approach for lateral unicompartmental knee arthroplasty: technique description and early outcome results. Arthroplast Today. 2021;9:129–33.
3. Keppler L, Klingbeil S, Navarre F, Michel B, Fulghum C, Reng W. Implantation accuracy of a lateral unicompartmental knee arthroplasty: a Hoffa's fat pad-preserving medial approach versus the transpatellar lateral approach. J Arthroplast. 2021;36:2752–8.
4. Fujita M, Hiranaka T, Mai B, Kamenaga T, Tsubosaka M, Takayama K, et al. External rotation of the tibial component should be avoided in lateral unicompartmental knee arthroplasty. Knee. 2021;30:70–7.
5. Bonanzinga T, Tanzi P, Altomare D, Dorotei A, Iacono F, Marcacci M. High survivorship rate and good clinical outcomes at mid-term follow-up for lateral UKA: a systematic literature review. Knee Surg Sports Traumatol Arthrosc. 2021;29:3262–71.
6. Xue L, Xue H, Wen T, Guan M, Yang T, Ma T, et al. Assessment of radiolucent lines in patients with lateral unicompartmental knee arthroplasty and the relationship between these lines and the outcome. Int Orthop. 2021;45:2017–23.
7. Hartman J, Dobransky J, Dervin GF. Midterm outcomes in lateral unicompartment knee replacement: the effect of patient age and bearing choice. J Knee Surg. 2022; https://doi.org/10.1055/s-0042-1743497. Online ahead of print.
8. Plancher KD, Briggs KK, Chinnakkannu K, Dotterweich KA, Commaroto SA, Wang KH, et al. Isolated lateral tibiofemoral compartment osteoarthritis: survivorship and patient acceptable symptom state after lateral fixed-bearing unicompartmental knee arthroplasty at mean 10-year follow-up. J Bone Joint Surg Am. 2022;104:1621–8.
9. Xue H, Ma T, Wen T, Yang T, Xue L, Tu Y. Predictors of satisfactory outcomes with fixed-bearing lateral unicompartmental knee arthroplasty: up to 7-year follow-up. J Arthroplast. 2021;36:910–6.
10. Zimmerer A, Navas L, Kinkel S, Weiss S, Hauschild M, Miehlke W, et al. Sports activity and patient-related outcomes after fixed-bearing lateral unicompartmental knee arthroplasty. Knee. 2021;28:64–71.
11. Murray JRD, Smith JRA, Bray R, Robinson JR, White P, Porteous AJ. Fixed bearing, all-polyethylene tibia, lateral unicompartmental arthroplasty - a final outcome study with up to 28 year follow-up of a single implant. Knee. 2021;29:101–9.

12. Fratini S, Meena A, Alesi D, Cammisa E, Zaffagnini S, Marcheggiani Muccioli GM. Does implant design influence failure rate of lateral unicompartmental knee arthroplasty? A meta-analysis. J Arthroplast. 2022;37:985–992.e3.
13. Heckmann ND, Antonios JK, Chen XT, Kang HP, Chung BC, Piple AS, et al. Midterm survivorship of robotic-assisted lateral unicompartmental knee arthroplasty. J Arthroplast. 2022;37:831–6.
14. Zambianchi F, Franceschi G, Banchelli F, Marcovigi A, Ensini A, Catani F. Robotic arm-assisted lateral unicompartmental knee arthroplasty: how are components aligned? J Knee Surg. 2022;35:1214–22.
15. Mohan T, Panicker J, Thilak J, Shaji D, Hari H. Short-term outcomes of robotic lateral unicompartmental knee arthroplasty: an Indian perspective. Indian J Orthop. 2021;56:655–63.
16. Tay ML, Matthews BG, Monk AP, Young SW. Disease progression, aseptic loosening and bearing dislocations are the main revision indications after lateral unicompartmental knee arthroplasty: a systematic review J ISAKOS 2022;S2059-7754(22)00067–0.

Total Knee Arthroplasty After Proximal Tibia Fracture

9

E. Carlos Rodríguez-Merchán,
Carlos A. Encinas-Ullán, Juan S. Ruiz-Pérez,
and Primitivo Gómez-Cardero

9.1 Introduction

When after proximal tibia fracture (PTF) a malunion with extensive joint involvement has been established or the initial cartilage damage has resulted in knee osteoarthritis (OA), the surgical alternative is total knee arthroplasty (TKA) (Fig. 9.1). It is reasonable to consider hardware removal months before TKA implantation, given that it seems to diminish infection percentages after TKA [1].

In 2009 Larson et al. stated that TKA carried out after PTF had a high percentage of adverse events [2]. In 2015 Scott et al. claimed that radiological evidence of posttraumatic OA (PT OA) of the knee after PTF was frequent but end-stage OA which needs TKA was much rarer [3].

According to Pander et al., PT OA following a PTF is a debilitating condition which frequently affects a young and active patient population for whom good knee function is crucial. Many times, TKA is the only surgical alternative [4]. In 2022 Tapper et al. stated that PT OA of the knee following PTF is a frequent complication that may lead to TKA as secondary treatment (S-TKA) [5]. The purpose of this chapter is to review recent developments on TKA after PTF.

E. C. Rodríguez-Merchán (✉) · C. A. Encinas-Ullán
J. S. Ruiz-Pérez · P. Gómez-Cardero
Department of Orthopedic Surgery, La Paz University
Hospital, Madrid, Spain

E. C. Rodríguez-Merchán (ed.), *Advances in Orthopedic Surgery of the Knee*,
https://doi.org/10.1007/978-3-031-33061-2_9

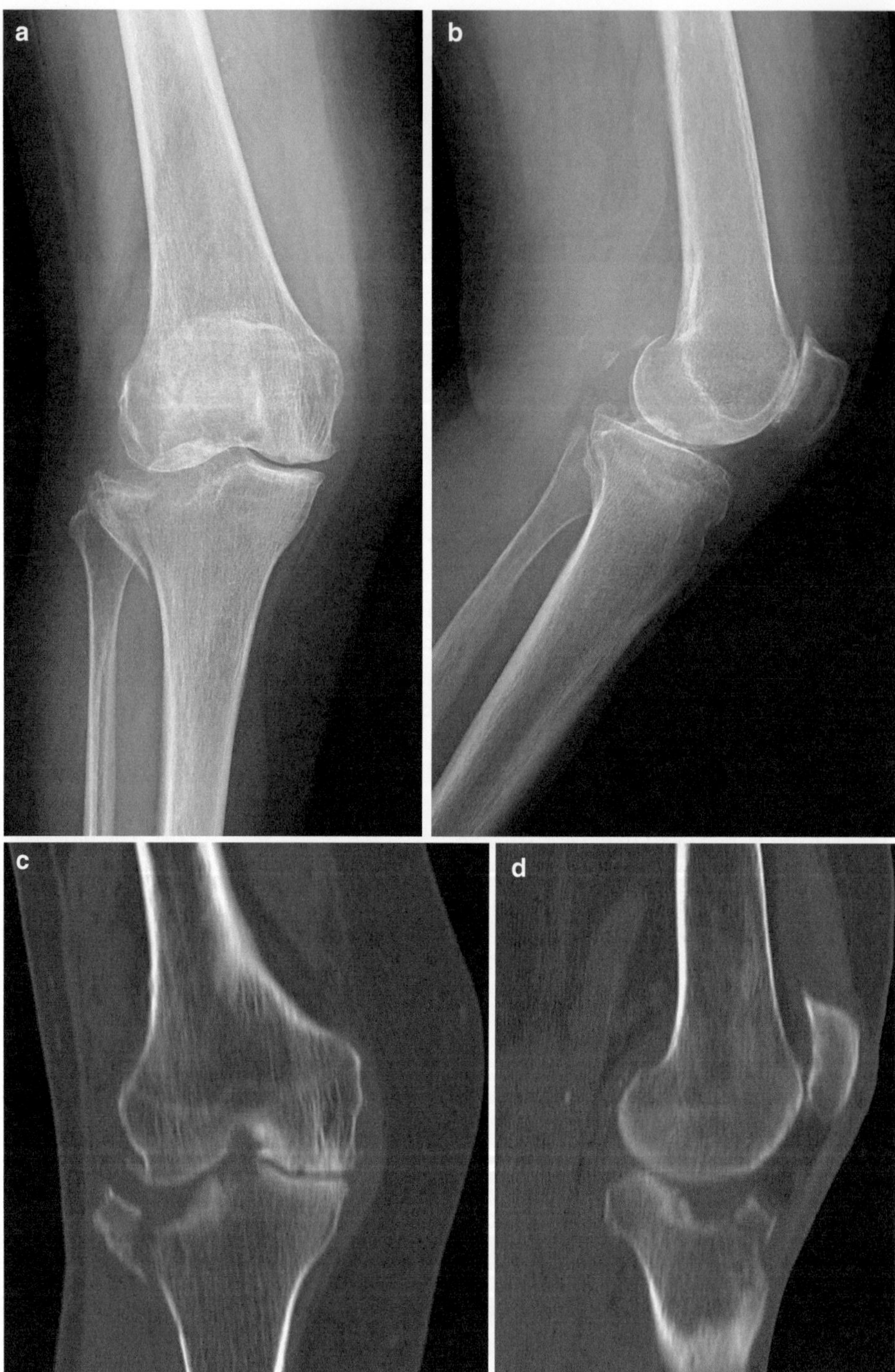

Fig. 9.1 (**a–k**) Tibial plateau fracture that was treated by open reduction and internal fixation (ORIF) with poor outcome and eventually required total knee arthroplasty (TKA) implantation to solve the problem: (**a**) preoperative anteroposterior (AP) radiograph. (**b**) Preoperative lateral radiograph. (**c**) Preoperative computed tomography (CT) scan (coronal view). (**d**) Preoperative CT scan (sagittal view). (**e**) Postoperative AP radiograph after ORIF. (**f**) Postoperative lateral view after ORIF. (**g**) Intraoperative image showing that the osteosynthesis plate had to be cut in order to remove it. (**h**) Intraoperative image showing the osteosynthesis plate already cut. (**i**) Removed osteosynthesis plate and screws. (**j**) AP radiograph of the TKA implanted. (**k**) Lateral view of the TKA

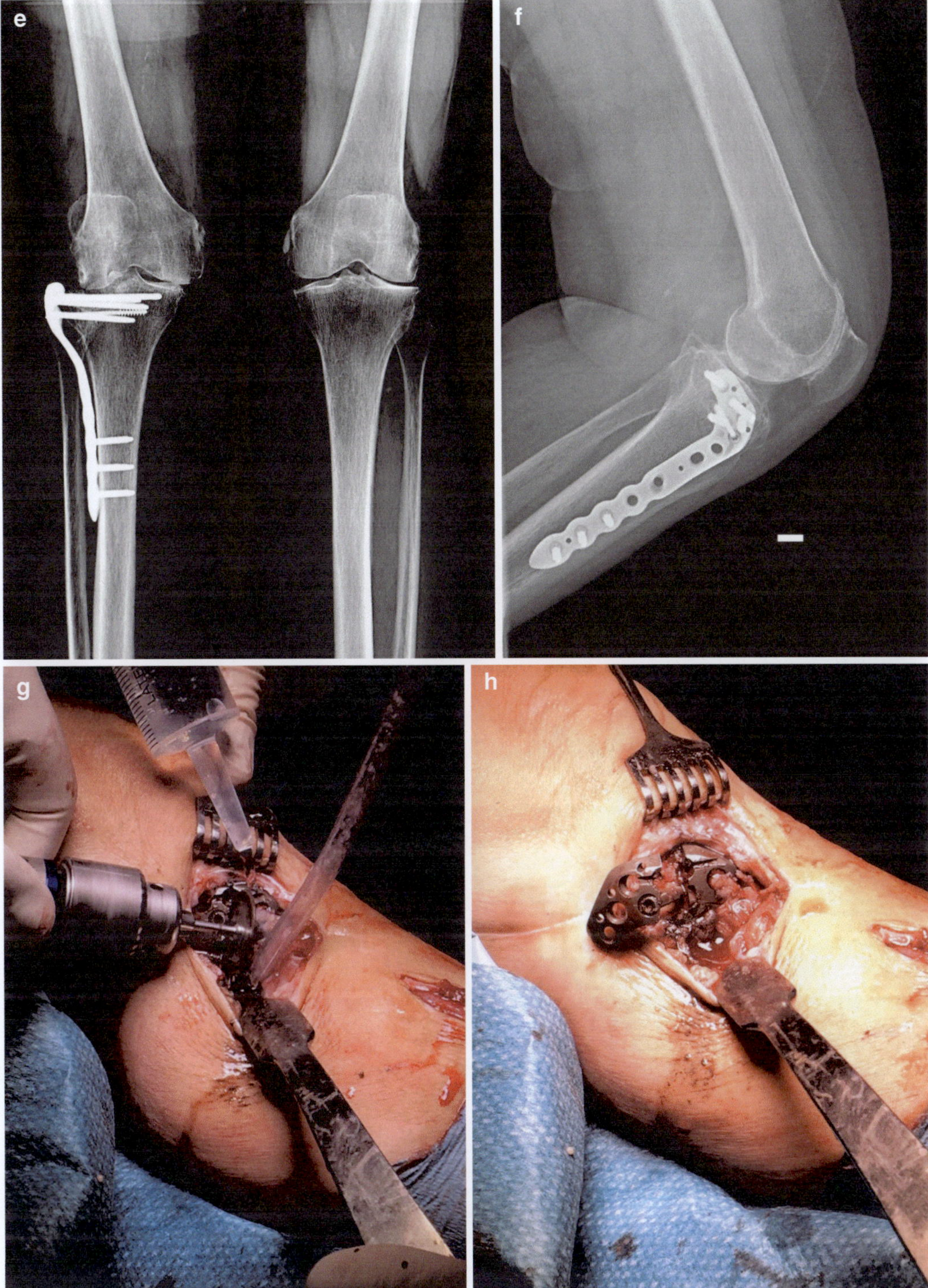

Fig. 9.1 (continued)

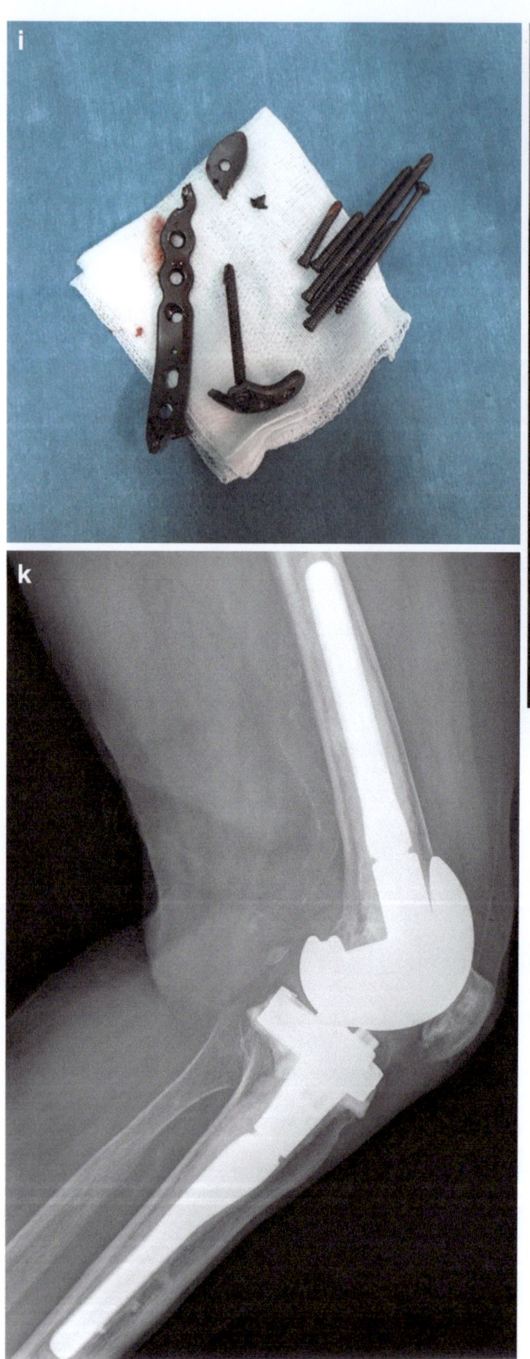

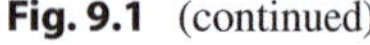

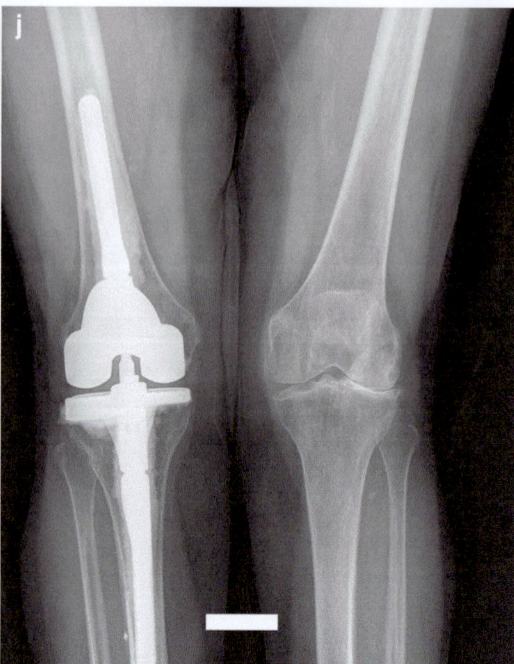

Fig. 9.1 (continued)

9.2 Risk of TKA After Proximal Tibia Fracture

In 2022 Tapper et al. determined the risk of S-TKA following PTF, whether treated nonoperatively or operatively and compared the outcomes with a 38-fold control group without prior PTF [5]. They recognized all subjects over 18 years of age in Finland with PTF treated during the period 2009–2018 from the Finnish Hospital Discharge Register (FHDR) and Finnish Arthroplasty Register (FAR). Age, sex, treatment method, follow-up time, and possible S-TKA were recorded. During the period 2009–2018, 7701 subjects were treated for PTF. Over the 5.1-year follow-up, S-TKA was carried out in 340 (4.3%) patients with a prior PTF after a mean of 2.1 years post-fracture. TKAS was required in 138 (3.7%) subjects in the nonoperatively treated group and in 202 (5%) individuals in the operatively treated group. Operative treatment, female sex, and high age were recognized as risk factors for S-TKA. The prevalence of S-TKA was highest during the first 2 years after fracture and remained elevated throughout the follow-up. Individuals with a prior PTF had a 1.8- to 3.2-fold higher risk of S-TKA compared with controls during the first 5 years post-fracture. Risk of S-TKA was associated with an operatively treated PTF, female sex, and high age. The subjects in the operative group likely sustained more complex fractures, while female sex and age might be explained by more osteoporotic bone quality [5].

9.3 Does Prior Infection Alter the Outcome of TKA After Tibial Plateau Fracture?

In 2009 Larson et al. stated that TKA carried out after PTF had a known high percentage of adverse events. In a therapeutic study with level 3 of evidence, Larson et al. hypothesized that TKAs carried out after infected PTFs would have an even higher adverse event percentage when compared with noninfected PTFs [2]. In a matched case-control study, they retrospectively reviewed 19 subjects who experienced primary TKAs after infected PTFs between 1971 and 2005. The mean time from the most recent infection to TKA was 5.6 years. The minimum clinical follow-up after TKA was 2 years. Case patients were matched for age, gender, and arthroplasty year with 19 control subjects who experienced TKAs for PTFs with no history of infections. After surgery, the Knee Society Scores for the study group improved from 45 to 63 for pain and from 37 to 63 for function. Ten case patients (53%) sustained adverse events, including surgery for wound breakdown (three), manipulation (one), aseptic loosening (two), definitive resection arthroplasty (two), and above-knee amputation (two). Recurrent infections happened in five subjects (26%) at a mean of 1.1 years. Previously infected knees were 4.1 times more likely to need additional procedures compared with knees with no previous infection [2].

9.4 Outcomes

In 2013 Piedade et al. analyzed the postoperative outcomes as well as adverse events and failures in two groups of subjects that had experienced knee surgery prior to primary TKA (bone surgery and soft tissue surgery) when compared to the no prior surgery group [6]. A retrospective and cohort series of 1474 primary TKA were assessed at a minimum follow-up period of 2 years: 1119 primary TKA experienced no prior surgery (1119 subjects) (group A), 85 primary TKA (85 subjects) (group B) had prior bone procedure (high tibial osteotomy [$n = 64$], tibial plateau fracture [$n = 10$], and patellar realignment [$n = 11$]), and the third group of 146 primary TKA (146 subjects) (group C) had experienced a soft tissue procedure (arthroscopy [$n = 60$] and meniscectomy [$n = 86$]) before primary TKA. All the subjects experienced a clinical and radiological assessment as well as International Knee Society (IKS) scores. Preoperatively, group B had 40% of cases classified as stage IV knee OA, while 57% of cases in group A showed higher levels of knee malalignment and group C had lower BMI. Intraoperative adverse events revealed no difference. Although group B had the poorest postoperative mean values of knee flexion, TKA procedure improved the preoperative mean values of knee flexion in all the study groups. The postoperative adverse events were more prevalent in group C, while the rate of revision TKA was similar for all study groups. At 120-month follow-up, the Kaplan-Meier survival curve percentages demonstrated no difference. This study confirmed that prior knee surgery could be considered a clinical condition that predisposed to higher postoperative complication rate in primary TKA compared to the no prior surgery group. After analyzing the three study groups, group C demonstrated a higher percentage of postoperative local adverse events and lower IKS knee scores, while group B demonstrated the poorest postoperative mean values of knee flexion as well as the need for extended surgical approach (tibial tubercle osteotomy [TTO] approach) was more prevalent in this study group. However, statistical analysis did not show a direct correlation between the type of prior knee surgery and TKA failures [6].

In 2015 Scott et al. examined the indications for, and results of, TKA after PTF and compared this with an age- and gender-matched cohort of TKAs performed for primary OA [3]. Between 1997 and 2011, 31 consecutive subjects (23 female, eight male) with a mean age of 65 years experienced TKA at a mean of 24 months after a PTF. Of these, 24 had experienced open reduction and internal fixation (ORIF) and seven had been treated nonoperatively. Subjects were evaluated preoperatively and at 6, 12, and >60 months using the Short Form-12 (SF-12), Oxford Knee Score (OKS), and a patient satisfaction score. Subjects with instability or nonunion needed TKA earlier (14 and 13.3 months postinjury) than those with intra-articular malunion (50 months). Primary cruciate-retaining implants were used in 27 (87%) individuals. Complication percentages were higher in the PT OA cohort and included wound complications (13% vs. 1%) and persistent stiffness (10% vs. 0%). Two (6%) PT OA subjects needed revision TKA at 57 and 114 months. The mean OKS was worse preoperatively in the cohort with primary OA (18 vs. 30) but there were no significant differences in postoperative OKS or patient satisfaction (primary OA 86%, PTOA 78%). TKA performed after PTF had a higher percentage of adverse events than that carried out for primary OA, but patient-reported outcomes (PROMs) and satisfaction were comparable [3].

A prospective matched cohort study was performed in 2015 by Lizaur-Utrilla et al. to compare outcomes of TKAs between 29 subjects with PT OA after a PTF and 58 individuals experienced routine TKA. Mean follow-up was 6.7 years. There were no significant differences in KSS (Knee Society Score), WOMAC (Western Ontario and McMaster Universities Osteoarthritis Index), and SF-12 scores or range of motion (ROM). In the control group there were no adverse events. In the posttraumatic group, adverse events happened in four subjects (13.7%) including partial patellar tendon detachment, superficial infection, skin necrosis, and knee stiffness. Only this last patient needed revision for manipulation under anesthesia (MUA). Also, there was a revision for tibial aseptic loosening in each group. TKA was an effective treatment for PT OA after PTF. Lizaur-Utrilla et al. recommended the prior removal of hardware, as well as TTO when necessary [6].

In 2015 Abdel et al. analyzed the 15-year results of 62 subjects who experienced a TKA after a prior PTF. Mean age at the index surgical intervention was 63 years. At most recent follow-up, there were 11 revisions. The 15-year survivorship free from revision for aseptic loosening was 96%. In unrevised cases, the components were radiographically well-fixed. There were a total of 21 adverse events, 90% of which happened at <2 years. While individuals experiencing TKA after a PTF had an increased percentage of adverse events, the 15-year outcomes indicated that subsequent survivorship was similar to that of subjects experiencing TKA for degenerative OA if early adverse events can be avoided [7].

In 2016 Houdek et al. stated that small studies had demonstrated that subjects who experience TKA following a distal femur and/or PTF have inferior outcomes. Houdek et al. assessed the mid-run results of a group of subjects experiencing TKA following periarticular knee fractures.

They recognized 531 subjects who experienced a TKA following a periarticular fracture from 1990 to 2012, comparing results to 19,641 subjects experiencing primary TKA for OA. Periarticular fracture significantly increased the risk of revision TKA, infection, and adverse events. There was no difference in the need for revision TKA or infection based on fracture location. Subjects with TKA following a periarticular fracture had worse overall revision-free survival compared to that with OA, with one in four subjects needing revision TKA by 15 years [8].

In 2020 Pinter et al. stated that PTF was routinely treated with ORIF; however, the long-run outcomes of ORIF were unclear [9]. In a retrospective study with level 3 of evidence, Pinter et al. assessed the results in a group of subjects, including the rate of conversion of ORIF to TKA, the relationship between elevated inflammatory markers after the initial ORIF and subsequent infection in TKA, and the rationale behind carrying out the conversion to TKA in one step vs. two steps. Utilizing current procedural terminology (CPT) codes, they assembled a group of 891 subjects (933 knees) who experienced ORIF for a PTF from 2007 to 2017. The subjects were then reviewed for pertinent demographic information and for the results of interest. Of the 933 knees, a total of 20 knees (2.15%) needed conversion from ORIF to TKA. Of the 20 knees that experienced conversion to TKA, three were carried out as a two-stage conversion. Of the 20 knees that experienced TKA, seven suffered from postoperative arthrofibrosis, four experienced postoperative infection, and four needed revision. This study suggested that the need for conversion to TKA was rare following ORIF of a PTF. Moreover, the conversion to TKA can be carried out as a one- or two-stage procedure. Pinter et al. suggested that there may be higher percentages of infection with the single stage conversion [9].

In 2020 Wang et al. investigated the results of TKA in subjects with a prior femoral or tibial fracture and recognized the risk factors for surgical site complications and reoperations [10]. Seventy-one TKAs carried out in 71 subjects with a prior tibial or femoral fracture between January 2005 and December 2016 were reviewed

retrospectively. Forty men (40 knees) and 31 women (31 knees) were included. The mean age at the time of TKA was 59.2 years. Results were evaluated utilizing the KSS before surgery and at the final follow-up visit. The subjects' satisfaction percentages were assessed. Adverse events and reoperations were recorded by clinical and radiographic evaluation. Logistic regression analysis was utilized to recognize the risk factors for surgical site complications and reoperations. The median follow-up period was 4.7 years. The median knee ROM increased from 90° preoperatively to 110° at the latest follow-up. The Knee Society knee score and function score improved from 35 and 40 to 90 and 90, respectively. The degree of overall satisfaction after TKA surgery was very satisfied in 41 subjects, satisfied in 20 subjects, neutral in four subjects, dissatisfied in four subjects, and very dissatisfied in two subjects. The overall satisfaction (very satisfied and satisfied) rate was 85.9% (61 knees). Twelve knees (16.9%) had 19 surgical site complications. Six knees (8.3%) experienced reoperations, including one revision due to periprosthetic joint infection (PJI), one debridement and implant retention for superficial infection, two debridements for delayed wound healing, one ORIF for supracondylar fracture, and one refixation and bone grafting for hardware failure after a combined femoral shaft osteotomy and TKA. Preoperative patella baja was diagnosed in 12 knees and was identified as a risk factor for surgical site complications and reoperations. TKA for PT OA significantly relieved pain and improved function, but the prevalence of surgical site complications and reoperations was high. Preoperative patella baja was a risk factor for surgical site complications and reoperations [10].

According to Pander et al., PT OA following a PTF is a debilitating condition which frequently affects a young and active patient population for whom good knee function is crucial. Many times, TKA is the only surgical alternative [4]. In a systematic review reported by Pander et al. in 2021, they assessed the functional result for TKA in PT OA patients, together with several secondary outcome parameters. In total, 162 subjects with a TKA for PT OA were included of whom 125

(77%) were managed operatively for their PTF. All studies reported improvements in functional outcome after TKA, with two studies demonstrating no significant differences between PT OA subjects and a matched group of primary OA individuals. Reported adverse events and reintervention percentages were higher for TKA subjects with PT OA. The outcomes of this study indicated the TKA for PT OA after a PTF provided satisfactory functional outcome, with results similar to those of matched primary OA subjects. Pander et al. concluded that TKA should be considered a viable treatment alternative to improve function, but both subjects and orthopedic surgeons should be aware of the higher adverse events percentages in this patient population [4].

9.5 Conclusions

Subjects with a prior proximal tibia fracture (PTF) have a 1.8- to 3.2-fold higher risk of secondary total knee arthroplasty (S-TKA) compared with controls during the first 5 years post-fracture. Risk of S-TKA is associated with an operatively treated PTF, female sex, and high age. Previously infected knees are 4.1 times more likely to need additional procedures compared with knees with no previous infection. TKA performed after PTF has a higher percentage of adverse events than that carried out for primary osteoarthritis (OA), but PROMs and satisfaction are comparable. While subjects experiencing TKA after a PTF have an increased percentage of adverse events, the 15-year outcomes indicate that subsequent survivorship is similar to that of individuals experiencing TKA for degenerative OA if early adverse events can be avoided. Around 2% need conversion from ORIF to TKA. The conversion to TKA can be carried out as a one- or two-stage procedure, although there may be higher percentages of infection with the single-stage conversion. TKA for posttraumatic (PT) OA significantly relieves pain and improves function, but the prevalence of surgical site complications and reoperations is high. Preoperative patella baja is a risk factor for surgical site complications and reoperations.

References

1. Galvez-Sirvent E, Ibarzabal-Gil A, Rodriguez-Merchan EC. Complications of the surgical treatment of fractures of the tibial plateau: prevalence, causes and management. EFORT Open Rev. 2022;7:554–68.
2. Larson AN, Hanssen AD, Cass JR. Does prior infection alter the outcome of TKA after tibial plateau fracture? Clin Orthop Relat Res. 2009;467:1793–9.
3. Scott CE, Davidson E, MacDonald DJ, White TO, Keating JF. Total knee arthroplasty following tibial plateau fracture: a matched cohort study. Bone Joint J. 2015;97-B:532–8.
4. Pander P, Fransen BL, Hagemans FJA, Keijser LCM. Functional outcome of total knee arthroplasty following tibial plateau fractures: a systematic review. Arch Orthop Trauma Surg. 2021; https://doi.org/10.1007/s00402-021-04188-1. Online ahead of print.
5. Tapper VS, Pamilo KJ, Haapakoski JJ, Toom A, Paloneva J. Risk of total knee replacement after proximal tibia fracture: a register-based study of 7841 patients. Acta Orthop. 2022;93:179–84.
6. Lizaur-Utrilla A, Collados-Maestre I, Miralles-Muñoz FA, Lopez-Prats FA. Total knee arthroplasty for osteoarthritis secondary to fracture of the tibial plateau. A prospective matched cohort study. J Arthroplast. 2015;30:1328–32.
7. Abdel MP, von Roth P, Cross WW, Berry DJ, Trousdale RT, Lewallen DG. Total knee arthroplasty in patients with a prior tibial plateau fracture: a long-term report at 15 years. J Arthroplast. 2015;30:2170–2.
8. Houdek MT, Watts CD, Shannon SF, Wagner ER, Sems SA, Sierra RJ. Posttraumatic total knee arthroplasty continues to have worse outcome than total knee arthroplasty for osteoarthritis. J Arthroplast. 2016;31:118–23.
9. Pinter Z, Jha AJ, McGee A, Paul K, Lee S, Dombrowsky A, et al. Outcomes of knee replacement in patients with posttraumatic arthritis due to previous tibial plateau fracture. Eur J Orthop Surg Traumatol. 2020;30:323–8.
10. Wang XS, Zhou YX, Shao HY, Yang DJ, Huang Y, Duan FF. Total knee arthroplasty in patients with prior femoral and tibial fractures: outcomes and risk factors for surgical site complications and reoperations. Orthop Surg. 2020;12:210–7.

E. Carlos Rodríguez-Merchán, Hortensia De la Corte-Rodríguez, and Juan M. Román-Belmonte

10.1 Introduction

It has been recently reported that one-third of adults are considered obese, and demand for total knee arthroplasty (TKA) is predicted to rise in these subjects. Also, surgeons are not eager to operate on obese subjects, but it is important to comprehend how obesity has affected TKA use [1]. In 2022 Baghbani-Naghadehi et al. affirmed that there was an existing opinion that obesity has a negative influence on adverse events after TKA. Also, information on the impact of obesity levels on patient-reported outcomes (PROMs) was rare [2].

In 2022 Muthusamy et al. stated that obesity was a recognized risk factor for severe knee osteoarthritis (OA). However, it remains unclear how obesity incidence trends in the current population experiencing TKA compared with those seen in subjects not experiencing this procedure [3]. It has also been published that obesity, a frequent risk factor for OA, accelerates articular deterioration resulting in the need for early TKA. Also, the role of obesity in the management of OA remains a debatable topic [4].

The purpose of this chapter is to review recent developments on TKA in subjects with severe obesity.

10.2 The Implications of an Aging Population and Increased Obesity for TKA Rates

In 2020 Overgaard et al. stated that TKA had increased considerably in Sweden [5]. This year Overgaard et al. quantified the relative risk for TKA in the Swedish community for various body mass index (BMI) categories and age groups. They examined whether the continued increase in TKA was attributable to increased incidence of obesity and elderly people in the population in order to put forward model forecasts for coming needs for TKA. They utilized the Swedish Nationwide Health Survey (SNHS) and the Swedish Knee Arthroplasty Register (SKAR) 2009–2015 to estimate the relative risk (RR) of TKA by age (middle-aged 45–64 years and elderly 65–84 years) and BMI (Fig. 10.1) [6]. BMI *is a person's weight in kilograms divided by the square of height in meters.* The RR for TKA was applied to the demographic predictions for the Swedish community as a forecasting model. Population size increased 5.2% from 2009 to

E. C. Rodríguez-Merchán (✉)
Department of Orthopedic Surgery, La Paz University Hospital, Madrid, Spain

H. De la Corte-Rodríguez
Department of Physical and Rehabilitation Medicine, La Paz University Hospital, Madrid, Spain

J. M. Román-Belmonte
Department of Physical and Rehabilitation Medicine, Cruz Roja San José y Santa Adela University Hospital, Madrid, Spain

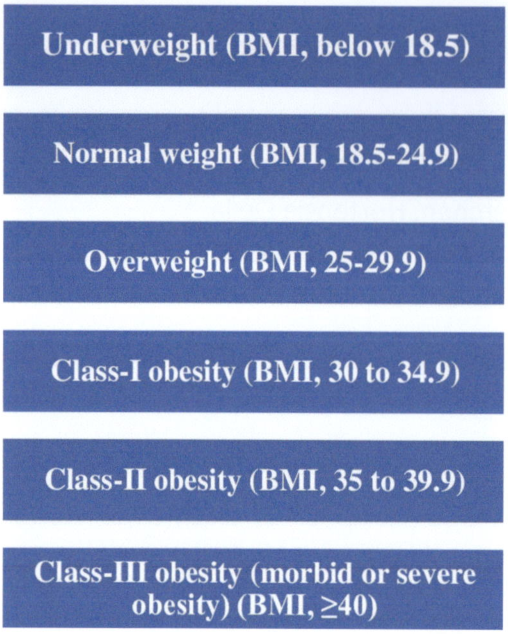

Underweight (BMI, below 18.5)

Normal weight (BMI, 18.5-24.9)

Overweight (BMI, 25-29.9)

Class-I obesity (BMI, 30 to 34.9)

Class-II obesity (BMI, 35 to 39.9)

Class-III obesity (morbid or severe obesity) (BMI, $\geq$40)

Fig. 10.1 World Health Organization (WHO) weight status. BMI = body mass index = body mass in kilograms divided by the square of the body height in meters, expressed in units of kg/m^2

2015 to 40,000 middle-aged and 250,000 elderly, and the incidence of obesity increased from 16% to 18% in these two age categories. Compared with those of normal weight, the RR for TKA was 2.7 higher for the overweight and 7.3 higher for the obese, aged 45–64 years. The corresponding figures for subjects aged 65–84 years were 2.1 and 4 higher, respectively. The changes in the incidence of obesity and an increase in the elderly population accounted for an estimated increase of 1700 TKAs over the 7 years. The increase in obesity incidence and the rise in the population of middle-aged and elderly might, to some extent, explain the rise in TKA use in Sweden [5].

10.3 The Rise of Obesity Among TKA Subjects

In 2022 Mohamed et al. stated that in the United States, one-third of adults were considered obese, and demand for TKA was predicted to rise in these subjects [1]. Also, surgeons were not eager to operate on obese subjects, but it was important to comprehend how obesity had affected TKA

use. In 2022 Mohamed et al. used a national database to assess prevalence, demographics, results, charges, and cost in nonobese, overweight, nonmorbidly obese, and morbidly obese TKA subjects. They queried the National Inpatient Sample from 2009 to 2016 for primary TKA subjects recognizing 4,053,037 nonobese subjects, 40,077 overweight subjects, 809,649 nonmorbidly obese subjects, and 428,647 morbidly obese subjects. Nonmorbidly obese and morbidly obese subjects represented 23.2% of all TKAs. TKA use increased 4.1% for nonobese subjects, 121.6% for overweight subjects, 73.6% for nonmorbidly obese subjects, and 83.9% for morbidly obese subjects. Morbidly obese subjects were younger, female, Black, and poor and used private insurance. They also had the longest length of stay and the highest mortality percentage. More morbidly obese subjects were discharged to other facilities, and they had the highest percentage of adverse events. Subjects with morbid obesity had the highest charges, but overweight subjects had the highest costs. The outcomes of this study showed the rise in obese and morbidly obese subjects seeking TKAs, which might be a reflection of the obesity epidemic in America. Although TKA use had increased for morbidly obese subjects, this BMI category also had the highest percentages of charges and adverse events, suggesting morbid obesity to be a changeable risk factor leading to worse surgical and economic results. Mohamed et al. concluded that obese subjects experiencing TKA may benefit from preoperative optimization of their weight, in an effort to diminish the risk of adverse results [1].

10.4 Does Obesity Affect PROMs Following TKA?

In 2022 Baghbani-Naghadehi et al. stated that there was an existing opinion that obesity has a negative influence on adverse events after TKA. Also, information on the impact of obesity levels on PROMs was rare. The aforementioned authors studied the association between different obesity classes with PROMs among subjects who experienced TKA [2]. They performed retrospective secondary analyses on data extracted from the total joint replacement data repository (Alberta, Canada) managed by the Alberta Bone and Joint Health Institute (ABJHI). Patients had WOMAC (Western Ontario and McMaster Universities Osteoarthritis Index) and ES-5D-5L (EuroQol five-dimensional questionnaire) scores measured at baseline in addition to 3 and/or 12 months after TKA. Subjects were stratified according to the World Health Organization (WHO) classification (Fig. 10.1) [6]. The association between BMI and mean changes in WOMAC subscales (pain, function, and stiffness) and EQ-5D-5L index over the time intervals of baseline to 3 months and 3–12 months following TKA was evaluated. Linear mixed-effects models were utilized, and the models were adjusted for age, sex, length of surgery, comorbidities, year of surgery, and geographical zone where the surgery was carried out. Mean age was 65.5 years. Postoperatively, there was a significant improvement in WOMAC subscales of patient-reported pain, function, and stiffness, as well as EQ-5D-5L regardless of the BMI group. Although subjects in BMI class II and class III reported significantly improved pain 3 months after TKA compared to those with normal BMI, all BMI groups obtained a similar level of pain decrease at 12 months following TKA. The greatest improvement in all WOMAC subscales, as well as EQ-5D-5L index, happened between baseline and 3 months. The findings of this study indicated that subjects reported improved pain, function, and stiffness across all BMI groups following TKA. Subjects with BMI classified as obese reported similar benefits to those with BMI classified as normal weight [2].

10.5 Trends of Obesity Percentage Between Subjects Experiencing Primary TKA and the General Population

In 2022 Muthusamy et al. stated that obesity was a recognized risk factor for severe knee OA. However, it remained unclear how obesity incidence trends in the current population experiencing TKA compared with those seen in sub-

jects not experiencing this procedure [3]. In a prognostic study with level 3 of evidence, Muthusamy et al. evaluated the annual trends in BMI and obesity percentages between subjects who have experienced primary TKA and those in the general population. They retrospectively reviewed all subjects ≥18 years of age from January 2013 through December 2020 who experienced primary, elective TKA and those who had a yearly routine physical examination at their institution within the same period. Baseline demographic characteristics were collected. A total of 11,333 subjects who experienced primary TKA and 1,158,168 subjects who experienced a yearly physical examination were included in the study. After adjusting for age, the aforementioned authors encountered the mean BMI for the TKA group to be significantly greater every year compared with the yearly physical group. The proportion of individuals who were categorized into any obesity class (BMI, ≥30 kg/m^2) was significantly higher for the TKA group each year compared with the yearly physical group. An analysis of trends over time demonstrated a significantly increasing trend in BMI and obesity percentages for the yearly physical group, but a stable trend for subjects experiencing TKA. Subjects who experienced TKA continued to have higher BMI than the general population, which demonstrated a steady increase over time. Muthusamy et al. concluded that physicians need to continue in their efforts to educate subjects on weight management and healthy lifestyles to potentially postpone the need for a surgical procedure [3].

10.6 Obesity, Comorbidities, and the Associated Risk Among Subjects Who Experience TKA

In 2022 Baghbani-Naghadehi et al. stated that obesity, a frequent risk factor for OA, accelerated articular deterioration resulting in the need for early TKA. Also, the role of obesity in the management of OA remained a debatable topic [4]. Baghbani-Naghadehi et al. analyzed whether obesity along with other comorbidities was associated with peri-/postoperative adverse events in subjects who experienced primary unilateral TKA. A retrospective secondary study was carried out on information extracted from data repository of patients ($n = 15{,}151$) who experienced TKA between 2012 and 2016. The sample was divided into five groups based on BMI classification developed by the WHO. The associations between dependent variable (presence or absence of an adverse event or comorbidity) with the independent variables (year of surgery, age, sex, length of surgery, and BMI groups) were analyzed utilizing binomial logistic regression. Results demonstrated that obese classes I, II, and III, irrespective of other covariates, were more likely to have diabetes and pulmonary embolism compared with the normal BMI group. Subjects with obese class III compared with subjects in the normal BMI group were more likely to have deep wound infection. Subjects with comorbidities were more likely to have a blood transfusion, infection, pulmonary embolism, and readmission. Subjects in higher BMI groups or with comorbidities were more likely to suffer perioperative and/or postoperative adverse events after TKA, although the level of risk depended on the severity of obesity [4].

10.7 TKA in Subjects with Severe Obesity Provides Value for Money in Spite of Increased Adverse Events

In 2022 Elcock et al. stated that access to TKA was sometimes restricted for subjects with class III obesity (morbid obesity) [7]. They compared the cost per quality-adjusted life year (QALY) associated with TKA in subjects with a BMI above and below 40 kg/m² to study whether this was supported. This single-center study compared 169 consecutive subjects with severe obesity (mean age 65.2 years, mean BMI 44.2 kg/m², 129/169 female) experiencing unilateral TKA to a propensity score-matched (age, sex, preoperative Oxford Knee Score [OKS]) cohort with a BMI < 40 kg/m² in a 1:1 ratio. Demographic data, comorbidities, and adverse events to one year were recorded. Preoperative and one-year

PROMs were completed: EuroQol five-dimension three-level questionnaire (EQ-5D-3L), OKS, pain, and satisfaction. Utilizing national life expectancy data with obesity correction and the 2020 National Health Service (NHS) National Tariff, QALYs (discounted at 3.5%) and direct medical costs accrued over a patient's lifetime were estimated. Probabilistic sensitivity analysis (PSA) was utilized to model variation in cost/QALY for each cohort across 1000 simulations. All PROMs improved significantly in both groups without differences between groups. Early adverse events were higher in patients with morbid obesity: 34/169 versus 52/169. A total of 16 (9.5%) individuals with morbid obesity were readmitted within one year with six reoperations (3.6%) including three (1.2%) revisions for infection. Assuming diminished life expectancy in severe obesity and revision costs, TKA in subjects with morbid obesity costs a mean of £1013/QALY more over a lifetime than TKA subjects with BMI < 40 kg/m². In PSA replicates, the maximum cost/QALY was £3921 in subjects with a BMI < 40 kg/m² and £5275 in subjects with morbid obesity. Higher complication percentages following TKA in severely obese subjects resulted in a lifetime cost/QALY that is £1013 greater than that for subjects with BMI < 40 kg/m², suggesting that TKA remained a cost-effective use of health care resources in severely obese subjects where the surgeon considered it adequate [7].

10.8 The Impact of Obesity on Achievement of a "Forgotten Joint" Following TKA

In a retrospective cohort study with level 3 of evidence published in 2022 by Singh et al., they analyzed the impact of BMI on improvement in results after TKA as evaluated by the Forgotten Joint Score-12 (FJS-12) [8]. They retrospectively reviewed 1075 subjects who experienced primary TKA from 2017 to 2020 with accessible postoperative FJS-12 scores. Subjects were stratified based on their BMI (kg/m²): <30, obese class I, obese class II, and obese class III. FJS-12 and KOOS-JR (Knee Injury and Osteoarthritis Outcome Score for Joint Replacement) scores were collected at various time points. Of the 1075 subjects included, there were 457 with a BMI < 30, 331 who were obese class I, 162 obese class II, and 125 obese class III. There were no statistical differences in FJS-12 scores between the BMI groups at 3 months (27.24 vs. 25.33 vs. 23.57 vs. 22.48), 1 year (45.07 vs. 41.86 vs. 40.51 vs. 36.22), and 2 years (51.31 vs. 52.86 vs. 46.17 vs. 44.97). Preoperative KOOS-JR scores significantly differed between the various BMI categories (49.33 vs. 46.63 vs. 44.24 vs. 39.33); however, 3-month and 1-year scores were not statistically significant. Mean improvement in FJS-12 scores from 3 months to 2 years was statistically greatest for obese class I subjects and lowest for obese class III subjects (24.07 vs. 27.53 vs. 22.60 vs. 22.49). KOOS-JR score improvement from baseline to 1 year was statistically greatest for obese class III subjects and lowest for nonobese subjects (22.34 vs. 25.49 vs. 23.77 vs. 27.58). While all groups showed postoperative improvement, those with higher BMI reported lower mean FJS-12 scores, but these differences were not encountered to be significant. This study demonstrated no significant influence of BMI on postoperative joint awareness, which implied that obese subjects, in all obesity classes, experienced similar functional improvement after TKA [8].

10.9 What Is the Influence of BMI Cutoffs on TKA Adverse Events?

In 2022 DeMik et al. stated that BMI cutoffs were usually utilized to decide whether to offer obese subjects elective TKA. Also, weight loss goals may be unachievable for many individuals who were consequentially denied complication-free surgery [9]. The aforementioned authors evaluated the influence of different BMI cutoffs on the percentages of complication-free surgery following TKA. Subjects experiencing elective, primary TKA from 2015 to 2018 were recog-

nized in the American College of Surgeons National Surgical Quality Improvement Program database utilizing Common Procedural Terminology code 27447. The BMI and percentages of any 30-day adverse event were collected. BMI cutoffs of 30, 35, 40, 45, and 50 kg/m^2 were applied to model the prevalence of adverse events if TKA would have been permitted or denied based on the BMI. A total of 314,719 subjects experienced TKA, and 46,386 (14.7%) had a BMI $\geq$40 kg/m^2. With a BMI cutoff of 40 kg/m^2, 268,333 (85.3%) subjects would have experienced TKA. A total of 282,552 (94.8%) would experience complication-free surgery, and 17.3% of all adverse events would be prevented. TKA would proceed for 309,479 (98.3%) subjects at a BMI cutoff of 50 kg/m^2. A total of 293,108 (94.7%) would not experience an adverse event, and 2.8% of adverse events would be prevented. A BMI cutoff of 35 kg/m^2 would prevent 36.6% of all adverse events while permitting 94.8% of complication-free surgeries to proceed. Lower BMI cutoffs can diminish adverse events but will limit access to complication-free TKA for many subjects. This study did not indicate that TKA should be carried out without consideration of risks from obesity [9].

10.10 Effect of BMI on the Results of Primary TKA Up to One Year

In 2022 Mishra et al. tried to establish a correlation between obesity and early results of TKA [10]. They carried out a prospective cross-sectional study in cases experiencing primary TKA between September 2019 and August 2020. Obesity was classified in all cases, and multiple variables like pain, functional status, range of motion (ROM), knee deformity, and PROMs were recorded. Mishra et al. studied 100 knees (37 bilateral and 26 unilateral) in 63 cases. Pain score diminished maximally in the normal and overweight group and minimal in class III obesity. Knee Society Score (KSS), Functional KSS (FKSS), and PROMs gradually ameliorated in all, except in morbidly obese. Even though the improvement in all variables was minimum in class III obesity compared to other classes of obesity, the margin of difference from the preoperative period was maximum in class III obese participants. All cases, irrespective of class of obesity, experienced a comparable improvement in their knee function and ameliorated quality of life. Besides, the TKA offered substantial benefits in terms of pain alleviation, knee stability, walking distance, ROM of the knee, and stair climbing [10].

10.11 The Impact of Obesity on TKA Revision Rate

In a prognostic study with level 3 of evidence published in 2022, Wall et al. studied the relationship of obesity with all-cause revision and revision for infection, loosening, instability, and pain after TKA [11]. Information for individuals experiencing primary TKA for OA from January 1, 2015, to December 31, 2020, was attained from the Australian Orthopedic Association National Joint Replacement Registry (AOANJRR). The percentages of all-cause revision and revision for infection, loosening, instability, and pain were compared for nonobese subjects, class-I and II obese subjects, and class-III obese subjects. The outcomes were adjusted for age, sex, tibial fixation, prosthesis stability, patellar component usage, and computer navigation utilization. During the study period, 141,673 individuals experienced primary TKA for OA in Australia; of these subjects, 48% were class I or II obese, and 10.6% were class III obese. The mean age was 68.2 years, and 54.7% of subjects were women. The mean follow-up period was 2.8 years. Of the 2655 revision procedures recognized, the reasons for revision TKA (rTKA) included infection in 39.7%, loosening in 14.8%, instability in 12%, and pain in 6.1% (Fig. 10.2). Class I and II obese subjects had a higher risk of all-cause revision (hazard ratio, 1.12) and revision for infection than nonobese subjects. Class III obese subjects had a higher risk of all-cause revision after 1 year, revision for infection after 3 months, and revision for loosening than nonobese subjects. The risks of

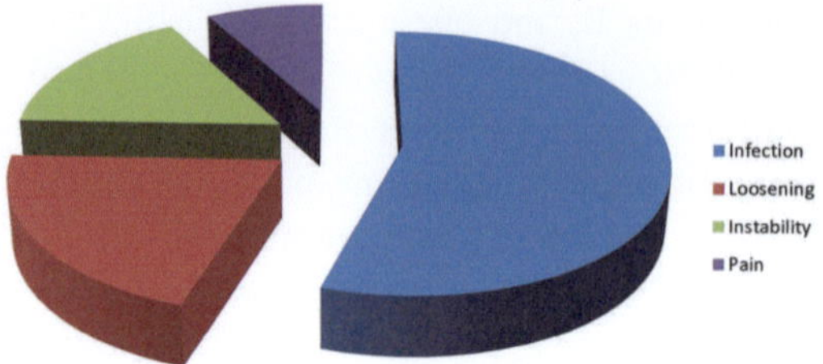

Fig. 10.2 Reasons for revision total knee arthroplasty (rTKA) in obese subjects

revision for instability and pain were similar among groups. Obese subjects with knee OA should be counseled with regard to the augmented risks associated with TKA, so they can make informed decisions about their health care [11].

10.12 Mid- to Long-Term Adverse Events and Result for Morbidly Obese Subjects After TKA

In 2022 van Tilburg and Rathsach Andersen reported a review article aimed to investigate mid- to long-run adverse events, revision percentages, and result for morbidly obese, compared with nonobese after TKA [12]. A systematic search was performed in May 2021. Included studies reported revision percentages for morbidly obese and nonobese with a mean follow-up of at least 2 years. Reported KSS was utilized to compare the functional result. From 12 studies that met the inclusion criteria, a total of 1031 cases of morbidly obese and 9797 cases of nonobese controls were included. The risk ratio for revision was 1.48 for the morbidly obese, compared with nonobese. Regarding aseptic and septic revision, the risk ratio was 1.44 and 2.22, respectively. The morbidly obese scored lower in Objective KSS (OKSS) and FKSS both preoperatively and postoperatively, compared with the nonobese; however, the two groups improved equally in function scores OKSS and FKSS. The overall risk ratio for adverse events was 1.56. The gained benefit in functional result surpassed the increase in risk of revision and adverse events for the morbidly obese in TKA surgery [12].

10.13 Cemented Versus Cementless TKA in Obese Subjects with BMI ≥35 kg/m²

In 2022 Goh et al. stated that cemented TKA had been demonstrated to have higher failure percentages in obese subjects, and cementless TKA might provide more durable fixation [13]. Goh et al. compared results and survivorship of obese subjects experiencing cemented and cementless TKA of the same modern design. They recognized a consecutive series of 406 primary cementless TKA carried out in obese subjects with BMI ≥35 kg/m² in 2013–2018. Each case was matched 1:1 with 406 cemented TKA based on age, sex, BMI, bearing surface, and year of surgery. KOOS-JR) and Short Form-12 (SF-12) were collected preoperatively, at 6 months and 2 years. Implant survivorship was recorded at mean 4 years. There was no difference in mean BMI between the cemented (38.6 kg/m²) and cementless groups (38.7 kg/m²). Both groups had similar final postoperative scores and improvement in scores at 2 years. Moreover, a similar percentage met the minimal clinically important difference (KOOS-JR, 70% versus 71.2%; SF-12 physical, 74.1% versus 70.4%). Both groups showed high 7-year survivorship free from aseptic revision (99% vs. 99.5%). Obese subjects with BMI ≥35 kg/m² experiencing cementless and cemented TKA of the same modern design had similar results and survivorship at early to mid-run follow-up [13].

10.14 Cementless TKA Utilizing a Highly Porous Tibial Baseplate in Morbidly Obese Subjects

In 2022 King et al. stated that morbidly obese subjects experiencing cemented TKA could pose a challenging problem with implant survivorship due to greater stress at the cement-bone interface. Also, with the advent of additive manufacturing (three-dimensional printing), highly porous implants were readily accessible [14]. In 2022 King et al. reviewed the outcomes of primary TKA in the morbidly obese subject utilizing a highly porous cementless tibial baseplate. This was a retrospective study of 167 TKAs in subjects with morbid obesity experiencing primary cementless TKA with a minimum 5-year follow-up. A total of 6 subjects passed away and 14 were lost to follow-up, leaving 147 TKAs in 136 subjects with a mean follow-up of 66 months. The average age was 59 years and average BMI was 45 kg/m². Clinical results, PROMs, radiographs, and adverse events were reviewed. There were 9 failures needing revision, including 3 for aseptic tibial loosening (2%), 2 for deep infection (1.4%), 2 for patellar resurfacing (1.4%), 1 for patella instability (0.7%), and 1 for extensor mechanism rupture (0.7%). KSS improved from 48 to 90 at 2- and 5-year follow-up. KSS function score improved from 49 to 68 and 79 at 2- and 5-year follow-up, respectively. Survivorship with aseptic loosening as the endpoint was 98% at 5 years. Cementless TKA utilizing a highly porous tibial baseplate in morbidly obese subjects showed excellent clinical outcomes with 98% survivorship at 5 years and seemed to offer durable long-run biologic fixation as an option to mechanical cement fixation in this challenging group of subjects [14].

10.15 Does BMI Influence the Results and Survivorship of Modern Cementless TKA?

According to Goh et al., higher BMI has been associated with higher percentages of aseptic loosening following cemented TKA [15]. Goh et al. stated that there was a paucity of evidence on the effect of BMI on the durability of modern cementless TKA. In 2022 they evaluated the association between BMI and clinical results after cementless TKA to determine if there was a BMI threshold beyond which the risk of revision significantly augmented. They recognized 1408 cementless TKAs of a modern design from an institutional registry. Subjects were classified into BMI categories: normal ($n = 136$), overweight ($n = 476$), obese class I ($n = 423$), obese class II ($n = 258$), and obese class III (n = 115). The KOOS-JR and SF-12 scores were collected preoperatively and 2 years postoperatively. Survivorship was recorded at minimum 2 years. BMI was analyzed as a continuous and categorical variable. The improvement in PROMs was similar across the groups. Thirty-four knees (2.4%) were revised and 14 (1%) were for aseptic failure. Mean time to revision was 1.2 years and did not differ across BMI categories. Survivorship free from all-cause and aseptic revision was 97.1% and 99% at mean 4 years, respectively. Using Cox regression to control for demographics and bilateral procedures, BMI had no association with all-cause revision or aseptic revision. No relationship between BMI and revision risk was found. BMI did not impact functional results and survivorship of modern cementless TKA, possibly due to improved biological fixation at the bone-implant interface [15].

10.16 Morbidly Obese Subjects Experiencing Primary TKA May Present Higher Percentages of VTE When Prescribed Direct Oral Anticoagulants Versus Aspirin

In 2022 Humphrey et al. stated that morbidly obese subjects experiencing total joint arthroplasty (TJA) were at high risk for postoperative venous thromboembolism (VTE); they also stated, however, that there was debate surrounding the optimal pharmacologic agent for prevention of VTE after TJA in this patient subset [16]. Current guidelines recommended against direct-acting oral anticoagulants (DOACS) in patients with BMI >40 kg/m^2 due to low-quality evidence justifying their utilization. Humphrey et al. assessed whether individuals with morbid obesity experiencing primary unilateral TJA would have augmented risk of postoperative VTE if prescribed DOACS compared to non-DOAC agents such as aspirin. The retrospective study analyzed 897 subjects with morbid obesity experiencing primary unilateral TJA. Demographic and comorbidity-related variables were collected.

The association between postoperative VTE and prophylactic pharmacologic drug prescribed was assessed by multivariate logistic regression. After controlling for comorbidities, Humphrey et al. encountered that the sole utilization of DOACS, specifically apixaban, for VTE prophylaxis was associated with an augmented risk of developing VTE compared to prophylaxis with aspirin alone in subjects with morbid obesity. Regardless of VTE prophylactic drug, individuals with morbid obesity experiencing TKA had at least 4.5-fold increased odds of developing VTE compared to subjects experiencing total hip arthroplasty (THA). In this retrospective study of subjects with morbid obesity, it was encountered that the utilization of DOACS, specifically apixaban, for VTE prophylaxis after TJA was associated with augmented odds of a VTE complication compared to the utilization of aspirin alone [16].

10.17 Conclusions

TKA use has increased around 4% for nonobese subjects, about 121% for overweight subjects, around 73% for nonmorbidly obese subjects, and about 84% for morbidly obese subjects. Subjects in higher BMI groups or with comorbidities were more likely to suffer perioperative and/or postoperative adverse events after TKA, although the level of risk depended on the severity of obesity. Morbid obesity is a changeable risk factor leading to worse surgical and economic results. Obese subjects experiencing TKA may benefit from preoperative optimization of their weight, in an effort to diminish the risk of adverse results. Obese individuals with knee OA should be counseled with regard to the augmented risks associated with TKA, so they can make informed decisions about their health care.

References

1. Mohamed NS, Wilkie WA, Remily EA, Dávila Castrodad IM, Jean-Pierre M, Jean-Pierre N, et al. The rise of obesity among total knee arthroplasty patients. J Knee Surg. 2022;35:1–6.
2. Baghbani-Naghadehi F, Armijo-Olivo S, Prado CM, Gramlich L, Woodhouse LJ. Does obesity affect

patient-reported outcomes following total knee arthroplasty? BMC Musculoskelet Disord. 2022;23(1):55.

3. Muthusamy N, Singh V, Sicat CS, Rozell JC, Lajam CM, Schwarzkopf R. Trends of obesity rates between patients undergoing primary total knee arthroplasty and the general population from 2013 to 2020. J Bone Joint Surg Am. 2022;104:537–43.

4. Baghbani-Naghadehi F, Armijo-Olivo S, Prado CM, Woodhouse LJ. Obesity, comorbidities, and the associated risk among patients who underwent total knee arthroplasty in Alberta. J Knee Surg. 2022; https://doi.org/10.1055/s-0042-1742646. Online ahead of print.

5. Overgaard A, Frederiksen P, Kristensen LE, Robertsson O, W-Dahl A. The implications of an aging population and increased obesity for knee arthroplasty rates in Sweden: a register-based study. Acta Orthop. 2020;91:738–42.

6. World Health Organization. A healthy lifestyle - WHO recommendations. https://www.who.int/europe/newsroom/fact-sheets/item/a-healthy-lifestyle%2D%2Dwho-recommendations. Accessed 15 Aug 2022.

7. Elcock KL, Carter TH, Yapp LZ, MacDonald DJ, Howie CR, Stoddart A, et al. Total knee arthroplasty in patients with severe obesity provides value for money despite increased complications. Bone Joint J. 2022;104-B:452–63.

8. Singh V, Yeroushalmi D, Lygrisse KA, Simcox T, Long WJ, Schwarzkopf R. The influence of obesity on achievement of a 'forgotten joint' following total knee arthroplasty. Arch Orthop Trauma Surg. 2022;142:491–9.

9. DeMik DE, Muffly SA, Carender CN, Glass NA, Brown TS, Bedard NA. What is the impact of body mass index cutoffs on total knee arthroplasty complications? J Arthroplast. 2022;37:683–7.e1.

10. Mishra AK, Vaish A, Vaishya R. Effect of body mass index on the outcomes of primary total knee arthroplasty up to one year - a prospective study. J Clin Orthop Trauma. 2022;27:101829.

11. Wall CJ, Vertullo CJ, Kondalsamy-Chennakesavan S, Lorimer MF, de Steiger RN. A prospective, longitudinal study of the influence of obesity on total knee arthroplasty revision rate: results from the Australian Orthopaedic Association National Joint Replacement Registry. J Bone Joint Surg Am. 2022;104:1386–92.

12. van Tilburg J, Rathsach AM. Mid- to long-term complications and outcome for morbidly obese patients after total knee arthroplasty: a systematic review and meta-analysis. EFORT Open Rev. 2022;7:295–304.

13. Goh GS, Fillingham YA, Sutton RM, Small I, Courtney PM, Hozack WJ. Cemented versus cementless total knee arthroplasty in obese patients with body mass index ≥35 kg/m²: a contemporary analysis of 812 patients. J Arthroplast. 2022;37:688–93.e1.

14. King BA, Miller AJ, Nadar AC, Smith LS, Yakkanti MR, Harwin SF, et al. Cementless total knee arthroplasty using a highly porous tibial baseplate in morbidly obese patients: minimum 5-year follow-up. J Knee Surg. 2022; https://doi.org/10.1055/s--0042-1748900. Online ahead of print.

15. Goh GS, Wells Z, Ong CB, Small I, Ciesielka KA, Fillingham YA. Does body mass index influence the outcomes and survivorship of modern cementless total knee arthroplasty? J Arthroplast. 2022; S0883-5403(22)00592-7.

16. Humphrey TJ, O'Brien TD, Melnic CM, Verrier KI, MGB Arthroplasty Outcomes Writing Committee, Bedair HS. Morbidly obese patients undergoing primary total joint arthroplasty may experience higher rates of venous thromboembolism when prescribed direct oral anticoagulants vs aspirin. J Arthroplast. 2022;37:1189–97.

Primary Total Knee Arthroplasty in Patients Younger than 55 Years

E. Carlos Rodríguez-Merchán, Hortensia De la Corte-Rodríguez, and Juan M. Román-Belmonte

11.1 Introduction

In 2017 Aujla and Esler claimed that the proportion of younger subjects experiencing total knee arthroplasty (TKA) was increasing and predictions stated that the <55-year age group will be the fastest-growing group by 2030 [1]. In 2018 Clement et al. affirmed that management of the young patient with end-stage osteoarthritis (OA) of the knee is difficult, with surgical options of osteotomy, unicompartmental knee arthroplasty (UKA), or TKA [2].

According to Egloff et al., the absolute number of TKAs continues to rise every year. In 2021 the aforementioned authors stated that around 10% of the subjects were less than 55 years of age, although it was known that functional outcomes and patient satisfaction were lower combined with an increased likelihood of revision compared to older subjects. Higher physical activity and patient expectations were a major challenge in this age group. At the same time, the prevalence of posttraumatic/postoperative alterations was high, including ligamentous or bony deficiencies, which can make the surgical procedure challenging. In view of these facts, conservative treatments and joint-sparing procedures should always be considered first. The potential correction of lower-limb deformities and UKAs need to be carefully assessed prior to considering TKA. Only in advanced cases of OA in more than one compartment of the knee with combined ligamentous instability can a TKA provide satisfactory outcomes in the young subject. However, the strongest predictor of satisfaction is a realistic expectation [3].

In 2021 Kim et al. expressed that methods to diminish the revision percentage of TKAs because of wear-related issues are important to examine, particularly because younger subjects had a disproportionately high risk of revision [4]. The purpose of this chapter is to review recent developments of TKA in patients younger than 55 years.

E. C. Rodríguez-Merchán (✉)
Department of Orthopedic Surgery, La Paz University Hospital, Madrid, Spain

H. De la Corte-Rodríguez
Department of Physical and Rehabilitation Medicine, La Paz University Hospital, Madrid, Spain

J. M. Román-Belmonte
Department of Physical and Rehabilitation Medicine, Cruz Roja San José y Santa Adela University Hospital, Madrid, Spain

11.2 Outcomes

In a study with level 2 of evidence published in 2017, Lizaur-Utrilla et al. compared outcomes after TKA for OA between subjects younger than 55 years and older subjects [5]. A group of 61 subjects aged 55 years or younger was prospectively matched for gender, body mass index

(BMI), and knee function with subjects with a median age of 66 years. Clinical evaluation was performed by the Knee Society Scores (KSSs), reduced Western Ontario and McMasters Universities (WOMAC), and Short-Form 12 (SF12) questionnaires. Radiological evaluation was also performed. The median follow-up was 12 years. Survival at 14 years was 96.7% in the younger group and 98.2% in the older group. There was no deep infection or loosening of femoral or patellar component in either group. In the younger group, two subjects needed revision (aseptic tibial loosening at 8 years and polyethylene [PE] wear at 10 years). In the older group, there was one revision (aseptic tibial loosening). Revision percentage was not significantly different. Multivariate analysis showed no significant relationship between revision and age, gender, or BMI. At 5-year follow-up, there were no significant differences between groups in KSS knee or function, WOMAC pain or function, or SF12 physical or mental, but in the last assessment there were better outcomes in younger subjects for KSS function, WOMAC function, SF12 physical, and SF12 mental, although these differences were not clinically relevant. A significant decline was noted for KSS function in either group from 5-year to the last follow-up. The TKA survival in younger subjects was comparable to older active subjects, without increased adverse events or revisions at a minimum follow-up of 10 years. Primary hybrid TKA can provide successful pain alleviation, function, and quality of life (QoL) in younger subjects than those at 55 years with OA. Lizaur-Utrilla et al. concluded that TKA was a suitable alternative for these young subjects with adequate surgical indications [5].

In 2017 Aujla and Esler published a systematic review assessing functional outcomes following TKA in patients <55 years of age. Across 13 studies the aforementioned authors were able to demonstrate 54-point improvement in clinical Knee Society Score (KSS) and a 46-point improvement on functional Knee Society Score. A 2.9° improvement in range of motion (ROM) was found at final follow-up. Satisfaction rate was 85.5%. Cumulative percentage all-cause revision rate was 5.4% across 1283 TKAs at a mean 10.8 years of follow-up. Ten-year survival, for aseptic loosening alone, was 98.2%. TKA was an excellent treatment option for the young osteoarthritic knee with a >50% improvement in functional knee scores. Satisfaction was high and the revision percentage remained 0.5% per year [1].

In 2018 Clement et al. assessed whether age less than 55 years was an independent predictor of functional outcome and satisfaction after TKA. The secondary aims were to identify preoperative differences in patient demographics, comorbidity, and function between subjects less than 55 years old compared to those 55 years old and over [2]. A retrospective cohort consisting of 2589 subjects experiencing a primary TKA was identified from an established arthroplasty database. Patient demographics, comorbidity, WOMAC, and Short Form (SF) 12 scores were collected preoperatively and 1 year postoperatively. In addition, patient satisfaction was evaluated at 1 year. Regression analysis was utilized to identify independent preoperative predictors of change in the WOMAC and SF-12 scores and patient satisfaction. Subjects less than 55 years old were significantly less likely to be satisfied with the overall result of their TKA. After adjusting for confounding variables, the age group was not an independent predictor of overall satisfaction with overall result. Independent predictors of an increased risk of dissatisfaction with the overall result at 1 year were depression and worse preoperative SF-12. Age less than 55 years was not an independent predictor of functional result or percentage of patient satisfaction after TKA. However, depression and poor mental health were significantly more prevalent in subjects less than 55 years old and were independently associated with a lower satisfaction percentage [2].

11.3 Oxidized Zirconium (OxZr) TKA Versus Cobalt-Chrome (CoCr) TKA

In a therapeutic study with level 1 of evidence published in 2019 by Kim et al., they tried to answer to the following questions: Are long-term Knee Society knee and function scores better in younger subjects with an oxidized zirconium (OxZr) TKA compared with those with a cobalt-chrome (CoCr) TKA? Are there any differences in radiographic signs of loosening or computed tomography (CT) findings of osteolysis between OxZr TKAs and CoCr TKAs? Are there fewer polyethylene (PE) wear particles in the OxZr TKA than CoCr TKA? Do the groups differ in terms of survivorship free from revision surgery at 13 years? [3]. From April 2003 to January 2007, the aforementioned authors enrolled 110 subjects younger than 55 years of age in a randomized, double-blind, prospective trial. Each subject served as his or her own control and each experienced an OxZr femoral component in one knee and a CoCr femoral component in the other. The minimum follow-up was 10 years; two died and nine were lost to follow-up before that time, leaving 99 subjects (198 knees) for analysis. There were 28 men and 71 women with a mean age of 53 years. They obtained Knee Society knee scores for each knee, but Knee Society function scores, WOMAC scores, and UCLA (University of California at Los Angeles) activity scores were obtained for each subject preoperatively and at each follow-up. Additionally, Kim et al. carried out radiographic examination preoperatively and at each follow-up. At a minimum of 10 years' (mean, 13 years) follow-up, they obtained computed tomography (CT) scans in all subjects. PE wear particles in the synovial fluid were analyzed at the final follow-up using thermogravimetric methods and scanning electron microscopy. Survivorship was ascertained using the Kaplan-Meier calculator. A sample size calculation determined that to detect a difference in the Knee Society knee score of 5 points, assuming a SD of 5 points, with an $\alpha = 0.05$ and $\beta = 0.80$, a total of 90 subjects would be required in each group. At the most recent follow-up, the mean Knee Society knee scores (92 versus 93 points), function scores (85 versus 85 points), WOMAC scores (23 versus 23 points), UCLA activity scores (6.5 versus 6.5 points), and ROM (125° versus 127°) were not different between the two groups. There was no radiographic evidence of loosening and no osteolysis visible on CT scan in either group. The weight of PE wear particles produced at the bearing surface was 0.046 g in 1 g of synovial fluid in subjects with an OxZr femoral component and 0.0448 g in subjects with a CoCr femoral component. Kaplan-Meier survivorship free from revision was 97% for the OxZr group and 98% for the CoCr group at

13 years after surgery. Given the absence of demonstrated superiority of either the CoCr implant or the OxZr implant, Kim et al. authors advised that surgeons and healthcare systems could reasonably choose the less expensive implant for routine use, unless there was some compelling reason in an individual subject to choose one over the other (such as severe, documented metal sensitivity) [3].

11.4 All-Cause Survivorship Rates and Reasons for Revision TKA

In a systematic review with level 4 of evidence published in 2022, Paul et al. evaluated all-cause survivorship, reasons for revision, patient-reported outcomes (PROMs), and return to physical activity and sport in 3095 subjects 55 years or younger experiencing primary TKA. Kaplan-Meier estimates of all-cause survivorship ranged from 90% to 98% at 5–10 years of follow-up after TKA and from 84% to 99% at 10 years to 20 years post-TKA. Common reasons for revision in TKA subjects were PE wear/loosening, aseptic tibial loosening, and infection. Return to physical activity and sport was reported variably; however, most subjects younger than 55 have improved physical activity levels after TKA relative to preoperative levels. To limit the frequency of revision in subjects younger than 55 years experiencing TKA, surgeons should be cautious of PE wear/loosening, aseptic tibial loosening, and infection, while knee pain and progression of knee OA are also common reasons for revision in subjects younger than 55 experiencing UKA [6].

11.5 Re-Revision-Free Survival and Risk Factors for Re-Revision in Patients Less than 55 Years Who Undergo Aseptic Revision TKA

In 2021 Chalmers et al. claimed that there were limited data on the results of revision TKA (rTKA) in young subjects. They sought to characterize the re-revision-free survival and risk factors for re-revision in subjects less than 55 years who experienced aseptic revision TKA [7]. They retrospectively reviewed 197 revision TKAs at a mean follow-up of 5 years. Mean age was 49 years; mean BMI was 31 kg/m². Twenty-seven (14%) subjects had at least one prior revision TKA. The most frequent indications for rTKA included instability (29%), arthrofibrosis (26%), and aseptic loosening (24%) (Fig. 11.1). Constraint included the following: 59 PS (30%), 123 varus-valgus constrained (62%), and 15 hinged (8%) (Fig. 11.2). Components revised included the following: 93 femur/tibia (47%), 68 PE only (35%), 19 femur only (10%), and 17 other (9%) (Fig. 11.3). Survivorship free from re-revision was calculated via the Kaplan-Meier method and a multivariate Cox proportional regression was utilized to identify risk factors for re-revision. Survivorship free from any re-revision at 5 years was 80%. In the multivariate analysis, subjects with a prior revision, an isolated PE exchange, and a hinged prosthesis were significant risk factors for lower revision-free survival. Forty-two subjects (21%) experienced re-revision, most frequently for periprosthetic joint infection (PJI) (7%), instability (6%), and aseptic loosening (5%). Re-revision happened in 18/68 (26%) subjects experiencing an isolated PE exchange. Subjects less than 55 years experiencing rTKA have a modest 5-year revision-free survival of 80%. Subjects with prior rTKAs, hinge-type prosthe-

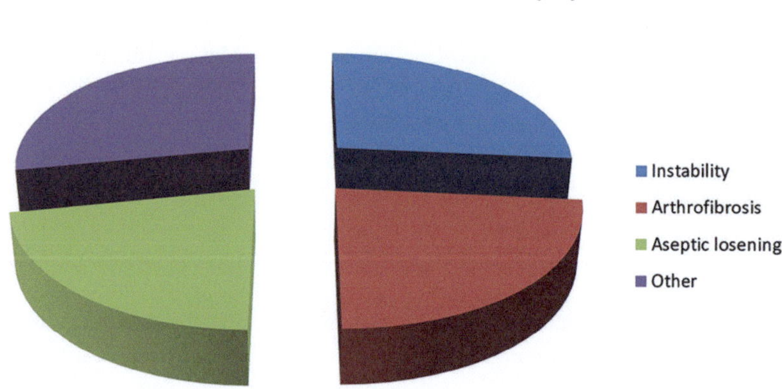

Fig. 11.1 Most frequent indications for revision total knee arthroplasty (rTKA) in patients younger than 55 years

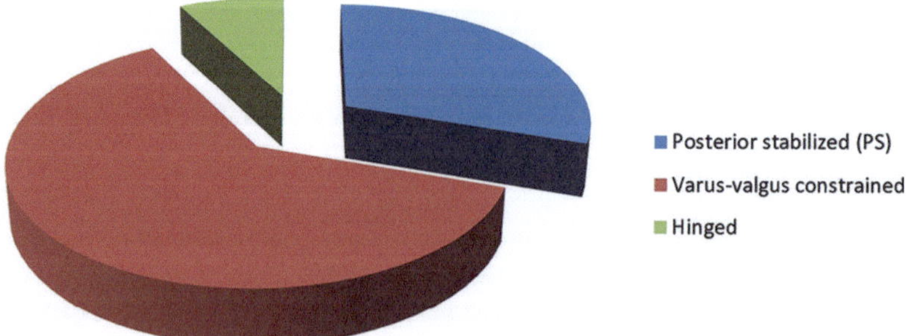

Fig. 11.2 Types of constraint used during revision total knee arthroplasty (rTKA) in patients younger than 55 years

Fig. 11.3 Components revised during revision total knee arthroplasty (rTKA) in patients younger than 55 years

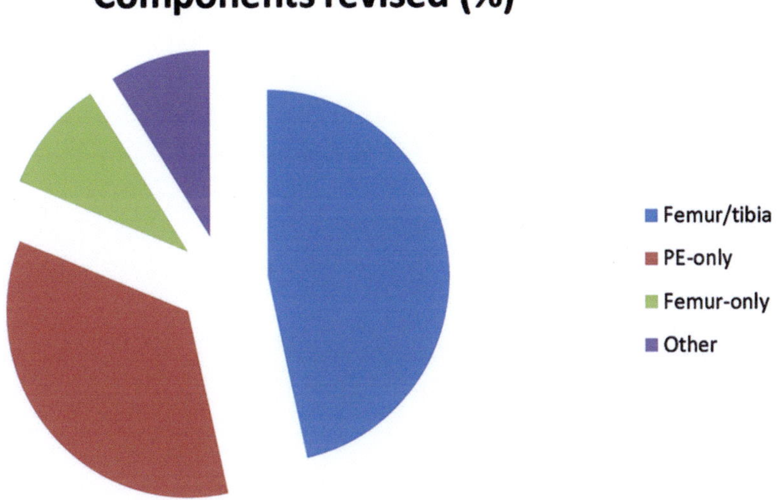

ses, and PE-only revisions had higher revision percentages [7].

11.6   Conclusions

Age less than 55 years is not an independent predictor of functional result or percentage of patient satisfaction after TKA. However, depression and poor mental health are significantly more prevalent in subjects less than 55 years old and are independently associated with a lower satisfaction percentage. Kaplan-Meier estimates of all-cause survivorship ranges from 90% to 98% at 5–10 years of follow-up after TKA and from 84% to 99% at 10 years to 20 years post-TKA. Common reasons for revision in TKA subjects are PE wear/loosening, aseptic tibial loosening, and infection. Subjects less than 55 years experiencing rTKA have a modest 5-year revision-free survival of 80%. Subjects with prior rTKAs, hinge-type prostheses, and PE-only revisions have higher revision percentages. In younger subjects with an oxidized zirconium (OxZr) TKA compared with those with a cobalt-chrome (CoCr) TKA, Kaplan-Meier survivorship free from revision is 97% for the OxZr group and 98% for the CoCr group at 13 years after surgery.

References

1. Aujla RS, Esler CN. Total knee arthroplasty for osteoarthritis in patients less than fifty-five years of age: a systematic review. J Arthroplast. 2017;32:2598–2603.e1.
2. Clement ND, Walker LC, Bardgett M, Weir D, Holland J, Gerrand C, et al. Patient age of less than 55 years is not an independent predictor of functional improvement or satisfaction after total knee arthroplasty. Arch Orthop Trauma Surg. 2018;138:1755–63.
3. Egloff C, Hirschmann MT, Moret C, Henle P, Ellenrieder M, Tischer T. Total knee arthroplasty in the young patient—an update. Orthopade. 2021;50:395–401.
4. Kim YH, Park JW, Kim JS. The 2018 Mark Coventry, MD award: does a ceramic bearing improve pain, function, wear, or survivorship of TKA in patients younger than 55 years of age? A randomized trial. Clin Orthop Relat Res. 2019;477:49–57.
5. Lizaur-Utrilla A, Martinez-Mendez D, Miralles-Muñoz FA, Marco-Gómez L, Lopez-Prats FA. Comparable outcomes after total knee arthroplasty in patients under 55 years than in older patients: a matched prospective study with minimum follow-up of 10 years. Knee Surg Sports Traumatol Arthrosc. 2017;25:3396–402.
6. Paul RW, Osman A, Clements A, Tjoumakaris FP, Lonner JH, Freedman KB. What are the all-cause survivorship rates and functional outcomes in patients younger than 55 years undergoing primary knee arthroplasty? A systematic review. Clin Orthop Relat Res. 2022;480:507–22.
7. Chalmers BP, Syku M, Joseph AD, Mayman DJ, Haas SB, Blevins JL. High rate of re-revision in patients less than 55 years of age undergoing aseptic revision total knee arthroplasty. J Arthroplast. 2021;36:2348–52.

Unilateral Primary Total Knee Arthroplasty Versus Simultaneous Bilateral Primary Total Knee Arthroplasty

E. Carlos Rodríguez-Merchán

12.1 Introduction

In 2006, two important questions remained in simultaneous bilateral total knee arthroplasty (sbTKA). Was sbTKA significantly more painful and was physical recovery significantly more difficult compared with staged bilateral TKA [1]? In 2015 Suleiman et al. claimed that sbTKA was potentially a cost-saving manner of caring for patients with bilateral symptomatic knee osteoarthritis (OA) [2]. In 2016 Bohm et al. claimed that there was no consensus about the outcome of simultaneous versus staged bilateral TKA [3]. In 2018 Masrouha et al. stated that sbTKA could offer certain benefits; however, its overall safety was still disputed [4].

In 2018 Kulshrestha et al. affirmed that sbTKA offered significant socioeconomic benefits. However, retrospective studies and public health data showed increased mortality and morbidity rates in patients undergoing sbTKA compared with those undergoing staged bilateral TKA, and there had been recommendations against the use of sbTKA. High-volume centers, which feature careful patient selection and fast-tracked surgery, continued to perform sbTKA and had published their results in favor of the procedure. However, the quality of evidence remained poor [5].

In 2022 Arif et al. expressed that sbTKA could save time, anesthesia, and cost of multiple procedures [6]. The purpose of this chapter is to review recent developments on staged bilateral TKA versus sbTKA.

12.2 Local Infiltration Analgesia

Ropivacaine is commonly used in local infiltration anesthesia (LIA) as pain management after TKA. Although considered safe, no studies evaluated the pharmacokinetics of high-dose ropivacaine infiltration in sbTKA. In 2021 Gromov et al. studied 13 subjects undergoing uTKA and 15 undergoing sbTKA [7]. A standard LIA technique was used with ropivacaine 0.2%, 200 mL (400 mg), injected periarticularly in each knee. Free and total plasma concentrations of ropivacaine were measured within 24 h using liquid chromatography-mass spectrometry. A population pharmacokinetic model was built using nonlinear mixed-effects models. Peak free ropivacaine concentration was 0.030 µg mL^{-1} versus 0.095 µg mL^{-1}, and peak total ropivacaine concentration was 0.756 µg mL^{-1} versus 1.695 µg mL^{-1} for uTKA and sbTKA, respectively. The pharmacokinetics was ascribed a one-compartment model with first-order absorption. The main identified covariates were protein binding, allometrically scaled body weight on clearance and volume, and unilateral or bilateral

E. C. Rodríguez-Merchán (✉)
Department of Orthopedic Surgery, La Paz University Hospital, Madrid, Spain

E. C. Rodríguez-Merchán (ed.), *Advances in Orthopedic Surgery of the Knee*,
https://doi.org/10.1007/978-3-031-33061-2_12

surgery on volume. This was the first study to investigate the pharmacokinetics of free and total ropivacaine after unilateral and bilateral TKA. A population model was successfully built and peak free ropivacaine concentration stayed below previously proposed toxic thresholds in subjects undergoing unilateral and bilateral TKA receiving LIA with high-dose ropivacaine [7].

12.3 Tranexamic Acid (TXA)

Despite the documented blood-saving effects of tranexamic acid (TXA) in TKA, the question whether clinical values of TXA are identical in uTKA and sbTKAs remains unclear. In 2014 Kim et al. studied the clinical values of TXA in uTKA and sBTKA under a contemporary blood-saving protocol in terms of efficacy (total blood loss and transfusion rate) and safety (the incidences of symptomatic deep vein thrombosis and pulmonary embolism) [8]. One hundred and eighty uTKA and 146 sbTKA subjects were randomized into the TXA group or control group. In uTKA subjects, TXA (10 mg/kg) was administered intravenously 20 min before tourniquet deflation and repeated 3 h after surgery. In sbTKA subjects, one more dose (10 mg/kg) was given before tourniquet deflation in the second TKA. A contemporary blood-saving protocol was applied to all subjects. The TXA and control groups were compared separately in uTKA and sbTKA subjects for the efficacy and safety variables. In uTKA subjects, the TXA group had less total blood loss (905 vs. 1018 mL) than the control group, but there was no difference in the allogenic transfusion rate (1 vs. 7%). In sbTKA subjects, the TXA group showed no differences in total blood loss (1282 vs. 1379 mL), but a significant reduction in the allogenic transfusion rate (7 vs. 27%). No symptomatic deep vein thrombosis or pulmonary embolism was found in all subjects. This study demonstrated that the use of TXA reduces total blood loss, but the effects on the transfusion rate can differ depending on the type of TKAs (unilateral vs. bilateral) and the blood-saving protocols [8].

12.4 Outcomes

In 2016 Bohm et al. examined this issue by analyzing 238,373 subjects [3]. Demographic, clinical, and outcome data were evaluated for TKA subjects (unilateral, 206,771; simultaneous bilateral, 6349; staged bilateral, 25,253) from the Canadian Hospital Morbidity Database for fiscal years 2006–2007 to 2012–2013. Outcomes were adjusted for age, sex, comorbidities, and hospital TKA volume. sbTKA subjects were younger than staged bilateral TKA subjects (median 64 years vs. 66 years), were more likely to be male (41% vs. 39%), and had a lower frequency of having ≥1 comorbid condition (2.9% vs. 4.2%). They also had a higher frequency of blood transfusions (41% vs. 19%), a shorter median length of stay (6 days vs. 8 days), a higher frequency of transfer to a rehabilitation facility (46% vs. 9%), and a lower frequency of knee infection (0.5% vs. 0.9%) than staged bilateral TKA patients, but they had a higher rate of cardiac complications within 90 days (2% vs. 1.7%). Simultaneous subjects had higher in-hospital mortality compared to the second TKA in staged subjects (0.16% vs. 0.06%), but they had similar rates of in-hospital mortality compared to unilateral patients (0.16% vs. 0.14%). The cumulative 3-year revision rate was highest in the unilateral group (2.3%), but it was similar in the staged and simultaneous bilateral groups (1.4%). This study found important differences between the outcomes of simultaneous and staged bilateral TKA. Further clarification of outcomes would be best determined in an adequately powered randomized trial, which would remove the selection bias inherent in this retrospective study design [3].

In 2021 Obaid-ur-Rahman et al. compared preoperative characteristics and perioperative findings in subjects undergoing uTKA and sbTKA. To work out safety criterion for selection of subjects for sbTKA, subjects undergoing uTKA (39) and sbTKA (36) from March 2014 to August 2014 were compared in terms of subject characteristics, underlying pathology, perioperative blood loss, transfusion requirements, and in-hospital complications. The mean age of subjects undergoing uTKA was 61 years and those undergoing sbTKA was 64 years, with similar male to female ratio (1:1.8) in both groups. Males undergoing sbTKA were significantly older than other subjects (71 years). Primary OA was the most common initial diagnosis (59% in uTKA and 89% in sbTKA) followed by rheumatoid arthritis. Average blood loss per knee was higher in simultaneous bilateral TKA procedures but the difference did not reach statistical significance. Blood transfusion requirements in sbTKA subjects not receiving antifibrinolytic agent were significantly higher than in similar uTKA subjects (75% vs. 17%) but were significantly reduced with perioperative administration of antifibrinolytic therapy (30% sbTKA). Complication rates, low in both, were more frequent in sbTKA subjects with comorbidities. In subjects requiring bilateral knee replacements, staged TKA (i.e., the two knees are replaced with a gap of at least 3 months) was a safe approach. uTKA was associated with lesser complications and blood transfusion requirements as compared to sbTKAs [9].

In 2022 Arid and Hafeez aimed to determine the frequency of uTKA and sbTKA and then compared their outcomes [6]. A total of 95 subjects were included and were divided into two groups, i.e., subjects undergoing uTKA were grouped as group A and subjects undergoing sbTKA were grouped as group B. Then subjects underwent surgery under general anesthesia. All subjects were followed up in the outpatient department (OPD). During follow-up, subjects were evaluated for the outcome, i.e., cardiac event, urinary tract infection, and surgical site infection. The mean age of subjects was 63 years. There were 50 (52.6%) males and 45 (47.4%) females. The mean body mass index (BMI) of females was 27.93 kg/m^2. There were 47 (49.5%) subjects who underwent sbTKA, while 48 (50.5%) underwent uTKA. It was observed that after surgery, the cardiac event occurred in one (1.1%) case and that case was from the unilateral surgery group; urinary tract infection occurred in four cases, two (4.3%) were from bilateral cases, while two (4.2%) were from the unilateral group, and surgical site infection occurred in four cases, and two (4.3%) were from bilateral cases, while two (4.2%) were from the unilateral group (Fig. 12.1). The difference was insignificant in both groups. There was no significant difference observed between both groups regarding complications after surgery [6].

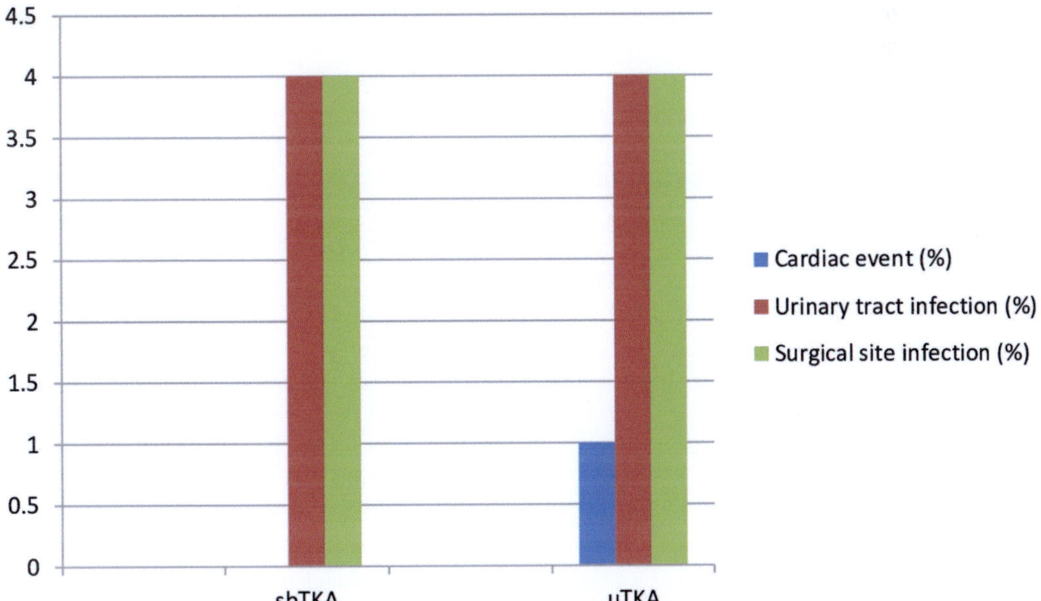

Fig. 12.1 Frequency of unilateral total knee arthroplasty (uTKA) and simultaneous bilateral total knee arthroplasty (sbTKA): comparative outcomes

12.4.1 Pain Levels and Recovery of Ambulatory Skills

In 2006 Powell et al. published a retrospective matched-pair analysis comparing 59 sbTKA and 59 uTKA subjects based on age, sex, diagnosis, surgeon, and surgery date [1]. Analog pain scores, narcotic use, ambulatory distances, and rehabilitative milestones were recorded. Bilateral patients' pain scores were 1 point higher during day 1 with subsequent equal scores. Narcotic use was 20% higher for the first 48 hours but equalized after that period. Ambulatory milestones lagged behind by 36 hours. Subjects wishing to pursue bilateral TKA could proceed without pain, use of narcotics, and walking distance significantly different than unilateral TKA [1].

12.4.2 Thrombosis Incidence

In 2013 Levy et al. compared the incidence of venous thromboembolic event (VTE) in 55 subjects (110 knees) undergoing sbTKA with 287 subjects (287 knees) undergoing uTKA using a mobile compression device as monotherapy prophylaxis in both groups [10]. All subjects were clinically evaluated 3 months after surgery with symptomatic confirmed VTE as an end point. Deep venous thrombosis (DVT) was documented by duplex ultrasound and pulmonary embolism (PE) was documented by spiral computed tomography (CT). The sbTKA group had 6 VTEs (10.9%) with 2 PEs (3.6%). The uTKA group had 9 VTEs (3.1%) and 0 PE. Subjects undergoing sbTKA yielded more than twice the rate of VTE compared with patients undergoing uTKA using a mobile compression device as sole thromboprophylactic modality [10].

12.4.3 Thirty-Day Risk of Venous Thromboembolism and Bleeding

A study published in 2018 by Masrouha et al. aimed at comparing the risk of thromboembolism and bleeding in subjects who underwent sbTKA versus uTKA [4]. The American College of Surgeons National Surgical Quality Improvement Program database from 2008 to 2015 was used to investigate the short-run postoperative complications and their risk factors following sbTKA as compared to uTKA. Demographics, comorbidities, and 30-day outcomes were analyzed. Complications with an increased incidence following sbTKA were stratified to identify subgroups of patients at high risk. A total of 155,022 subjects were identified, of which 150,581 underwent uTKA and 4441 underwent sbTKA. The sbTKA group was found to be at a higher risk of venous thromboembolism (VTE), bleeding, and composite morbidity. Stratification analysis revealed that sbTKA subgroups at higher risk of VTE include subjects of black or Asian origin, obese subjects, and those who underwent anesthesia other than general or spinal/epidural. sbTKA subgroups at higher risk of bleeding included subjects older than 85 years, those with race other than white, underweight and obese subjects, and subjects who underwent anesthesia other than spinal/epidural. Although none of the subgroups were protected from bleeding, subjects who underwent spinal/epidural anesthesia had a lower risk of bleeding compared to other types of anesthesia. sbTKA conferred an increased risk of postoperative VTE, bleeding, and composite morbidity at 30 days, with no increase in mortality [4].

12.4.4 Perioperative Outcomes

In 2015 Suleiman et al. performed a retrospective analysis using the 2010–2012 American College of Surgeons National Surgical Quality Improvement Program (ACS-NSQIP) to evaluate the risk of perioperative complication following sbTKA. Demographic characteristics, comorbidities, and 30-day complication rates were studied using a propensity score-matched analysis comparing subjects undergoing uTKA and sbTKA. A total of 4489 subjects met the inclusion criteria, of which 973 were sbTKA. sbTKA was associated with increased overall complications, medical complications, and reoperation. Further, the total length of hospital stay (4 vs. 3.4 days) was significantly longer following bilateral surgery [2].

12.4.5 Ninety-Day Morbidity and Mortality

In 2018 Kulshrestha et al. prospectively examined the 90-day morbidity and mortality of sbTKA compared with uTKA [5]. A total of 1200 consecutive subjects were recruited in each arm. Ninety-day mortality was higher in sbTKA subjects than in uTKA subjects (0.58% vs. 0.42%, respectively). Overall procedure-related complications were significantly higher in the sbTKA group (7.25% vs. 4.42%, respectively). The relative risk of cardiovascular complications in sbTKA subjects was 6.5 times higher than that in uTKA subjects (1.08% vs. 0.17%, respectively). Neurological complications were 9.5 times more common in the sbTKA group (1.58% vs. 0.17%, respectively) (Fig. 12.2). All other complications were comparable in the two groups. Risk screening and preoperative optimization reduced mortality and overall complication rates in sbTKA

subjects; however, overall procedure-related complications, specifically cardiovascular and neurological, remained significantly high in sbTKA subjects, for which a guarded approach was recommended [5].

12.4.6 Component Alignment

In 2019 Qadir et al. investigated differences in component alignment between the first and second knees in sbTKA and uTKA [11]. Two hundred and seventy-four sbTKAs and 198 uTKAs were included in study. Subjects were divided into three groups as sbTKA on the right knee (group A), sbTKA on the left knee (group B), and uTKA (group C). Femoral and tibial component alignment was checked in both coronal plane (alpha [α] and beta [β] angles) and sagittal plane (gamma [γ] and delta [δ] angles) radiographs. There were no statistically significant differences among groups in the preoperative anatomical varus angle and Kellgren-Lawrence OA classification grade. In the coronal plane, the alignment of femoral component (α-angle) and tibial component (β-angle) was similar in all

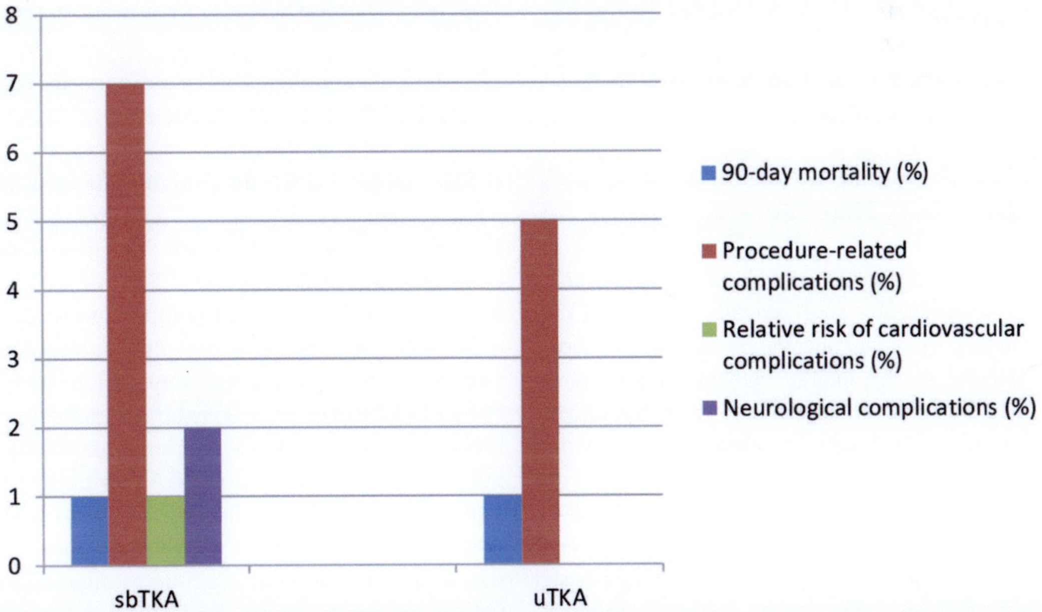

Fig. 12.2 Frequency of complications of unilateral total knee arthroplasty (uTKA) versus simultaneous bilateral total knee arthroplasty (sbTKA)

three groups (α-angle, 95.01 vs. 95.14 vs. 94.9, p = 0.945; β-angle, 90.03 vs. 89.67 vs. 89.98). The sagittal plane alignment of femoral component (γ-angle) and tibial component (δ-angle) did not show significant differences (γ-angle, 7.04 vs. 6.98 vs. 7.00; δ-angle, 86.56 vs. 87.41 vs. 86.73). The angular alignment of components was similar between sbTKA and uTKA [11].

12.5 Risk Factors Increasing Morbidity

Because surgeons are electing to perform sbTKA, it is important to identify which subjects are at increased risk. In 2011 Fabi et al. performed a retrospective cohort analysis of 150 subjects with uTKA versus 150 subjects with sbTKA. The bilateral group demonstrated a 2.1 times greater mean overall complication rate as well as increased transfusion rates. Subjects older than 70 years exhibited significantly higher complication rates. Having a preexisting pulmonary disorder in the bilateral cohort carried nearly a threefold risk of complications. Subjects with BMIs greater than 30 displayed a complication rate of 0.97 in the bilateral group as opposed to 0.44 in the control group. This study demonstrated that age, BMI, and a preexisting pulmonary disorder resulted in increased complications [12].

12.6 Cost-Effectiveness

Although studies have compared the claims costs of simultaneous and staged bilateral TKA, whether a simultaneous procedure is cost-effective to the facility remains unknown. In 2022 Goh et al. compared facility costs and perioperative outcomes of simultaneous versus staged bilateral TKA [13]. They reviewed a consecutive series of 777 bilateral TKA (163 staged and 451 simultaneous). Itemized facility costs were calculated using time-driven activity-based costing. Ninety-day outcomes were compared. Margin was standardized to unadjusted Medicare Diagnosis-Related Group payments (simultaneous, $18,523; staged, $22,386). Multivariate regression was used to determine the independent association between costs/clinical outcomes and treatment strategy (staged vs. simultaneous). Simultaneous bilateral subjects had significantly lower personnel, supply, and total facility costs compared with staged subjects with no difference in 90-day complications between the groups. Multivariate analyses showed that overall facility costs were $704 lower in TKA. Despite lower costs, margin for the facility was lower in the simultaneous group ($6718 vs. $10,067 for TKA). Simultaneous bilateral TKA had lower facility costs than staged procedures because of savings associated with a single hospitalization. With the increased Medicare reimbursement for two unilateral procedures, however, margin was higher for staged procedures. In the era of value-based care, policymakers should not penalize facilities for performing cost-effective simultaneous bilateral arthroplasty in appropriately selected subjects [13].

12.7 Conclusions

Ninety-day mortality is higher in sbTKA subjects than in uTKA subjects (0.58% vs. 0.42%, respectively). Overall procedure-related complications are significantly higher in the sbTKA group (7.25% vs. 4.42%, respectively). The relative risk of cardiovascular complications in sbTKA subjects is 6.5 times higher than that in uTKA subjects (1.08% vs. 0.17%, respectively). Neurological complications are 9.5 times more common in the sbTKA group (1.58% vs. 0.17%, respectively). The bilateral group demonstrates a 2.1 times greater mean overall complication rate as well as increased transfusion rates. Patients older than 70 years exhibit significantly higher complication rates. Having a preexisting pulmonary disorder in the sbTKA carries nearly a threefold risk of complications. Patients with BMIs greater than 30 display a complication rate of 0.97 in the bilateral group as opposed to 0.44 in the control group. Age, BMI, and a preexisting pulmonary disorder result in increased complications. sbTKA confers an increased risk of postoperative VTE, bleeding, and composite morbidity at 30 days, with no increase in mortality. Subjects undergoing sbTKA yielded more than twice the rate of VTE compared with subjects undergoing uTKA using a mobile compression device as sole thromboprophylactic modality.

References

1. Powell RS, Pulido P, Tuason MS, Colwell CW Jr, Ezzet KA. Bilateral vs unilateral total knee arthroplasty: a patient-based comparison of pain levels and recovery of ambulatory skills. J Arthroplast. 2006;21:642–9.
2. Suleiman LI, Edelstein AI, Thompson RM, Alvi HM, Kwasny MJ, Manning DW. Perioperative outcomes following unilateral versus bilateral total knee arthroplasty. J Arthroplast. 2015;30:1927–30.
3. Bohm ER, Molodianovitsh K, Dragan A, Zhu N, Webster G, Masri B, et al. Outcomes of unilateral and bilateral total knee arthroplasty in 238,373 patients. Acta Orthop. 2016;87(Suppl 1):24–30.
4. Masrouha KZ, Hoballah JJ, Tamim HM, Sagherian BH. Comparing the 30-day risk of venous thromboembolism and bleeding in simultaneous bilateral vs unilateral total knee arthroplasty. J Arthroplast. 2018;33:3273–80.e1.
5. Kulshrestha V, Kumar S, Datta B, Sinha VK, Mittal G. Ninety-day morbidity and mortality in risk-screened and optimized patients undergoing two-team fast-track simultaneous bilateral TKA compared with unilateral TKA-A prospective study. J Arthroplast. 2018;33:752–60.
6. Arif MA, Hafeez S. Comparison of frequency and morbidity of unilateral total knee replacement versus simultaneous bilateral total knee replacement. Cureus. 2022;14(1):e21655.
7. Gromov K, Grassin-Delyle S, Foss NB, Pedersen LM, Nielsen CS, Lamy E, et al. Population pharmacokinetics of ropivacaine used for local infiltration anaesthesia during primary total unilateral and simultaneous bilateral knee arthroplasty. Br J Anaesth. 2021;126:872–80.
8. Kim TK, Chang CB, Kang YG, Seo ES, Lee JH, Yun JH, et al. Clinical value of tranexamic acid in unilateral and simultaneous bilateral TKAs under a contemporary blood-saving protocol: a randomized controlled trial. Knee Surg Sports Traumatol Arthrosc. 2014;22:1870–8.
9. Obaid-ur-Rahman, Hafeez S, Amin MS, Ameen J, Adnan R. Unilateral versus simultaneous bilateral total knee arthroplasty: a comparative study. J Pak Med Assoc. 2021;71((Suppl 5)(8)):S21–5.
10. Levy YD, Hardwick ME, Copp SN, Rosen AS, Colwell CW Jr. Thrombosis incidence in unilateral vs. simultaneous bilateral total knee arthroplasty with compression device prophylaxis. J Arthroplast. 2013;28:474–8.
11. Qadir I, Shah B, Waqas M, Ahmad U, Javed S, Aziz A. Component alignment in simultaneous bilateral versus unilateral total knee arthroplasty. Knee Surg Relat Res. 2019;31:31–6.
12. Fabi DW, Mohan V, Goldstein WM, Dunn JH, Murphy BP. Unilateral vs bilateral total knee arthroplasty risk factors increasing morbidity. J Arthroplast. 2011;26:668–73.
13. Goh GS, Sutton RM, D'Amore T, Baker CM, Clark SC, Courtney PM. A time-driven activity-based costing analysis of simultaneous versus staged bilateral total hip arthroplasty and total knee arthroplasty. J Arthroplast. 2022;37(8S):S742–7.

Mobile-Bearing Versus Fixed-Bearing for Total Knee Arthroplasty

13

E. Carlos Rodríguez-Merchán,
Carlos A. Encinas-Ullán, Juan S. Ruiz-Pérez,
and Primitivo Gómez-Cardero

13.1 Introduction

In 2015 Bailey et al. affirmed that mobile-bearing (MB) in total knee arthroplasty (TKA) (Fig. 13.1) could confer benefits with regard to range of motion (ROM) and have improved clinical outcome scores in comparison with an arthroplasty with a fixed-bearing (FB) design [1]. The same year Hofstede et al. claimed that it was unclear whether there were differences in benefits and harms between MB and FB prostheses for TKA [2].

In 2020 Killen et al. stated that TKA with FB implants had demonstrated impressive functional results and survival rates. Meanwhile, MB implants had biomechanically been shown to reduce polyethylene (PE) wear, lower the risk of component loosening, and better replicate anatomic knee motion. However, there was growing question of the clinical impact these design changes have in the long run [3]. In 2020 Sappey-Marinier et al. expressed that TKA was the treatment of choice for severe osteoarthritis (OA) of the knee. They also stated that many studies had been carried out comparing MB and FB designs; however, there were insufficient data regarding the patellar position in either system [4]. The purpose of this chapter is to review recent developments on MB versus FB for TKA.

E. C. Rodríguez-Merchán (✉) · C. A. Encinas-Ullán
J. S. Ruiz-Pérez · P. Gómez-Cardero
Department of Orthopedic Surgery, La Paz University
Hospital, Madrid, Spain

© The Author(s), under exclusive license to Springer Nature Switzerland AG 2023
E. C. Rodríguez-Merchán (ed.), *Advances in Orthopedic Surgery of the Knee*,
https://doi.org/10.1007/978-3-031-33061-2_13

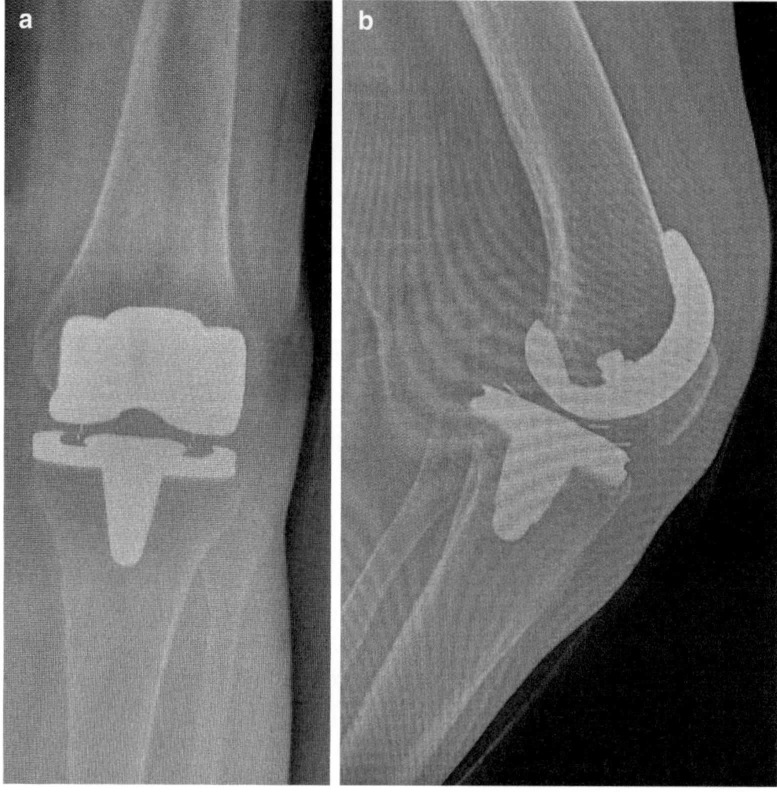

Fig. 13.1 (a, b) Mobile-bearing total knee arthroplasty: (**a**) anteroposterior radiograph; (**b**) lateral view

13.2 Clinical, Radiological, and General Health Results

A series of individuals undergoing TKA utilizing either an MB or an FB implant was reported in 2004 by Woolson et al. [5]. Forty-four individuals experienced 57 MB implants, and 40 individuals experienced 45 FB posterior stabilized (PS) implants. At an average 41-month follow-up, no significant differences were observed between the groups with respect to Knee Society ratings or pain scores. Postoperative flexion was not different between the groups (116° for MB and 118° for FB). Three MB knees were revised for implant-related adverse events. There was no difference between these MB or FB knee implants clinically or radiographically at early follow-up. However, more subjects with an MB knee required early revision for failure of rotating patellar or tibial PE implants [5].

In 2012 Shemshaki et al. compared clinical, radiological, and general health results of two prostheses (MB vs. FB devices) that were utilized in TKA with a 5-year follow-up (level 1 of evidence) [6]. This randomized controlled study was conducted from 2004 to 2010. Three hundred individuals with expected TKA without severe deformity (a fixed varus or valgus deformity greater than 20°) experienced FB design ($n = 150$) or MB design ($n = 150$). Clinical, radiological, and quality of life (QoL) results were compared between the two groups at 6-month intervals for the first year, after which the comparisons were made yearly for the next 4 years. Both groups had similar baseline characteristics. Although there was significant improvement in both groups, there was no significant difference between the groups with regard to the means of the Knee Society Scores (KSS), which were 92 for the FB device and 93 for the MB device (n.s.) at the final follow-up point. Radiographs showed that there was no significant difference in prosthetic alignment and no evidence of loosening. After TKA, the Medical Outcomes Short Form-36 (SF-36) score increased in both groups, but there was no statistical difference between the groups in QoL at the final follow-up (62 vs. 64). There was no revision after 5 years. In terms of clinical, radiological, or general health outcomes for people who underwent TKA, the results of this study showed no clear advantage of MB over the FB prosthesis at the five-year follow-up [6].

In 2016 Baktir et al. compared long-term clinical and radiographic outcomes of MB and FB TKAs [7]. A randomized controlled study compared the clinical and radiographic outcomes of MB and FB prostheses in 93 subjects who underwent primary TKA for knee OA. Mean follow-up of the subjects was 100.9 months in the MB group and 93.7 months in the FB group. The clinical results were graded according to the Knee Society Knee Score (KSKS) and the Knee Society Functional Score (KSFS). Secondary outcomes included pain, patellofemoral joint function, QoL, and radiologic outcomes (Knee Society's radiologic assessment system). Even though there was significant improvement in both groups, there were no significant differences between the groups with respect to mean KSFS and radiologic outcomes. However, mean pain score of the MB group was significantly higher than that of the FB group (48.83 vs. 47.39, respectively), and mean KSKS was significantly higher than that of the FB group (93.5 vs. 89.7, respectively). TKA clinical outcomes were satisfactory in both the MB and FB groups. KSKS and pain scores were significantly better in the MB than in the FB group. However, no differences were encountered in other assessments. Thus, Batkir et al. concluded that the best design was the one with which the surgeon was most comfortable and most able to implant reproducibly [7].

In a meta-analysis published in 2021 by Hao et al., the benefits and risks of FB and MB designs for TKA were compared, and the long-run (9 years of follow-up) functional, clinical, and radiological outcomes were analyzed. Primary outcome measures were Knee Society Scores (KSSs), range of motion (ROM) in knee joint values, complication rates, and revision percentages. The KSSs include the KSKSs (Knee Society Knee Scores), which are mainly used to

evaluate pain, ROM, and knee stability, and the KSFSs (Knee Society Function Scores), which are used to evaluate a patient's ability to walk and climb stairs. A total of 451 individuals with 612 knees met the inclusion criteria. There was no significant difference in the KSSs, ROM values, revision percentages, or adverse event rates between the two bearing design groups. After about 10 years of follow-up, the MB design had advantages in KSFSs over the FB design. Hao et al. affirmed that the MB design could also have advantages in the revision percentages over the FB design when the posterior cruciate ligament (PCL) was substituted. There was no clear difference in KSSs, ROM values, or complication percentages between these two designs [8].

In a meta-analysis with level 2 of evidence reported in 2022, Chen et al. compared the clinical and radiographic outcomes between MB TKA and FB TKA at a minimum 10-year follow-up. This meta-analysis showed no significant difference between the two groups with respect to the KSS, KSS function score, the Western Ontario and McMaster Universities Osteoarthritis index (WOMAC), ROM, radiolucent line, femoral and tibial component positions in the coronal plane, revision prevalence, and survivorship percentages. Meanwhile, it showed a slight difference between the two groups in the tibial component position in the sagittal plane. According to this meta-analysis, the current best available evidence suggested no significant difference between the MB TKA and FB TKA groups with respect to the clinical results, radiographic outcomes, revision, and survivorship at a minimum 10-year follow-up [9].

13.3 Function and Implant Longevity

In an experimental study, randomize controlled trial (RCT) with level 1 of evidence published in 2020, Killen et al. compared function and implant survival in individuals who experienced either FB or RP press-fit condylar Sigma (PFC Sigma, DePuy, Warsaw, IN) TKAs at a minimum follow-up of 12 years [3]. Patient-reported outcome measures (PROMs) utilized included the functional KSS, WOMAC scores, SF-36 score, and satisfaction assessment on a four-point Likert scale. The data was collected preoperatively, two years after, and at the final encounter (mean 13.95 years). A total of 28 RP and 19 FB knees (58.8%) were analyzed at the final follow-up. Among all subjects, KSS and WOMAC scores statistically improved from preop to 2 years, while KSS statistically worsened from 2 years to the final follow-up. The MB group averaged better follow-up scores in all assessments at the final follow-up with exception of overall satisfaction. There was no statistically significant difference in the functional KSS, SF-36, WOMAC scores, patient satisfaction, or implant survival between the two groups at any measured period. The use of an FB or MB design did not convey significant superiority in terms of function or implant longevity at a minimum 12 years after TKA [3].

13.4 Patellar Position

In 2020 Sappey-Marinier et al. claimed that TKA was the treatment of choice for severe osteoarthritis (OA) of the knee and that many studies had been performed comparing MB and FB designs; however, there were insufficient data regarding the patellar position in either system [4]. In a prospective randomized study with level 1 of evidence, Sappey-Marinier et al. compared the resultant patellar position with an MB versus an FB TKA and the influence of both designs on clinical results. In this prospective randomized study, between 2007 and 2009, 160 TKA individuals were assessed; 79 experienced an MB and 81 experienced an FB implant, for medial compartment OA. A PS, HLS Noetos knee prosthesis (Tornier, Saint-Ismier, France) was utilized in all cases. The only difference between the groups was whether the tibial component incorporated a fixed or mobile bearing. The patella was resurfaced in all cases. The International KSS and the patellar tilt and translation were compared postoperatively. Patellar

translation and patellar tilt analyses were subdivided into two subgroups (<5 mm vs. >5 mm and <5° vs. >5°). The KSS was not statistically different between the groups at a mean follow-up of 7.4 years. Patellar translation and patellar tilt were not statistically different between the groups. When considering the patellar translation subgroup analysis, a significantly increased risk of patellar translation, greater than 5 mm, was encountered in the MB group compared to the FB group without generating any meaningful difference in clinical results. The theoretical advantages of MB implants compared to FB implants were not demonstrated in this study, at mid-run follow-up. In daily practice, the choice between MB and FB designs should be based on the experience and clinical judgment of the surgeon [4].

13.5 Fixed- Versus Mobile-Bearing Cruciate-Retaining TKA

In 2015 Bailey et al. compared clinical results between individuals who experienced TKA with either an MB or FB using a PCL design (level 1 of evidence). Three hundred and thirty-one individuals were randomized to receive either an MB (161 subjects) or an FB (170 subject) implant. All individuals were assessed preoperatively and at 1 and 2 years postoperatively using standard tools (ROM, Oxford Knee Score [OKS], American KSS, SF12, and Patella Score). There was no difference in pre- to 2-year postoperative outcomes between the groups with regard to improvement in ROM (10° vs. 9°), improvement in OKS (−17.6 vs. −19.1), improvement in American KSS (49.5 vs. 50.7), function (23.6 vs. 25) and pain (34.9 vs. 35.8) subscores, improvement in SF-12 Score (10 vs. 12.3), or improvement in Patella Score (9.7 vs. 10.6). No difference was demonstrated in clinical outcome between individuals with an MB and FB PCL-retaining TKA at 2-year follow-up [1].

13.6 Postoperative Functional Status in Patients with Osteoarthritis and Rheumatoid Arthritis

In a Cochrane Database Systematic Review published in 2015, Hofstede et al. assessed the benefits and harms of MB compared with FB PCL-retaining TKA for functional and clinical results in subjects with OA or rheumatoid arthritis (RA). They calculated the standardized mean difference (SMD) for pain, using the KSS and visual analogue scale (VAS) in 11 studies (58%) and 1531 knees (68%). No statistically significant differences between groups were found. Moderate- to low-quality evidence suggested that MB prostheses may have similar effects on knee pain, clinical and functional scores, health-related QoL, revision surgery, mortality, reoperation percentage, and other serious adverse events compared with FB prostheses in PCL-retaining TKA. Therefore, these authors could not draw firm conclusions. Most (98.5%) participants had OA, so the findings primarily reflect results reported in participants with OA [2].

13.7 Radiostereometric Analysis

In a randomized, single-blind, controlled trial with level 1 of evidence published in 2017, Schotanus et al. investigated two types of cemented TKA, the MB or FB variant from the same family, with the use of radiostereometric analysis. This prospective, patient-blinded RCT was designed to investigate early migration of the tibia component after 2 years of follow-up with use of radiostereometric analysis. A total of 50 individuals were randomized to receive an MB or FB TKA from the same family. Individuals were evaluated during 2-year follow-up, including radiostereometric analysis, physical and clinical examination, and PROMs. At two-year follow-up, the mean maximum total point motion (MTPM) in the FB group was 0.82 versus 0.92 mm in the MB group with the largest migration seen during the first 6 weeks (0.45 vs. 0.54). The clinical outcome and PROMs significantly improved within each group, not between both groups. The results of this study demonstrated that early migration of the MB was similar to that of the FB component at 2 years and was mainly seen in the first weeks after implantation [10].

13.8 Activities of Daily Living and Pain

In a RCT with level 1 of evidence published in 2017, Amaro et al. analyzed whether there were middle-run differences in knee function and pain in individuals experiencing FB and MB TKA. Eligible subjects were randomized into two groups: the first group experienced TKA implantation with a fixed tibial platform (group A); the second group experienced TKA with a mobile tibial platform (group B). Individuals were followed up (2 years), and their symptoms and limitations in daily living activities were evaluated using the Knee Outcome Survey-Activities of Daily Living Scale (ADLS), in addition to pain evaluation assessed using the pain VAS. There were no significant differences in function and symptoms in the ADLS and VAS between the study groups. The type of platform utilized in TKA (fixed vs. mobile) did not change the symptoms, function, or pain of individuals 2 years post-surgery. Although mobile TKAs may have better short-run outcomes, at medium- and long-run follow-up, they did not present important clinical differences compared with fixed-platform TKAs [11].

13.9 High-Flexion Fixed-Bearing Versus High-Flexion Mobile-Bearing TKAs

In 2018 Kim et al. studied whether clinical results, radiographic and computed tomography (CT) scan results, and the survival percentage of a high-flexion MB TKA were better than that of a high-flexion FB TKA. The study consisted of 92 individuals (184 knees) who experience same-day bilateral TKA. Of those, 17 were men and 75 were women. The mean age at the time of index arthroplasty was 61.5 years. The mean body mass index (BMI) was 26.2 kg/m². The mean follow-up was 11.2 years. The KSS scores (93 vs. 92 points) and function scores (80 vs. 80 points), WOMAC scores (14 vs. 15 points), and UCLA (University of California at Los Angeles) activity scores (6 vs. 6 points) were not different between the two groups at 12 years' follow-up. There were no differences in any radiographic CT scan parameters between the two groups. Kaplan-Meier survivorship of the TKA component was 98% in the high-flexion FB TKA group and 99% in the high-flexion MB TKA group 12 years after the operation. These authors found no benefit to MB TKA in terms of pain, function, radiographic and CT scan results, and survivorship [12].

13.10 Fixed- Versus Mobile-Bearing TKA Using Titanium-Nitride-Coated Posterior-Stabilized Prostheses

In a study with level 2 of evidence published in 2019, Park et al. prospectively compared the clinical and radiographic results between MB and FB TKAs utilizing ceramic titanium nitride (TiN)-coated prostheses. Seventy MB and 70 FB TKAs using TiN-coated prostheses (ACS®) were evaluated. There were no differences in demographic characteristics between the two groups. Clinically, the Knee Society knee and function scores, WOMAC, and ROM were compared. Considering the possibility of a kinematic change in the PE insert and a decrease in ROM following MB TKA, serial changes in the ROM were also compared. The thickness of the PE insert was compared according to the size of the femoral component. Radiographically, the alignment and positions of the components were compared. There were no differences between the two groups in clinical scores or ROM. The maximum

flexion increased from 133.5° to 137.6° across all time points in the MB group. The serial maximum flexion angles did not differ between the two groups over time (n.s.). The average thickness of the PE insert was greater in the MB group (12.0 vs. 11.2 mm, respectively), especially when a large femoral component was utilized (12.7 vs. 11 mm). The pre- and postoperative mechanical axes and positions of the components did not differ between the two groups. TiN-coated MB TKA showed no significant advantage over FB TKA. The selection of bearing design would be clinically insignificant when utilizing the TiN-coated TKA prosthesis [13].

13.11 Simultaneous High-Flexion Mobile-Bearing and Fixed-Bearing TKAs Performed in the Same Patients

In 2019 Kim et al. determined the long-run clinical, radiographic, and CT scanning results of high-flexion MB and fixed-bearing TKAs in the same younger individuals. In addition, the survivorship and complication percentages of both groups were assessed. Bilateral simultaneous sequential TKAs were carried out in 164 subjects (328 knees). There were 142 women and 22 men with a mean age of 63 years, who received a high-flexion MB prosthesis in one knee and a high-flexion FB prosthesis in the other. The mean follow-up was 16.9 years. At the latest follow-up, the mean Knee Society knee scores (94 vs. 95 points), WOMAC (20 vs. 20 points), ROM (125° vs. 127°), and UCLA activity scores (7.8 vs. 7.8 points) were below the level of clinical significance between the two groups. The survival rate of high-flexion MB TKA was 98.2% and that of high-flexion FB TKA was 97% at 16 years. No osteolysis was identified in either group. After a minimum duration of follow-up of 13 years, these authors found no significant difference between these two groups with regard to functional outcome, knee motion, prevalence of osteolysis, or survivorship. This study did not clearly direct the surgeon toward either arm of treatment [14].

13.12 Mobile-Bearing TKA with Unique Ball and Socket Post-Cam Mechanism Versus Established Fixed-Bearing Prosthesis

An MB posterior-stabilized (PS) TKA system with ball and socket post-cam mechanism had been developed with the aims of better prosthesis fit and enhanced stability. However, the data are limited to compare its clinical outcomes with an already established FB implant design. In a prospective randomized study with level 1 of evidence, Tawari et al. compared 260 individuals in the MB group and 133 individuals in the FB group with a minimum 2 years of follow-up. Intraoperative variables, postoperative functional outcomes, and incidence of adverse events were compared. The MB group showed better prosthesis fit as the incidence of overhang of femoral component at junction and trochlea was less than the FB group. The MB group also showed better gap balancing as the incidence of mediolateral gap difference more than 2 mm was less in flexion and extension (Table 13.1). Postoperative functional outcomes and incidence of adverse events showed no difference between the two groups at 2 years. New MB design offered similar functional outcomes and stability along with better intraoperative prosthesis fit and gap balancing compared to an established fixed-bearing design. Hence, this new MB design could be an alternative prosthesis of choice for PS TKA [15].

13.13 Ceramic Titanium-Nitride-Coated Mobile-Bearing Prosthesis Versus Fixed-Bearing Prosthesis

In a study with level 3 of evidence, Song et al. compared the prevalence of aseptic component loosening and subsequent revision, and the survival rate between ceramic titanium-nitride-coated MB and FB TKAs carried out in individuals with moderate to severe varus deformities. In total, 200 TKAs utilizing advanced coated system PS (posterior stabilized) prostheses in varus deformity of mechanical axis > 8° between 2012 and 2016 were retrospectively reviewed. One hundred MB (ceramic-m group) and 100 fixed-bearing (ceramic-f group) prostheses were included. The matches were made according to preoperative demographics, ROM, and severity of deformity. The results are shown in Table 13.2.

Table 13.1 Mobile-bearing (MB) posterior stabilized (PS) total knee arthroplasty (TKA) system with unique ball and socket post-cam mechanism versus established fixed-bearing (FB) prosthesis (minimum 2 years follow-up) [15]

			Mobile-bearing	Fixed-bearing
Over-hang of femoral component	At junction	Medial	1%	5%
Over-hang of femoral component	At junction	Lateral	2%	4%
Over-hang of femoral component	At trochlea	Medial	2%	30%
Over-hang of femoral component	At trochlea	Lateral	13%	21%
Incidence of medio-lateral gap difference > 2 mm		Flexion	2.3%	16%
Incidence of medio-lateral gap difference > 2 mm		Extension	3.1%	9.8%

Table 13.2 Ceramic titanium-nitride-coated posterior stabilized (PS) mobile-bearing (MB) TKA versus titanium-nitride-coated PS fixed-bearing (FB) TKA in individuals with moderate to severe varus deformity (mechanical axis >8°)

	Ceramic titanium-nitride-coated mobile-bearing prosthesis	Ceramic titanium-nitride-coated fixed-bearing prosthesis
Mean follow-up	4.8 years	5.1 years
Incidence of revision TKA due to aseptic component loosening[a]	7%	1%
Overall survival rate	91.3%	98.9%

[a]All cases of aseptic loosening happened at the tibial component. *PS* posterior stabilized, *TKA* total knee arthroplasty

Considering the higher revision incidence and lower survival percentage due to tibial component loosening, caution should be taken in tibial component fixation when utilizing advanced coated system MB prosthesis in moderate to severe varus deformity [16].

13.14 Axial Tibiofemoral Rotation and Functional Outcomes

In 2020 Amaro et al. tried to establish in vivo knee kinematics and clinical results of subjects who experienced FB and MB TKA at 1- and 2-year follow-up. This prospective double-blinded randomized controlled trial was carried out from November 2011 to December 2012. A total of 64 individuals were randomized to FB and MB TKA groups (32 patients in each group). All individuals were assessed with the following: three-dimensional in vivo knee kinematics analysis during gait, stepping up, and stepping down stair steps and getting up from and sitting on a chair and knee ROM and patient-reported outcome measures (Knee Outcome Survey Activities of Daily Living Scale [KOS-ADLS] and pain VAS) at 1- and 2-year follow-up. The mean axial tibiofemoral rotation in subjects who experienced MB TKA was significantly higher during gait (13.3 vs. 10.7), stepping up (12.8 vs. 10) stair steps, and getting up (16.1 vs. 12.1) from a chair compared with FB TKA subjects at 1-year follow-up. The KOS-ADLS function score was significantly higher in the MB compared with the FB TKA group (32 vs. 27.7) at 1-year follow-up. No significant difference in kinematics and clinical results between the FB and MB TKA groups was found at 2-year follow-up. Based on the outcomes of this study, MB TKA permitted a higher degree of rotation when walking, stepping up stair steps, and standing up from a chair and had higher functional results compared with FB TKA at 1-year follow-up. However, no difference in in vivo kinematics or in clinical results was encountered between FB and MB prostheses at 2-year follow-up [17].

13.15 Mobile-Bearing Versus Fixed-Bearing TKAs in Individuals <60 Years of Age with Osteoarthritis

In 2021 Kim et al. studied long-run (up to 27 years) outcomes of FB versus MB TKAs in subjects <60 years with OA. This study included 291 individuals (582 knees; mean age 58 years), who experienced an MB TKA in one knee and an FB TKA in the other. The mean duration of follow-up was 26.3 years. At the latest follow-up, the mean Knee Society knee scores (91 vs. 89 points), WOMAC (35 vs. 37 points), ROM (128° vs. 125°), and UCLA activity score (6 vs. 6 points) were below the level of clinical significance between the two groups. Revision of MB and FB TKA happened in 16 (5.5%) and 20 knees (6.9%), respectively. The percentage of survival at 27 years for MB and FB TKA was 94.5% and 93.1%, respectively, and no significant differences were observed between the groups. Osteolysis was observed in four knees (1.4%) in each group. There were no significant differences in functional results, percentage of loosening, osteolysis, or survivorship between the two groups [18].

13.16 Anatomic Versus Dome Patella

It has been hypothesized that the patella, working in conjunction with both medial and lateral femoral condyles, can impact kinematic parameters such as posterior femoral rollback and axial rotation. In 2021 Smith et al. determined the in vivo kinematics of subjects implanted with an FB or MB PS TKA, with a specific focus on assessing the influence that anatomic and medialized dome patellar components have on tibiofemoral kinematic patterns. Tibiofemoral kinematics was assessed for 40 individuals: 20 with an anatomic patella and 20 with a dome patella. Within these groups, 10 individuals experienced an FB PS TKA and 10 individuals experienced an MB PS TKA. All individuals were analyzed using fluoroscopy while performing a deep knee bending activity. Kinematics was collected during specific intervals to determine similarities and differences in regard to patella and bearing type. The greatest variation in kinematics was detected between the two anatomic patellar groups. Specifically, the MB-anatomic individuals experienced greater translation of the lateral condyle, the highest magnitude of axial rotation, and the highest ROM compared to the FB-anatomic individuals. Subjects with a dome patella displayed much variability among the average kinematics, with all parameters between FB and MB cohorts being similar. The findings in this study suggested that individuals with an anatomic patellar component could have more normal kinematic patterns with an MB PS TKA as opposed to an FB PS TKA, while individuals with a dome patella could achieve similar kinematics regardless of TKA type [19].

13.17 Postmortem Analysis of Polyethylene Damage and Periprosthetic Tissue in Rotating Platform and Fixed-Bearing Tibial Inserts

In 2022 Chen et al. stated that MB designs were intended to diminish wear, but mixed outcomes were published from retrieval analyses and that postmortem (PM) assessment provided the opportunity to assess polyethylene (PE) damage in successful implants. Chen et al. compared damage configurations, magnetic resonance imaging (MRI) presentation, and histology between MB and fixed tibial inserts retrieved at PM and compared these results to their prior findings from implants retrieved at revision. Eleven PM knees with rotating platform (RP) implants and 13 with FB implants were examined. All were MRI scanned, and tissue samples were collected from standardized regions for histology. PE inserts were subjectively scored to assess articular, backside, and PS post surfaces for damage modes and severity. The average duration of

implantation was 9.3 years. Surface burnishing was the most common PE damage mode. Average damage scores were higher for RP (53.4) compared to FB inserts (34.4) due to greater backside damage (13.4 for RP vs. 1.4 for FB). A minimal difference in damage was observed on the articular surfaces (37.4 RP vs. 30 FB). Mild innate macrophage reactions were seen in eight (72.7%) RP and five (45.5%) FB specimens. Polyethylene particles were identified in seven (63.6%) RP and three (27.7%) FB specimens [20].

13.18 Conclusions

No significant difference has been found between the mobile-bearing (MB) total knee arthroplasty (TKA) and fixed-beating (FB) TKA implants with respect to the clinical outcomes, radiographic outcomes, revision, and survivorship at a minimum 10-year follow-up. The percentage of survival at 27 years for MB and FB TKA is 94.5% and 93.1%, respectively. Osteolysis occurs in 1.4% in each type of implant. There are no significant differences in functional results, percentage of loosening, osteolysis, or survivorship between the two types of designs. This review of recent literature does not clearly direct the orthopedic surgeon toward either type of design.

References

1. Bailey O, Ferguson K, Crawfurd E, James P, May PA, Brown S, et al. No clinical difference between fixed- and mobile-bearing cruciate-retaining total knee arthroplasty: a prospective randomized study. Knee Surg Sports Traumatol Arthrosc. 2015;23:1653–9.
2. Hofstede SN, Nouta KA, Jacobs W, van Hooff ML, Wymenga AB, Pijls BG, et al. Mobile bearing vs fixed bearing prostheses for posterior cruciate retaining total knee arthroplasty for postoperative functional status in patients with osteoarthritis and rheumatoid arthritis. Cochrane Database Syst Rev. 2015;2:CD003130.
3. Killen CJ, Murphy MP, Hopkinson WJ, Harrington MA, Adams WH, Rees HW. Minimum twelve-year follow-up of fixed- vs mobile-bearing total knee arthroplasty: Double blinded randomized trial. J Clin Orthop Trauma. 2020;11:154–9.
4. Sappey-Marinier E, de Abreu FGA, O'Loughlin P, Gaillard R, Neyret P, Lustig S, et al. No difference in

patellar position between mobile-bearing and fixed-bearing total knee arthroplasty for medial osteoarthritis: a prospective randomized study. Knee Surg Sports Traumatol Arthrosc. 2020;28:1542–50.

5. Woolson ST, Northrop GD. Mobile- vs. fixed-bearing total knee arthroplasty: a clinical and radiologic study. J Arthroplast. 2004;19:135–40.

6. Shemshaki H, Dehghani M, Eshaghi MA, Esfahani MF. Fixed versus mobile weight-bearing prosthesis in total knee arthroplasty. Knee Surg Sports Traumatol Arthrosc. 2012;20:2519–27.

7. Baktır A, Karaaslan F, Yurdakul E, Karaoğlu S. Mobile- versus fixed-bearing total knee arthroplasty: a prospective randomized controlled trial featuring 6-10-year follow-up. Acta Orthop Traumatol Turc. 2016;50:1–9.

8. Hao D, Wang J. Fixed-bearing vs mobile-bearing prostheses for total knee arthroplasty after approximately 10 years of follow-up: a meta-analysis. J Orthop Surg Res. 2021;16(1):437.

9. Chen P, Huang L, Zhang D, Zhang X, Ma Y, Wang Q. Mobile bearing versus fixed bearing for total knee arthroplasty: meta-analysis of randomized controlled trials at minimum 10-year follow-up. J Knee Surg. 2022;35:135–44.

10. Schotanus MGM, Pilot P, Kaptein BL, Draijer WF, Tilman PBJ, Vos R, et al. No difference in terms of radiostereometric analysis between fixed- and mobile-bearing total knee arthroplasty: a randomized, single-blind, controlled trial. Knee Surg Sports Traumatol Arthrosc. 2017;25:2978–85.

11. Amaro JT, Arliani GG, Astur DC, Debieux P, Kaleka CC, Cohen M. No difference between fixed- and mobile-bearing total knee arthroplasty in activities of daily living and pain: a randomized clinical trial. Knee Surg Sports Traumatol Arthrosc. 2017;25:1692–6.

12. Kim YH, Park JW, Kim JS. Comparison of high-flexion fixed-bearing and high-flexion mobile-bearing total knee arthroplasties—a prospective randomized study. J Arthroplast. 2018;33:130–5.

13. Park CH, Kang SG, Bae DK, Song SJ. Mid-term clinical and radiological results do not differ between fixed- and mobile-bearing total knee arthroplasty using titanium-nitride-coated posterior-stabilized prostheses: a prospective randomized controlled trial. Knee Surg Sports Traumatol Arthrosc. 2019;27:1165–73.

14. Kim YH, Park JW, Kim JS. The long-term results of simultaneous high-flexion mobile-bearing and fixed-bearing total knee arthroplasties performed in the same patients. J Arthroplast. 2019;34:501–7.

15. Tiwari V, Meshram P, Park CK, Bansal V, Kim TK. New mobile-bearing TKA with unique ball and socket post-cam mechanism offers similar function and stability with better prosthesis fit and gap balancing compared to an established fixed-bearing prosthesis. Knee Surg Sports Traumatol Arthrosc. 2019;27:2145–54.

16. Song SJ, Lee HW, Bae DK, Park CH. High incidence of tibial component loosening after total knee arthroplasty using ceramic titanium-nitride-coated mobile bearing prosthesis in moderate to severe varus deformity: a matched-pair study between ceramic-coated mobile bearing and fixed bearing prostheses. J Arthroplast. 2020;35:1003–8.

17. Amaro JT, Novaretti JV, Astur DC, Cavalcante ELB, Rodrigues Junior AG, Debieux P, et al. Higher axial tibiofemoral rotation and functional outcomes with mobile-bearing compared with fixed-bearing total knee arthroplasty at 1- but not at 2-year follow-up—a randomized clinical trial. J Knee Surg. 2020;33:474–80.

18. Kim YH, Park JW, Jang YS. Long-term (up to 27 years) prospective, randomized study of mobile-bearing and fixed-bearing total knee arthroplasties in patients <60 years of age with osteoarthritis. J Arthroplast. 2021;36:1330–5.

19. Smith LA, LaCour MT, Dennis DA, Komistek RD. Anatomic vs dome patella: is there a difference between fixed- vs mobile-bearing posterior-stabilized total knee arthroplasties? J Arthroplast. 2021;36:3773–80.

20. Chen JB, Baral EC, Hopper RH Jr, McDonald JF 3rd, Koff MF, Potter HG, et al. A postmortem analysis of polyethylene damage and periprosthetic tissue in rotating platform and fixed bearing tibial inserts. J Arthroplast. 2022;37:1203–9.

E. Carlos Rodríguez-Merchán

14.1 Introduction

Fast-track surgery has reduced the hospital length of stay (LOS), morbidity, and convalescence in primary total knee arthroplasty (pTKA) [1]. In 2020 Rodriguez-Merchan claimed that some authors had published that outpatient TKA was a successful, safe, and cost-effective treatment for advanced osteoarthritis (OA). The success attained had been attributed to the coordination of the multidisciplinary team, standardized perioperative protocols, optimal hospital discharge planning, and careful selection of subjects [2]. Besides, limited data exist on fast-track protocols in relation to revision TKA (rTKA) [3]. The purpose of this chapter is to review recent developments on fast-track pTKA and rTKA.

14.2 Fast-Track Primary TKA

14.2.1 Outcomes

In 2020 Ascione et al. described an advanced pTKA fast-track program and determined discharge parameters during hospitalization, as well as subject satisfaction, results, and adverse events within the first 12 months after surgery [4]. This prospective study was based on subjects selected consecutively for elective pTKA, experiencing surgery between 2014 and 2017 in an established fast-track setting. Hospitalization-related parameters were collected: demographics, body mass index (BMI), surgical time, ischemia time, hemoglobin values, blood transfusions, hospital length of stay (LOS), weight-bearing and stair-climbing time, opioid administration, preoperative and discharge loss of extension and maximum active flexion of the knee, visual analog scale (VAS) score, 12-month follow-up satisfaction rate and range of motion (ROM), any adverse events, and hospital readmission and reoperation within the first 12 months. Differences were determined using t-tests. A total of 704 pTKAs implanted in 481 subjects were included in the study and 223 patients had a bilateral pTKA. Their mean age was 69.8 years. At the 12-month follow-up, 623 subjects (88.5%) reported being satisfied or very satisfied and 15 (2.1%) were dissatisfied with their pTKA, and the mean active flexion and loss of extension were 104.4° and 2.3°, respectively. A total of 15 adverse events happened (2%): five painful knees, three knee stiffness, three hematomas, two infections, one hospital readmission, and one deep venous thrombosis (DVT). No cases of pulmonary embolism and death related to surgery were encountered [4].

According to Rodriguez-Merchan, a higher risk of perioperative surgical and medical results had been reported in outpatient pTKA than inpa-

E. C. Rodríguez-Merchán (✉)
Department of Orthopedic Surgery, La Paz University Hospital, Madrid, Spain

tient pTKA, including component failure, surgical site infection, knee stiffness, and deep vein thrombosis (DVT). Besides, there remained a lack of universal criteria for subject selection. Outpatient pTKA had thus far been carried out in relatively young subjects with few comorbidities. It was not yet clear whether outpatient pTKA was worth considering, except in very exceptional cases (young subjects without associated comorbidities). In 2020 Rodriguez-Merchan concluded that outpatient pTKA should not be generally recommended [2].

Early functional result following pTKA has been reported before, but without focus on the presence of certain functional recovery patterns. Van Egmond et al. investigated patterns of functional recovery during the first 3 months after pTKA and determined characteristics for nonresponders in functional result [5]. All pTKAs in a fast-track setting with complete patient-reported outcome measures (PROMs) preoperatively, at 6 weeks, and 3 months postoperatively, were included. Included PROMs were Oxford Knee Score (OKS), Knee disability and Osteoarthritis Outcome Score Physical Function Short-Form (KOOS-PS), and EuroQol 5 dimensions (EQ-5D) including the self-rated health visual analog scale (VAS). Patients with improvement on OKS less than the minimal clinically important difference (MCID) were determined as nonresponders at that time point. Characteristics between groups of responders and nonresponders in functional recovery were tested for differences: Van Egmond et al. defined four groups a priori, based on the responder status at each time point. Six hundred and twenty-three subjects were included. At 6 weeks OKS, KOOS-PS, and EQ-5D self-rated health VAS scores were statistically significantly improved compared with preoperative scores. The mean improvement was clinically relevant at 6 weeks for KOOS-PS and at 3 months for OKS. Subject characteristics in nonresponders were higher BMI and worse scores on EQ-5D items: mobility, self-care, usual activities, and anxiety/depression. Both statistically significant and clinically relevant functional improvement was encountered in most subjects during the first 3 months after pTKA. Presumed modifiable subject characteristics in nonresponders on early functional result were BMI and anxiety/depression [5].

In 2021 Jenny et al. assessed the influence of fast-track procedures (FTPs) on LOS after pTKA in a prospective, national, multicentric analysis. The innovative point was that no patient selection was utilized [6]. The hypothesis was that FTPs reduce hospital stay after pTKA for nontraumatic conditions compared with the national database. An observational prospective study was conducted in ten centers throughout France. A total of 839 subjects included in FTPs were followed up for 3 months. The average LOS, direct return home percentage, unscheduled readmission percentage, and reintervention percentage were compared with those in the national database (93,329 pTKAs). The Knee Society and Oxford scores were collected. The mean LOS was 4.4 days, while the national base LOS was 6.4 days. A total of 560 subjects (66.7%) were able to return home, compared with 47,617 (49.6%) in the national database. Thirty-five subjects (4.2%) were readmitted within 90 days of the intervention, compared with 10,399 (10.8%) in the national database. Seventeen subjects (2%) were reoperated upon within 90 days after the pTKA, compared with 529 (0.5%) in the national database (Fig. 14.1). The FTPs used by unselected subjects permitted a significant reduction in the mean LOS and in the percentage of readmission and a significant increase of the percentage of direct home return after pTKA compared with the national database. Jenny et al. claimed that the significant increase in the reoperation rate warranted further investigation. However, FTP should become the standard of care after this intervention [6].

14.2.2 Clinical Outcomes for Patients Aged >80 Years

In 2022 Leung et al. affirmed that because of the ageing population in Hong Kong, there was an increasing prevalence of pTKAs implanted in subjects aged >80 years [7]. This retrospective case-control study enrolled all subjects who were aged >80 years and experienced fast-track pTKA

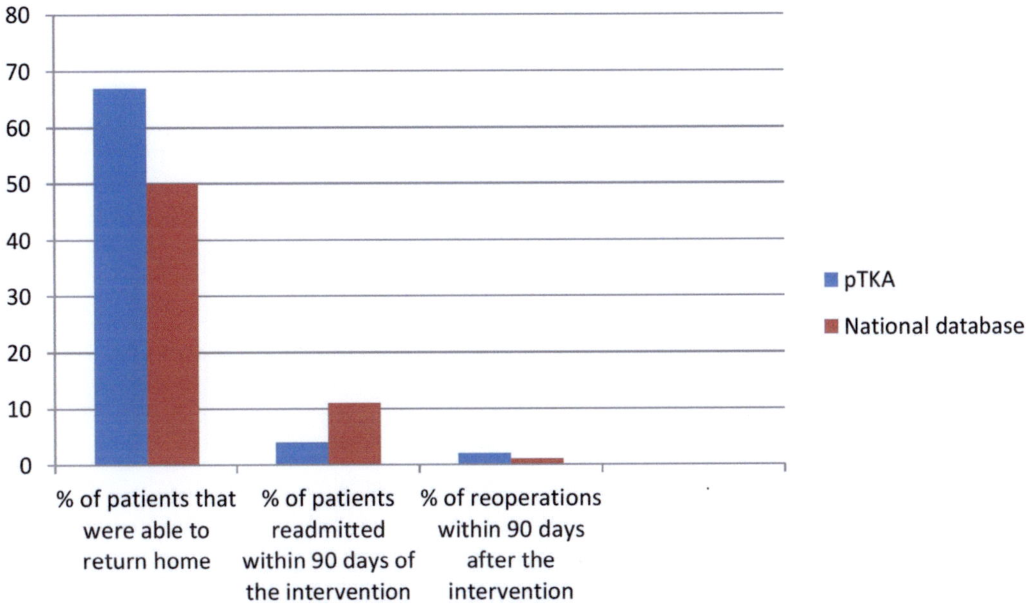

Fig. 14.1 Fast-track primary TKA (pTKA) compared to a national database

between 2011 and 2015. Their results were compared with the results of a matched control group of younger subjects who experienced fast-track TKA in the same period. In total, 220 subjects were included in this study with a follow-up period of at least 2 years (mean = 3.2 years; range, 2–5 years); 112 (51%) were octogenarians and 108 (49%) were non-octogenarians. Greater improvement in Knee Society Score (KSS) was encountered in the octogenarian group at 1 year after surgery (46 vs 39). The prevalence of adverse events was higher in the octogenarian group (15.2% vs 4.6%). There were no significant differences in the prevalence of major adverse events, the percentage of intensive care unit admission, or the 1-year mortality percentage between the two groups. After adjustment for confounding factors, Charlson Comorbidity Index >5, history of major cerebrovascular accident, and history of peptic ulcer disease were predictive of adverse events following fast-track pTKA; octogenarian status was not predictive of adverse events. Octogenarians had greater improvement in KSS at 1 year after fast-track pTKA, compared with non-octogenarians, but there were no significant differences in the incidences of mortality or major adverse events [7].

14.2.3 Bleeding Complications

In 2022 Moisander et al. claimed that fast-track total joint replacement (TJR) had become increasingly frequent and also that routine thromboprophylaxis for pulmonary embolism and deep venous thrombosis (DVT) prevention lasted from 2 to 5 weeks [8]. In a retrospective registry study they focused on clinically relevant bleeding adverse events 90 days after fast-track primary TJR. All fast-track primary total hip (pTHA) and pTKA carried out between 2015 and 2016 were extracted from the Finnish Arthroplasty Register and Finnish Hospital Discharge Register. The type of arthroplasty and indication for the surgical procedure were combined with diagnoses of clinically relevant bleeding adverse events within 90 days of surgery. The prevalence of these bleedings was the primary outcome measure. Of the total of 8511 subjects (mean age 67 years; 60% female), 45% experienced unilateral pTHA, 52% unilateral pTKA, and 3% bilateral pTKA. The prevalence of clinically relevant bleeding adverse events within 90 days was 1%. No difference was found in the bleeding prevalence between the groups. The 87 bleedings comprised 57 operative site bleedings, 17 gastrointestinal bleedings, 6 intracranial nontraumatic bleedings, 5 bleedings from the nose or another undetermined site, and 2 intraocular bleedings. One death due to intracranial bleeding was observed, and hence, clinically relevant bleeding-specific 90-day mortality was 0.01%. The prevalence of clinically relevant bleeding adverse events was low. However, they cause subject discomfort, increase the utilization of healthcare services, and can be life-threatening and even fatal [8].

14.2.4 Postoperative Morbidity and Discharge Destinations in Patients Older than 85 Years

In 2016 Pitter et al. stated that elderly subjects were at risk of increased LOS, postoperative adverse events, readmission, and discharge to destinations other than home after elective pTHA and pTKA. Also, recent studies had encountered that enhanced recovery protocols or fast-track surgery can be safe for elderly subjects experiencing these procedures and may result in reduced LOS. However, detailed studies on preoperative comorbidity and differentiation between medical and surgical postoperative morbidity in elderly subjects were scarce [9]. In 2016 Pitter et al. performed a descriptive, observational study in 522 subjects ≥85 years experiencing fast-track pTHA/pTKA. The median age was 87 years and median LOS of 3 days. In 27.3% procedures, LOS was >4 days, with 82.7% due to medical causes, most frequently related to anemia needing blood transfusion and mobilization issues. Utilization of walking aids was associated with LOS >4 days, whereas preoperative anemia demonstrated borderline significance. Thirty-eight subjects (6.9%) were not discharged directly home, of which 68.4% had LOS >4 days. Readmission percentages were 14.2% and 17.9% within 30 and 90 days, respectively, and 75.5% of readmissions within 90 days were medical, mainly due to falls and suspected but disproved venous thromboembolic events. Preoperative anemia was associated with increased risk of 90-day readmissions. Ninety-day mortality was 2%, with 1% happening during primary admis-

sion. Pitter et al. concluded that fast-track pTHA and pTKA with an LOS of median 3 days and discharge to home were feasible in most subjects ≥85 years. However, further attention to pre- and postoperative anemia and the pathogenesis of medical complications was needed to improve postoperative results and diminish readmissions [9].

14.3 Fast-Track Revision TKA

14.3.1 Outcomes

In 2011 Husted et al. assessed whether patients undergoing rTKA for nonseptic indications might also benefit from fast-track surgery [1]. Twenty-nine subjects were operated with 30 revision arthroplasties. Median age was 67 years. All patients followed a standardized fast-track setup designed for pTKA. Husted et al. determined the outcome regarding LOS, morbidity, mortality, and satisfaction. Median LOS was 2 days excluding one patient, who was transferred to another hospital for logistical reasons (10 days). None of the patients died within 3 months, and three patients were readmitted (two for suspicion of DVT, which was not found, and one for joint mobilization). Patient satisfaction was high. Patients undergoing rTKA for nonseptic reasons may be included in fast-track protocols. Outcome appeared to be similar to that of pTKA regarding LOS, morbidity, and satisfaction. These findings called for larger confirmatory studies and studies involving other indications (rTHA, one-stage septic revisions) [1].

In 2022 Lindberg-Larsen et al. reported LOS, risk of LOS > 5 days, and readmission ≤90 days after revision knee arthroplasty in centers with a well-established fast-track protocol in both primary and revision surgery [3]. It was an observational cohort study from the Centre for Fast-track Hip and Knee Replacement and the Danish Knee Arthroplasty Register. They included elective aseptic major component revision knee arthroplasties consecutively from six dedicated fast-track centers from 2010 to 2018. Moreover, 1439 revision knee arthroplasties were analyzed, including 900 total revisions, 171 large partial revisions (revision of either femoral or tibia component), and 368 revisions of unicompartmental knee arthroplasty (rUKA) to TKA. Mean age was 65 years and 66% were females. Mean LOS was 3.7 days in the study period but decreased to 2.4 days in 2018. Risk factors for LOS > 5 days was ≥1 previous revision, use of walking aid, BMI > 35, and ages <50, 70–79, and ≥ 80 years, whereas rUKA to TKA and large partial revision were negatively associated. The 90-day readmission and mortality risk was 9.1% and 0.5%, respectively. Cardiac disease and use of walking aid were associated with increased risk of readmission ≤90 days. Elective aseptic major component revision knee arthroplasty using similar fast-track protocols as in pTKA was safe with short and decreasing LOS [3].

14.3.2 Venous Thromboembolism

In 2021 Petersen et al. affirmed that venous thromboembolism (VTE) prophylaxis was much debated within THA/TKA. Also, revision hip and knee arthroplasties are more extensive procedures, but information on the risk of postoperative VTE was conflicting and there were no specific guidelines for thromboprophylaxis. Furthermore, data on revision THA/revision TKA within a fast-track protocol was sparse [10]. In 2021 Petersen et al. evaluated the incidence and time course of VTE in unselected elective revision THA/revision TKA within their established multicenter fast-track collaboration with in-hospital only thromboprophylaxis if length of stay (LOS) ≤ 5 days. They used an observational study design of unselected consecutive fast-track elective major component rTHA/rTKA from six dedicated fast-track centers between 2010 and 2018. They obtained information on revisions through Danish hip and knee arthroplasty registers and complete (>99%) 90 days of follow-up through the Danish National Patient Registry in combination with chart review. They included 2814 procedures with median LOS of 3 days and 21% had LOS >5 days. The 90-day incidence of VTE was 0.42% (*n* = 12), with 8 (0.28%) DVT

and 4 (0.14%) pulmonary embolism, after median 14 days with the latest on day 31. The 90-day incidence of VTE after elective fast-track rTHA and rTKA was about 0.4% which is comparable to the 90-day VTE incidence after fast-track pTHA, pTKA, and pUKA. Future investigations should focus on the identification of high-risk patients while the surgical trauma per se may be less important [10].

14.4 Conclusions

Fast-track pTKA utilized by unselected subjects seems to permit a significant reduction in the mean LOS and in the percentage of readmission and a significant increase of the percentage of direct home return after pTKA. Octogenarians had greater improvement in KSS at 1 year, compared with non-octogenarians, but there were no significant differences in the incidences of mortality or major adverse events. In patients older than 85 years, LOS was >4 days and 6.9% of subjects were not discharged directly to home. Readmission percentages were 14.2% and 17.9% within 30 and 90 days, respectively, and 75.5% of readmissions within 90 days were medical, mainly due to falls and suspected but disproved VTE. Preoperative anemia was associated with increased and living alone with diminished risk of 90-day readmissions. Ninety-day mortality was 2%, with 1% happening during primary admission. Elective aseptic fast-track rTKA using similar fast-track protocols as in pTKA has been reported to be safe, with short and decreasing LOS and a 90-day incidence of VTE of about 0.4%, which is comparable to the 90-day VTE incidence after fast-track pTKA.

References

1. Husted H, Otte KS, Kristensen BB, Kehlet H. Fast-track revision knee arthroplasty. A feasibility study. Acta Orthop. 2011;82:438–40.
2. Rodriguez-Merchan EC. Outpatient total knee arthroplasty: is it worth considering? EFORT Open Rev. 2020;5:172–9.

3. Lindberg-Larsen M, Petersen PB, Corap Y, Gromov K, Jørgensen CC, Kehlet H, Centre for Fast-track Hip and Knee Replacement Collaborating Group. Fast-track revision knee arthroplasty. Knee. 2022;34:24–33.

4. Ascione F, Braile A, Romano AM, di Giunta A, Masciangelo M, Senorsky EH, et al. Experience-optimised fast track improves outcomes and decreases complications in total knee arthroplasty. Knee. 2020;27:500–8.

5. Van Egmond JC, Hesseling B, Verburg H, Mathijssen NMC. Short-term functional outcome after fast-track primary total knee arthroplasty: analysis of 623 patients. Acta Orthop. 2021;92:602–7.

6. Jenny JY, Courtin C, Boisrenoult P, Chouteau J, Henky P, Schwartz C, Société Française de Chirurgie Orthopédique et Traumatologique (SOFCOT), et al. Fast-track procedures after primary total knee arthroplasty reduce hospital stay by unselected patients: a prospective national multi-centre study. Int Orthop. 2021;45:133–8.

7. Leung TP, Lee CH, Chang EWY, Lee QJ, Wong YC. Clinical outcomes of fast-track total knee arthroplasty for patients aged >80 years. Hong Kong Med J. 2022;28:7–15.

8. Moisander A, Pamilo K, Eskelinen A, Huopio J, Kautiainen H, Kuitunen A, et al. Low incidence of clinically relevant bleeding complications after fast-track arthroplasty: a register study of 8511 arthroplasties. Acta Orthop. 2022;93:348–54.

9. Pitter FT, Jørgensen CC, Lindberg-Larsen M, Kehlet H, Lundbeck Foundation Center for Fast-track Hip and Knee Replacement Collaborative Group. Postoperative morbidity and discharge destinations after fast-track hip and knee arthroplasty in patients older than 85 years. Anesth Analg. 2016;122:1807–15.

10. Petersen PB, Lindberg-Larsen M, Jørgensen CC, Kehlet H, Lundbeck Foundation Centre for Fast-track Hip and Knee Arthroplasty Collaborating Group. Venous thromboembolism after fast-track elective revision hip and knee arthroplasty - a multicentre cohort study of 2814 unselected consecutive procedures. Thromb Res. 2021;199:101–5.

Repeat Two-Stage Revision for Knee Periprosthetic Joint Infection

E. Carlos Rodríguez-Merchán

15.1 Introduction

A two-stage reimplantation procedure is a well-accepted procedure for the treatment of first-time infected total knee arthroplasty (TKA). However, there is a lack of consensus on the management of subsequent reinfections [1]. Two-stage exchange arthroplasty after a previous, failed two-stage exchange procedure is fraught with difficulties, and there are no clear recommendations for management or prognosis given the heterogeneous group of subjects in whom this procedure has been carried out. The Musculoskeletal Infection Society (MSIS) staging system was developed in an attempt to stratify subjects according to infection type, host status, and local soft-tissue status [2].

The gold-standard method in North America for the treatment of infected TKA is two-stage revision arthroplasty. This has provided generally a high success percentage. However, persistent infection after two-stage revision TKA does happen [3]. Joint infection following TKA has significant consequences on both the subject and healthcare system. Two-stage revision TKA is viewed as the gold standard in treatment. However, recurrence of infection following this procedure is a growing clinical problem for many

reasons. Despite several surgical alternatives for management of failure of two-stage revision TKA, the potential for adverse events and functional limitation remains high, and the optimal strategy is yet to be established [4].

Two-stage revision TKA is a commonly chosen approach to manage chronic periprosthetic joint infection (PJI). However, management of recurrent infection after a two-stage exchange remains debated and the result of a repeat two-stage procedure is not clear [5]. The result of repeat septic revision after a failed one-stage exchange for PJI in TKA remains unknown [6]. Two-stage revision TKA is the gold standard for the management and eradication of knee PJI, but the literature is limited on the results of repeat two-stage TKA after PJI recurrence [7]. The purpose of this chapter is to review recent development on repeat two-stage revision for knee (PJI).

15.2 Arthrodesis Should Be Considered

In 2014 Wu et al. carried out a decision analysis to establish the treatment method likely to yield the highest quality of life for a subject after a failed two-stage revision TKA [1]. They carried a systematic review to determine the expected success percentages of a two-stage reimplantation procedure, chronic suppression, arthrodesis, and amputation for the management of infected

E. C. Rodríguez-Merchán (✉)
Department of Orthopedic Surgery, La Paz University Hospital, Madrid, Spain

TKA. Overall, the composite success percentage for two-stage revision TKA was 79.1%. Knee arthrodesis was the treatment most likely to yield the highest expected utility (quality of life) after initially failing a two-stage revision. Based on best available evidence, knee arthrodesis should be strongly considered as the treatment of choice for subjects who have persistent infected TKA after a failed two-stage reimplantation procedure. Wu et al. recognized that particular circumstances such as severe bone loss can preclude or limit the applicability of arthrodesis as an alternative and that individual clinical circumstances must always dictate the best treatment, but where arthrodesis is practical, their model supported it as the best approach [1].

15.3 Risk Factors for Failure

In 2017 Fehring et al. reported the results of two-stage exchange arthroplasty following a previous, failed two-stage exchange protocol for knee PJI and identified risk factors for failure (therapeutic study with level 4 of evidence) [2]. They retrospectively identified 45 subjects who had experienced two or more two-stage exchange arthroplasties for knee PJI from 2000 to 2013. Subjects were stratified according to the Musculoskeletal Infection Society-MSIS (McPherson et al.) system, and risk factors for failure were analyzed (Figs. 15.1 and 15.2) [3]. The minimum follow-up was 2 years. At the time of follow-up, 22 (49%) of the subjects had experienced another revision due to infection and 28 (62%) had experienced another revision for any reason. The infection recurred in six (75%) of eight substantially immunocompromised hosts (MSIS type C) and in three (30%) of ten uncompromised hosts (type A) following the second two-stage exchange arthroplasty. The infection recurred in four (80%) of nine subjects with compromise of the extremity (MSIS type 3) and three (33%) of nine subjects with an uncompromised limb (type 1). Both extremely compromised hosts with an extremely compromised limb (type C3) had recurrence of the infection, whereas three (30%) of the ten uncompromised subjects with no or less compromise of the limb (type A1 or A2) did. Five subjects in the failure group experienced a third two-stage exchange arthroplasty following reinfection, and three of them were infection-free at the time of the latest follow-up. Uncompromised hosts (MSIS type A) with an acceptable wound (MSIS type 1 or 2) had a 70% rate of success (7 of 10) after a repeat two-stage exchange arthroplasty, whereas type-B2 hosts had a 50% success rate (10 of 20).

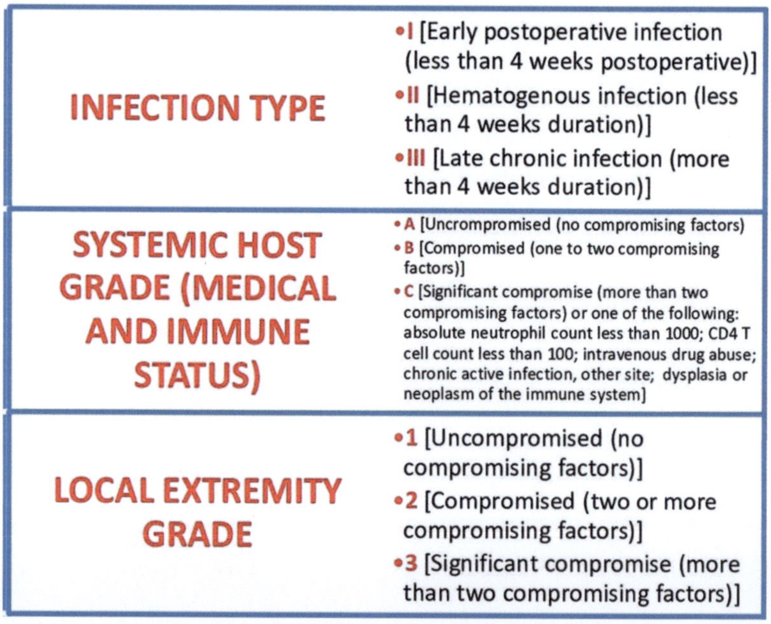

Fig. 15.1 Staging system for periprosthetic joint infection (PJI)

INFECTION TYPE	•I [Early postoperative infection (less than 4 weeks postoperative)] •II [Hematogenous infection (less than 4 weeks duration)] •III [Late chronic infection (more than 4 weeks duration)]
SYSTEMIC HOST GRADE (MEDICAL AND IMMUNE STATUS)	•A [Uncrompromised (no compromising factors) •B [Compromised (one to two compromising factors)] •C [Significant compromise (more than two compromising factors) or one of the following: absolute neutrophil count less than 1000; CD4 T cell count less than 100; intravenous drug abuse; chronic active infection, other site; dysplasia or neoplasm of the immune system]
LOCAL EXTREMITY GRADE	•1 [Uncompromised (no compromising factors)] •2 [Compromised (two or more compromising factors)] •3 [Significant compromise (more than two compromising factors)]

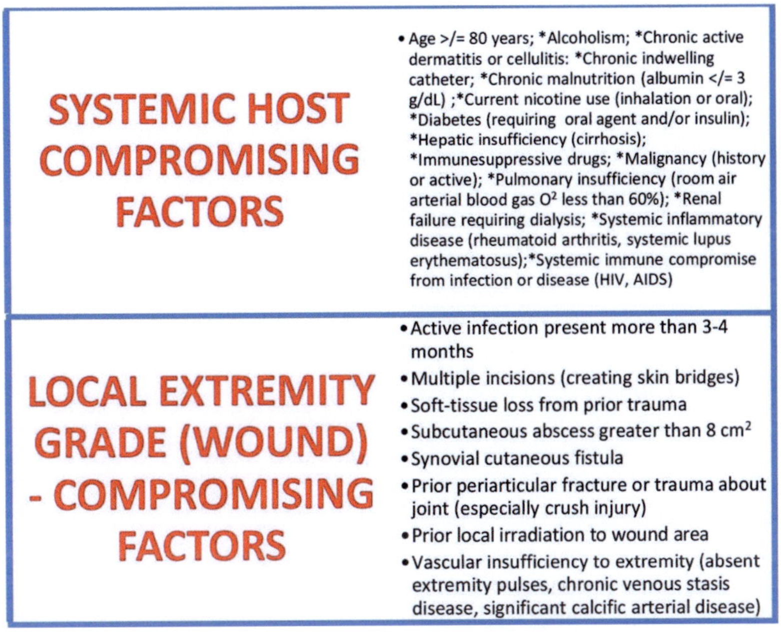

Fig. 15.2
Compromising factors
for periprosthetic joint
infection (PJI)

SYSTEMIC HOST COMPROMISING FACTORS	• Age >/= 80 years; *Alcoholism; *Chronic active dermatitis or cellulitis: *Chronic indwelling catheter; *Chronic malnutrition (albumin </= 3 g/dL) ;*Current nicotine use (inhalation or oral); *Diabetes (requiring oral agent and/or insulin); *Hepatic insufficiency (cirrhosis); *Immunesuppressive drugs; *Malignancy (history or active); *Pulmonary insufficiency (room air arterial blood gas O^2 less than 60%); *Renal failure requiring dialysis; *Systemic inflammatory disease (rheumatoid arthritis, systemic lupus erythematosus);*Systemic immune compromise from infection or disease (HIV, AIDS)
LOCAL EXTREMITY GRADE (WOUND) - COMPROMISING FACTORS	• Active infection present more than 3-4 months • Multiple incisions (creating skin bridges) • Soft-tissue loss from prior trauma • Subcutaneous abscess greater than 8 cm^2 • Synovial cutaneous fistula • Prior periarticular fracture or trauma about joint (especially crush injury) • Prior local irradiation to wound area • Vascular insufficiency to extremity (absent extremity pulses, chronic venous stasis disease, significant calcific arterial disease)

The repeat two-stage exchange technique failed in both type-C3 hosts; thus, alternative salvage techniques should be considered for such subjects [2].

15.4   Effectiveness

In a study published in 2019, Vadiee et al. tried to predict the success percentage of second, two-stage revision arthroplasty [4]. All infected TKAs treated between 2000 and 2015 that were operated by a single senior surgeon were reviewed retrospectively. Subjects were stratified according to general health and extremity status according to the MSIS scoring system. A statistical relationship between the higher stage of MSIS score, type of microorganism, flap surgery, and reinfection percentage after reimplantation of second two-stage surgery was found. There was not any statistically significant correlation between age, gender, constraint pattern of prosthesis, number of spacers, and time interval between the first and second stages of second two-stage surgery. Another two-stage knee revision was an effective method of treatment. However, Vadiee et al. found a higher prevalence of failure in those subjects with poor general health based on the MSIS score, inadequate soft tissue envelope and resistant bacteria.

The success of second, two-stage protocol was best in subjects with optimized general health, soft tissue coverage, and antibiotic-sensitive microorganism. According to Vadiee et al., subjects who cannot be optimized are most likely to need amputation or knee arthrodesis than another futile two-stage surgery [4].

15.5   Outcomes

In 2021 Maden et al. carried out a systematic review of the results of the surgical management of failure of two-stage revision arthroplasty published up to and including January 2020 [5]. Nine articles with a total of 273 subjects were encountered and analyzed. All surgical procedures had mixed results in terms of clinical and functional results, and the percentage of adverse events was high in all studies. Knee arthrodesis had a lower risk of failure than repeat two-stage revision. Poor subject immunological status and extremity status were weakly associated with increased risk of failure. Knee arthrodesis seemed to provide the best outcomes for improving quality of life and diminishing infection recurrence, although the complication percentage was high and the functional results seemed to be worse [5].

15.6 What Are the Chances for Success?

In 2022 Steinicke et al. investigated the success percentages of repeat two-stage exchange arthroplasty and analyzed possible risk factors for failure [6]. They retrospectively identified 55 subjects (23 hips, 32 knees) who were treated with repeat resection arthroplasty and planned delayed reimplantation for recurrent PJI between 2010 and 2019 after a prior two-stage revision. The minimum follow-up was 12 months with a median follow-up time of 34 months. Seventy-eight percent (43/55) experienced reimplantation after a repeat implant removal. Of those who completed the second-stage surgery, 37% (16/43) experienced additional revision for infection and 14% (6/55) experienced amputation. The reinfection-free implant survivorship amounted to 77% after 1 year and 38% after 5 years. Subjects with a higher comorbidity score were less likely to experience second-stage reimplantation (median 5 vs. 3). Furthermore, obese subjects and diabetics had a higher risk for further infection. Most frequently, cultures yielded polymicrobial growth at the repeat two-stage exchange (27%, 15/55) and at re-reinfection (32%, 9/28). Pathogen persistence was found in 21% (6/28) of re-reinfected patients [6].

15.7 Revision Rates

In 2022 Neufeld et al. reported the infection-free and all-cause revision-free survival of repeat septic revision after a failed one-stage exchange and determined whether the MSIS stage was associated with subsequent infection-related failure [7]. They retrospectively reviewed all repeat septic revision TKAs which were performed after a failed one-stage exchange between 2004 and 2017. A total of 33 repeat septic revisions (29 one-stage and four two-stage) met the inclusion criteria. The mean follow-up from repeat septic revision was 68.2 months. At the most recent follow-up, 17 repeat septic revisions (52%) had a subsequent infection-related failure and the five-year infection-free survival was 59%. A total of 19 experienced a subsequent all-cause revision (58%) and

the five-year all-cause revision-free survival was 47%. The most frequent indication for the first subsequent aseptic revision was loosening. The MSIS stage of the host status and extremity status were not significantly associated with subsequent infection-related failure. Repeat septic revision after a failed one-stage exchange TKA for PJI was associated with a high percentage of subsequent infection-related failure and all-cause revision. The host and extremity status according to the MSIS staging system were not associated with subsequent infection-related failure [7].

15.8 Failure Rates

In 2022 Christener et al. published the results of repeat two-stage revision TKA and investigated potential factors contributing to success or failure [8]. A retrospective study was performed investigating all two-stage revision TKA carried out at one institution between 2005 and 2020. Twenty cases experienced repeat two-stage revision TKA. Subject results and factors contributing to management success or failure were analyzed. PJI was diagnosed according to MSIS criteria. Of the 20 cases, 14 were classified as failed management (70%) due to a failure to eradicate infection, further surgical intervention, or death. In this series, there were no statistically significant differences between the groups regarding factors contributing to management success or failure. In the success group, subject-reported functional outcomes were variable. This study demonstrated that subjects experiencing a repeat two-stage TKA have very poor results. This study did not identify any factors that predicted failure. Subjects need to be counselled regarding poor results with repeat two-stage TKA, and other treatment alternatives such as early amputation or lifelong suppression should be considered [8].

15.9 Conclusions

All surgical procedures used for the surgical management of failure of two-stage revision arthroplasty have mixed results in terms of clinical and functional results, and the percentage of adverse events is high. Uncompromised hosts (Musculoskeletal Infection Society-MSIS type A) with an acceptable wound (MSIS type 1 or 2) have a 70% rate of success after a repeat two-stage exchange arthroplasty, whereas type-B2 hosts have a 50% success rate. The repeat two-stage exchange technique fails in both type-C3 hosts; thus, alternative salvage techniques should be considered for such subjects. Another two-stage knee revision is an effective method of treatment. However, there is a higher prevalence of failure in those subjects with poor general health based on the MSIS score, inadequate soft tissue envelope, and resistant bacteria. The success of second, two-stage protocol is best in subjects with optimized general health, soft tissue coverage, and antibiotic-sensitive microorganism. Seventy-eight percent of subjects experience reimplantation after a repeat implant removal. Of those who complete the second-stage surgery, 37% experience additional revision for infection and 14% experience amputation. The reinfection-free implant survivorship amounts to 77% after 1 year and 38% after 5 years. Subjects with a higher comorbidity score are less likely to experience second-stage reimplantation. Moreover, obese subjects and diabetics have a higher risk for further infection. Most frequently, cultures yield polymicrobial growth at the repeat two-stage exchange (27%) and at re-reinfection (32%). Pathogen persistence is found in 21% of re-reinfected subjects. Repeat septic revision after a failed one-stage exchange total knee arthroplasty (TKA) for periprosthetic joint infection (PJI) is associated with a high percentage of subsequent infection-related failure and all-cause revision. The host and extremity status according to the MSIS staging system are not associated with subsequent infection-related failure. Subjects experiencing a repeat two-stage TKA have very poor results. Knee arthrodesis has the lower risk of failure than repeat two-stage revi-

sion. Poor subject immunological status and extremity status are associated with increased risk of failure. Knee arthrodesis seems to provide the best outcomes for improving quality of life and diminishing infection recurrence, although the complication percentage is high and the functional results seem to be worse. Knee arthrodesis should be strongly considered as the treatment of choice for subjects who have persistent infected TKA after a failed two-stage reimplantation procedure.

References

1. Wu CH, Gray CF, Lee GC. Arthrodesis should be strongly considered after failed two-stage reimplantation TKA. Clin Orthop Relat Res. 2014;472:3295–304.
2. Fehring KA, Abdel MP, Ollivier M, Mabry TM, Hanssen AD. Repeat two-stage exchange arthroplasty for periprosthetic knee infection is dependent on host grade. J Bone Joint Surg Am. 2017;99:19–24.
3. McPherson EJ, Tontz W Jr, Patzakis M, Woodsome C, Holton P, Norris L, et al. Outcome of infected total knee utilizing a staging system for prosthetic joint infection. Am J Orthop (Belle Mead NJ). 1999;28:161–5.
4. Vadiee I, Backstein DJ. The effectiveness of repeat two-stage revision for the treatment of recalcitrant total knee arthroplasty infection. J Arthroplast. 2019;34:369–74.
5. Maden C, Jaibaji M, Konan S, Zagra L, Borella M, Harvey A, et al. The outcomes of surgical management of failed two-stage revision knee arthroplasty. Acta Biomed. 2021;92(3):e2021197.
6. Steinicke AC, Schwarze J, Gosheger G, Moellenbeck B, Ackmann T, Theil C. Repeat two-stage exchange arthroplasty for recurrent periprosthetic hip or knee infection: what are the chances for success? Arch Orthop Trauma Surg. 2022; https://doi.org/10.1007/s00402-021-04330-z. Online ahead of print.
7. Neufeld ME, Liechti EF, Soto F, Linke P, Busch SM, Gehrke T, et al. High revision rates following repeat septic revision after failed one-stage exchange for periprosthetic joint infection in total knee arthroplasty. Bone Joint J. 2022;104-B:386–93.
8. Christiner T, Yates P, Prosser G. Repeat two-stage revision for knee prosthetic joint infection results in very high failure rates. ANZ J Surg. 2022;92:487–92.

Revision Knee Arthroplasty for "Pain Without Loosening" Versus "Aseptic Loosening"

16

E. Carlos Rodríguez-Merchán

16.1 Introduction

The number of revision total knee arthroplasties (TKA) that is carried out is expected to increase. However, previous reports of the causes of failure after TKA are limited in that they report the causes at specific hospitals, which are frequently dependent on referral patterns. In 2016 Abdel et al. published the most frequent indications for reoperations and revisions in a large series of posterior-stabilized (PS) TKAs performed at a single hospital, excluding referrals from elsewhere, which may bias the causes of failure [1]. A total of 5098 TKAs which were carried out between 2000 and 2012 were included in the study. Reoperations, revisions with modular component exchange, and revisions with non-modular component replacement or removal were identified from the medical records. The mean follow-up was 5 years. The Kaplan-Meier 10-year survival without a reoperation, modular component revision, and nonmodular component revision was 95.7%, 99.3%, and 95.3%, respectively. The most frequent indications for a reoperation were postoperative stiffness (58%), delayed wound healing (21%), and patellar clunk (11%). The indications for isolated modular component revision were acute periprosthetic joint

infection (PJI) (64%) and instability (36%). The most frequent indications for nonmodular component revision were chronic PJI (52%), aseptic loosening (17%), periprosthetic fracture (10%), and instability (10%). Postoperative stiffness remains the most frequent indication for reoperation after TKA. Infection is the most frequent indication for modular and nonmodular component revision. Aseptic loosening was not an uncommon cause of failure; however, it was much less common than in national registry and non-registry data. Focusing on PS TKAs initially carried out permitted for an accurate evaluation of the causes of failure in a contemporary specialty practice [1]. Subjects having a knee arthroplasty revision for the indication "pain without loosening" may have a higher risk of re-revisions than subjects revised for other indications [2].

16.2 Revision for Unexplained Pain Following UKA and TKA

According to Baker et al., unicompartmental knee arthroplasty (UKA) has been associated with consistently worse implant survival percentages than TKA in worldwide arthroplasty registers. The percentage of revision and the proportion of revisions carried out for unexplained knee pain after either a UKA or TKA were analyzed to evaluate if there is evidence to support

E. C. Rodríguez-Merchán (✉)
Department of Orthopedic Surgery, La Paz University Hospital, Madrid, Spain

the hypothesis that the numbers of revisions carried out for unexplained knee pain differ between these two implant types [3]. Utilizing information from the National Joint Registry (NJR) of England and Wales, Baker et al. identified 402,714 primary knee arthroplasties (366,965 TKAs and 35,749 UKAs) that were consecutively entered from April 2003 to December 2010. The status of all implants was evaluated as of December 2010, at which time 6075 implants (4503 TKAs and 1572 UKAs) had been revised at a maximum of eight years. Survival analysis and Cox regression analysis with adjustment of differences in age, sex, American Society of Anesthesiologists (ASA) grade, and indication for arthroplasty were carried out with use of the end points of revision for any reason, revision for unexplained pain, and revision for other reasons. Revision for unexplained pain was more frequent after UKA than after TKA (representing 23% of revisions as compared with 9% of revisions). The 5-year rate of revision for unexplained pain was 1.6% for the UKA group and 0.2% for the TKA group. With the use of Cox regression, the hazard ratio (HR) for UKA relative to TKA with the end points of revision for any reason, revision for unexplained pain, and revision for all other reasons was 2.82, 6.76, and 2.39, respectively. The mean time from primary implantation to revision was similar for both implant types. While more UKAs than TKAs were revised for unexplained pain, when these revisions for unexplained pain were discounted, UKA still had a significantly greater risk of revision from other reasons than did TKA. The revision rate in isolation may not be a reliable way to compare different implant designs and should instead be considered in the context of the reason for failure [3].

16.3 Outcomes of UKA After Aseptic Revision to TKA

The general recommendation for a failed primary UKA is revision to a TKA. In 2016 Leta et al. compared the results, intraoperative infor-

mation, and mode of failure of primary UKAs and primary TKAs revised to TKAs [4]. The study was based on 768 failed primary TKAs revised to TKAs (TKA → TKA) and 578 failed primary UKAs revised to TKAs (UKA → TKA) reported to the Norwegian Arthroplasty Register between 1994 and 2011. Patient-reported outcome measures (PROMs) including the EuroQol (EQ)-5D, the Knee Injury and Osteoarthritis Outcome Score (KOOS), and visual analog scale (VAS) evaluating satisfaction and pain were utilized. Leta et al. carried out Kaplan-Meier and Cox regression analyses adjusting for propensity score to evaluate the survival percentage and the risk of re-revision and multiple linear regression analyses to estimate the differences between the two groups in mean PROM scores. Overall, 12% in the UKA → TKA group and 13% in the TKA → TKA group experienced re-revision between 1994 and 2011. The ten-year survival rate of UKA → TKA versus TKA → TKA was 82% versus 81%, respectively. There was no difference in the overall risk of re-revision for UKA → TKA versus TKA → TKA, or in the PROMs. However, the risk of re-revision was two times higher for TKA → TKA subjects who were greater than 70 years of age at the time of revision. A loose tibial component (28% versus 17%), pain alone (22% versus 12%), instability (19% versus 19%), and deep infection (16% versus 31%) were major causes of re-revision for UKA → TKA versus TKA → TKA, respectively, but the observed differences were not significant, with the exception of deep infection, which was significantly greater in the TKA → TKA group. The surgical procedure of TKA → TKA took a longer time (mean of 150 versus 114 min) and more of the procedures required stems (58% versus 19%) and stabilization (27% versus 9%) compared with UKA → TKA. Despite TKA → TKA appearing to be a technically more difficult surgical procedure, with a higher rate of re-revisions due to deep infection compared with UKA → TKA, the overall results of UKA → TKA and TKA → TKA were similar [4].

16.4 Complications and Failures of Nontumoral Hinged TKA in Primary and Aseptic Revision Surgery

Hinged TKA implants are a frequently used alternative during revision or even primary surgery, but their adverse events are not as well known, due to the quick adoption of gliding implants. The literature is inconsistent on this topic, with studies having a small sample size, varied follow-up duration, and very different indications. This led Caron et al. to carry out a large multicenter study in 2016 (retrospective cohort study with level 4 of evidence), with a minimum follow-up of 5 years, to assess the adverse events after hinged TKA in a nontumoral context based on the indications of primary arthroplasty, aseptic surgical revision, or fracture treatment around the knee [5]. **The hypothesis was that** hinged TKA was associated with a high complication percentage, no matter the indication. Two hundred and ninety patients (290 knees) were included retrospectively between January 2006 and December 2011 at 17 sites, with a minimum follow-up of 5 years. The subjects were separated into three groups: primary surgery (111 subjects), aseptic revision surgery (127 subjects), and surgery following a recent (<3 months) fracture (52 subjects: 13 around the TKA and 39 around the knee treated by hinged TKA). Subjects who had an active infection of the knee of interest were excluded. All the subjects were reviewed based on a standardized computer questionnaire validated by the French Society of Orthopedic Surgery and Traumatology (SOFCOT). The mean follow-up was 71 months. Of the 290 subjects included in the study, 108 subjects (37%) suffered at least one adverse event and 55 subjects (19%) had to experience revision surgery: 16 in the primary TKA group (16/111, 14% of primary TKA), 28 in the revision surgery group (28/127, 22% of revision TKA), and 11 in the fracture treatment group (11/52, 21% of fracture TKA). The adverse events due to the hinged TKA for the entire series from most to least common were stiffness (41/290, 14%), chronic postopera-

tive pain (37/290, 13%), infection (32/290, 11%), aseptic loosening (23/290, 8%), general adverse events (20/290, 7%), extensor mechanism complications (19/290, 6%), periprosthetic fracture (9/290, 3%), and mechanical failure (2/290, 0.7%). In the primary TKA group, the main complication leading to reoperation was infection (12/111, 11%), while it was loosening for the revision TKA group (15/127, 12%) and infection (8/52, 15%) for the fracture TKA group. The 37% complication rate for hinged TKA implants was high, with 19% of them needing reoperation. The rate of adverse events differed depending on the context in which the hinged implant was utilized (primary, revision, fracture). The adverse events needing revision surgery were major ones that prevented subjects from preserving their autonomy (infection, symptomatic loosening, fracture, implant failure). The most encountered adverse events – stiffness and chronic pain – rarely led to revision [5].

16.5 Subjects Who Experience Early Aseptic Revision TKA Within 90 Days of Surgery Have a High Risk of Re-Revision and Infection at 2 Years

Early aseptic revision within 90 days after primary TKA is a devastating adverse event. The causes, complications, and re-revision risks of aseptic revision TKA carried out during this period are poorly described. In a therapeutic study with level 3 of evidence published in 2022, Shen et al. tried to answer to the following questions [6]: What was the likelihood of re-revision within 2 years after early aseptic TKA revision within 90 days compared with that of a control group of subjects experiencing primary TKA? What were the indications for early aseptic TKA revision within 90 days? What were the differences in revision risk between different indications for early aseptic revision TKA? Subjects who experienced unilateral aseptic revision TKA within 90 days of the index procedure were identified in a national insurance claims database (PearlDiver Technologies) utilizing administrative codes. The exclusion criteria comprised revision for infection, history of bilateral TKA, and age younger than 18 years. The PearlDiver database was selected for its large and geographically diverse patient base and the availability of outpatient follow-up data that are unavailable in other databases focused on inpatient care. A total of 481 subjects met criteria for early aseptic revision TKA, with 14% (67) loss to follow-up at 2 years. This final cohort of 414 subjects was compared with a control group of subjects who experienced primary TKA without revision within 90 days. For the control group, 137,661 subjects experienced primary TKA without early revision, with 13% (18,138) loss to follow-up at 2 years. Among these subjects, 414 controls were matched utilizing a one-to-one propensity score method; no differences in age, gender, and Charlson comorbidity index score were found between the groups. Indications for initial revision and 2-year re-revision were recorded. The Kaplan-Meier method was utilized to evaluate survival between the early revision and control groups. Two-year survivorship free from additional revision surgery was lower in the early aseptic revision cohort compared with the control (78% versus 98%). Among early revisions, 10% (43 of 414) of the subjects experienced re-revision for periprosthetic infection with an antibiotic spacer within 2 years. The reasons for early aseptic revision TKA were instability/dislocation (37%), periprosthetic fracture (23%), aseptic loosening (23%), pain (11%), and arthrofibrosis (6%). Early revision for pain was associated with higher odds of re-revision than early revisions carried out for all other reasons (44% versus 29%). Acute early aseptic revision TKA carries a high risk of re-revision at 2 years and a high risk of subsequent PJI. Subjects who experience an early revision should be carefully counseled regarding the very high risk of repeat revision and discouraged from having early revision unless the indications are clear and compelling. Early aseptic revision for pain alone carries an unacceptably high risk of repeat revision and should not be carried out. Adjunctive measures for infection prophylaxis should be strongly considered. Specific interventions to diminish surgical adverse events in this subset of subjects have not been adequately studied; additional investigation of strategies to minimize the risk of reoperation or infection is warranted [6].

## 16.6	Prosthesis Survival After Revision Knee Arthroplasty for "Pain Without Loosening" Versus "Aseptic Loosening"

In 2022 Ardnt et al. compared the survival of knee arthroplasties revised for "pain without loosening" compared with "aseptic loosening." They also investigated the prosthesis survival rates in three surgical subgroups: TKA-TKA, partial revision (revision of tibial or femoral component), and UKA-TKA. They also compared the prosthesis survival rates for 1997–2009 and 2010–2018 [2]. In the period 1997–2018 from the Danish Knee Arthroplasty Register, 4299 revisions were identified. Of these, 1111 (26%) were carried out due to "pain without loosening" without any other indications, 674 (16%) due to "pain without loosening" combined with other indications, and 2514 (59%) due to "aseptic loosening" (Fig. 16.1). Survival analysis was carried out by a Cox multivariate analysis and Kaplan-Meier curves were presented. The cumulated proportions of re-revision after 2, 5, and 20 years were 12%, 18%, and 23% for "pain without loosening" versus 11%, 16%, and 19% for "aseptic loosening," respectively (Fig. 16.2). There were no statistically significant differences between the two indications in repeated analyses for each of the surgical subgroups. The hazard ratio for re-revision comparing "pain without loosening" with "aseptic loosening" was 1.03. The 8-year risk of re-revision for "pain without loosening" was 22% versus 22% for "aseptic loosening" in the period from 1997 to 2009 and 18% versus 14% in the period from 2010 to 2018.

Fig. 16.1 Causes of revision

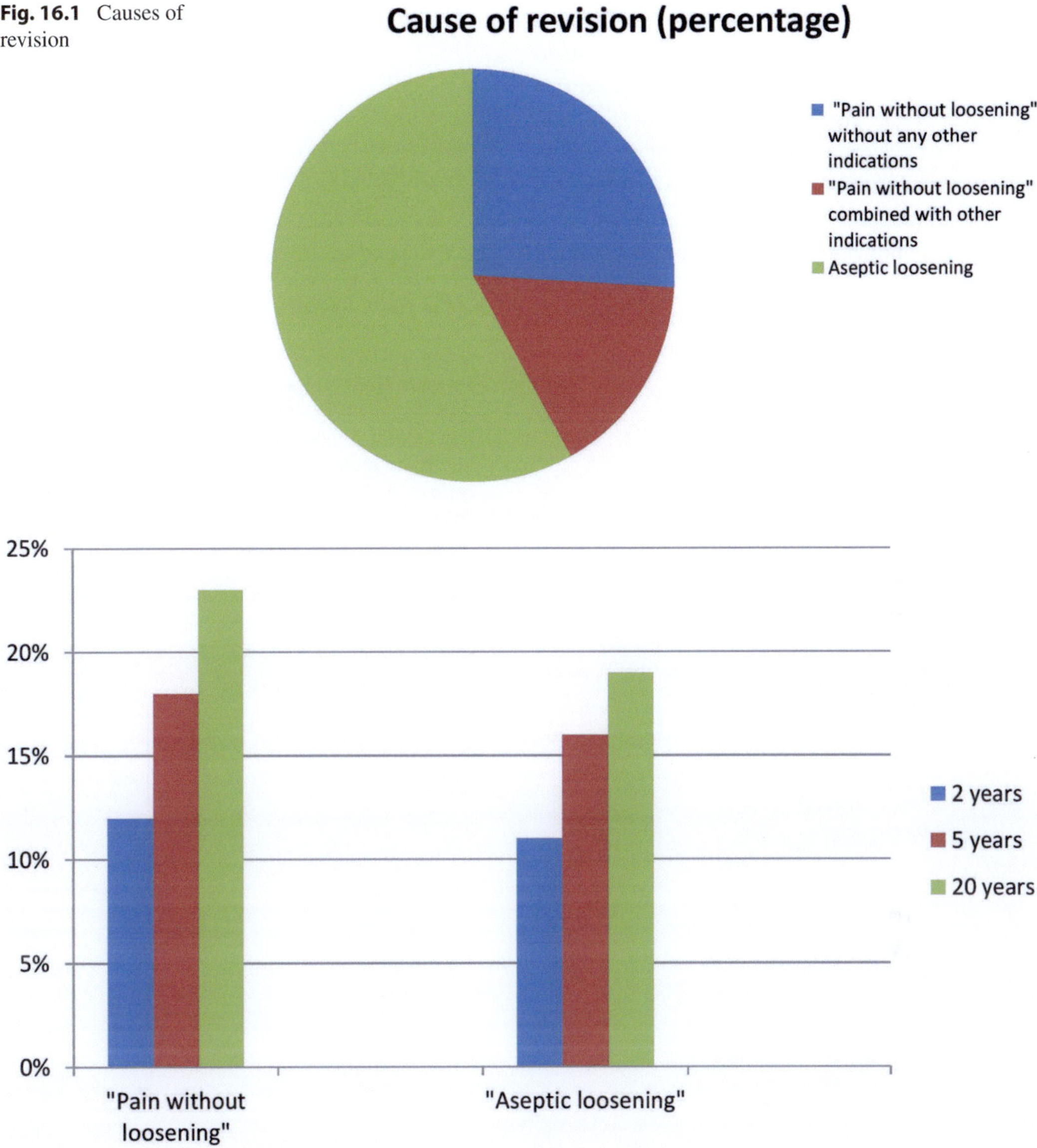

Fig. 16.2 Cumulated proportions of re-revision

The risk of re-revision was similar for subjects having a knee arthroplasty revision for the indication "pain without loosening" compared with "aseptic loosening." However, a slight improvement of prosthesis survival rates after revisions for both indications from 1997–2009 to 2010–2018 was observed. Arndt et al. could not advise for or against revision in cases with "pain without loosening" based on this information alone [2].

16.7   Conclusions

It has been reported that revision for unexplained pain is more frequent after UKA than after TKA (representing 23% of revisions as compared with 9% of revisions). The 5-year rate of revision for unexplained pain was 1.6% for the UKA group and 0.2% for the TKA group. Regarding revision knee arthroplasty for "pain without loosening" versus "aseptic loosening," contradictory results have been published. Some authors have claimed that early aseptic revision for pain alone carries an unacceptably high risk of repeat revision and should not be carried out. However, other authors have reported that the risk of re-revision was similar for subjects having a knee arthroplasty revision for the indication "pain without loosening" compared with "aseptic loosening." Thus, recent literature cannot advise for or against revision in cases with "pain without loosening."

References

1. Abdel MP, Ledford CK, Kobic A, Taunton MJ, Hanssen AD. Contemporary failure aetiologies of the primary, posterior-stabilised total knee arthroplasty. Bone Joint J. 2017;99-B:647–52.
2. Arndt KB, Schrøder HM, Troelsen A, Lindberg-Larsen M. Prosthesis survival after revision knee arthroplasty for "pain without loosening" versus "aseptic loosening": a Danish nationwide study. Acta Orthop. 2022;93:103–10.
3. Baker PN, Petheram T, Avery PJ, Gregg PJ, Deehan DJ. Revision for unexplained pain following unicompartmental and total knee replacement. J Bone Joint Surg Am. 2012;94(17):e126.
4. Leta TH, Lygre SH, Skredderstuen A, Hallan G, Gjertsen JE, Rokne B, et al. Outcomes of unicompartmental knee arthroplasty after aseptic revision to total knee arthroplasty: a comparative study of 768 TKAs and 578 UKAs revised to TKAs from the Norwegian Arthroplasty Register (1994 to 2011). J Bone Joint Surg Am. 2016;98:431–40.
5. Caron É, Gabrion A, Ehlinger M, Verdier N, Rubens-Duval B, Neri T, French society of orthopedic surgery and traumatology (SOFCOT), et al. Complications and failures of non-tumoral hinged total knee arthroplasty in primary and aseptic revision surgery: a review of 290 cases. Orthop Traumatol Surg Res. 2021;107(3):102875.
6. Shen TS, Gu A, Bovonratwet P, Ondeck NT, Sculco PK, Su EP. Patients who undergo early aseptic revision TKA within 90 days of surgery have a high risk of re-revision and infection at 2 years: a large-database study. Clin Orthop Relat Res. 2022;480:495–503.

Robotic-Assisted Primary Unicompartmental Knee Arthroplasty and Total Knee Arthroplasty

17

E. Carlos Rodríguez-Merchán, Carlos A. Encinas-Ullán, Juan S. Ruiz-Pérez, and Primitivo Gómez-Cardero

17.1 Introduction

It has been reported that femorotibial alignment is crucial for the result of unicompartmental knee arthroplasty (UKA) and that robotic-assisted systems are useful to increase the accuracy of alignment in UKA [1]. In 2022 Yeroushalmi et al. stated that UKA, as an alternative to total knee arthroplasty (TKA), had been demonstrated to be an efficacious option for subjects with single-compartment end-stage knee osteoarthritis (OA) [2].

In 2022 St Mart et al. expressed that robotic-assisted UKA (RA-UKA) was associated with improved component positioning and comparable short- and mid-run implant survivorship with conventional (jig-based manual) UKA (C-UKA) [3]. Dobelle et al. have claimed that UKA is a procedure with low morbidity and fast recovery [4].

According to Haffar et al., poor ergonomics and acute stress can affect surgical accomplish-ment and produce work-related injuries. Robotic assistance might optimize these psychophysiological factors during UKA [5]. In 2022 Goh et al. affirmed that the cost-effectiveness of RA-UKA remained unclear [6]. Heckmann et al. claimed that lateral UKA (L-UKA) is a popular option to TKA for subjects with isolated lateral compartment OA [7].

According to Vaidya et al., precise positioning and alignment of the prosthesis is a very relevant factor for endurance of prosthesis and implant survival which is improved with the utilization of technology in TKA. However, the long-run functional results and survivorship are indeterminate [8]. Robotic-assisted total knee arthroplasty (RA-TKA) was introduced to improve surgical accuracy and patient outcomes (Fig. 17.1). However, RA-TKA may also increase operating time and add cost to TKA [9]. The purpose of this chapter is to review recent development on robotic-assisted primary UKA and TKA.

E. C. Rodríguez-Merchán (✉) · C. A. Encinas-Ullán
J. S. Ruiz-Pérez · P. Gómez-Cardero
Department of Orthopedic Surgery, La Paz University Hospital, Madrid, Spain

E. C. Rodríguez-Merchán (ed.), *Advances in Orthopedic Surgery of the Knee*,
https://doi.org/10.1007/978-3-031-33061-2_17

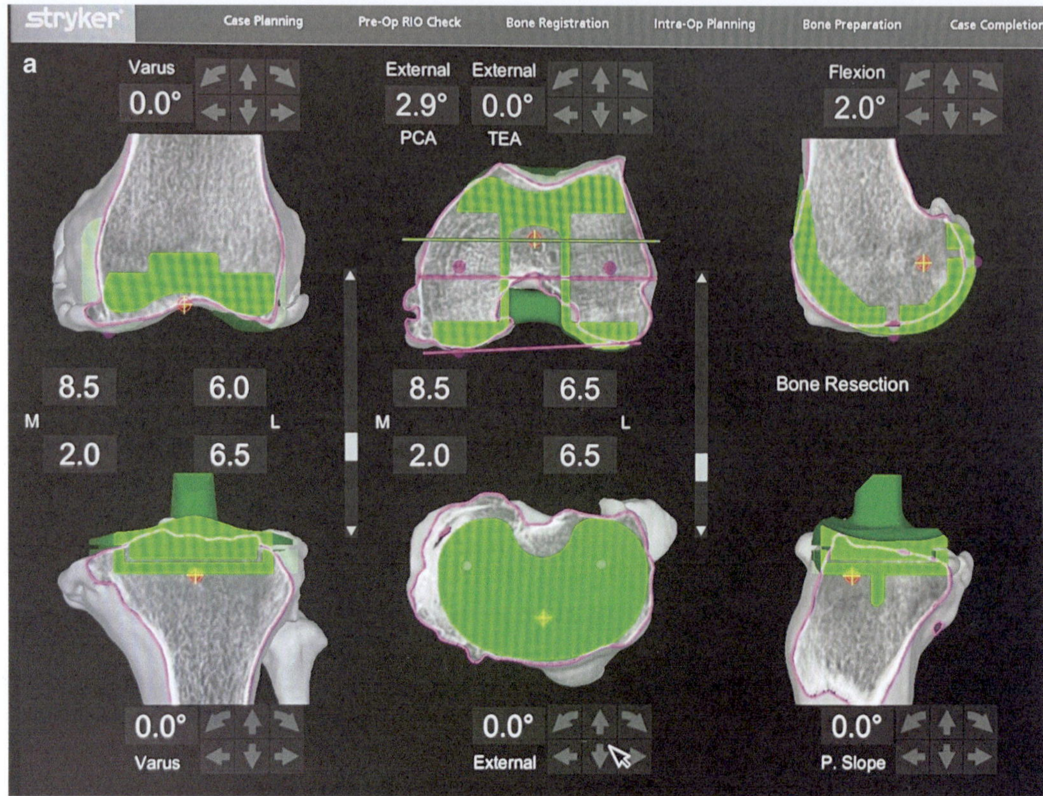

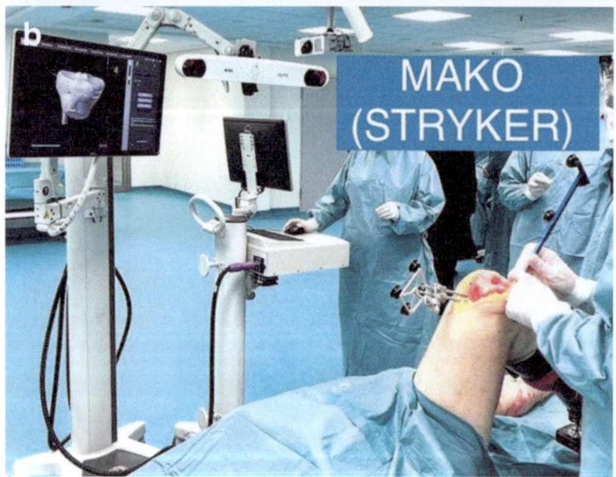

Fig. 17.1 (**a**, **b**) MAKO-assisted total knee arthroplasty (TKA) (MAKO Surgical Corporation [Stryker], Fort Lauderdale, FL, USA): (**a**) preoperative planning. (**b**) Verification of tibial plateau recordings

17.2 Robotic-Assisted UKA

17.2.1 Clinical Results

St Mart et al. assessed clinical and radiological results following RA-UKA as well as any potential learning curves associated with the introduction of such new technology. It was a prospective study of subjects experiencing RA-UKA [3]. Outcome measures were PROMs including Western Ontario and McMaster Universities Osteoarthritis Index (WOMAC), Knee Society Score (KSS) and Oxford Knee Score (OKS), adverse events, implant survivorship, component positioning, and learning curve. Eighty-five subjects comprising 100 knees were recruited and followed up for 21 months. At 2 years, there were significant and sustained improvements in patient-reported outcomes (PROMs) and 100% implant survivorship percentage. A high grade of implant accuracy was accomplished with the robotic system. A cumulative learning curve of 20 cases was noted. The conclusion was that RA-UKA achieved excellent implant accuracy and clinical results in the short run. Long-run follow-up was required to assess this relationship [3].

17.2.2 Dependability of Intraoperative Measurements of the Frontal Femorotibial Axis Robotic-Assisted Medial UKA

Deroche et al. tried to determine whether measurement of the mechanical femorotibial axis (mFTA) in the coronal plane with handheld robotic assistance during surgery was equivalent to a static measurement on radiographs and to a dynamic measurement during walking [1]. Twenty subjects scheduled for robotic-assisted medial UKA (RA-M-UKA) using handheld technology were included in this prospective study. Three measurements of the frontal femorotibial axis were compared: intraoperative acquisition by computer assistance (dynamic, non-weightbearing position), radiographic measurements on long leg X-ray (static, weightbearing position), and gait analysis during walking (dynamic, weightbearing position). There was no significant difference in the mFTA between computer (174.4°), radiological (173.9°), and gait analysis (172.9°) measurements. There was a strong positive correlation between robotic-assisted measurements and gait analysis. There was no significant difference in the femorotibial axis measured by the image-free robotic assistance, from the preoperative radiographs or by gait analysis. The dependability of intraoperative measurements of the frontal femorotibial axis by these robotic-assisted systems was acceptable [1].

17.2.3 Facility Costs Between RA-UKA and C-UKA

Goh et al. performed a study to compare true facility costs between RA-UKA and C-UKA [6]. They analyzed 265 consecutive UKAs (133 RA-UKAs, 132 C-UKAs) carried out at a specialty hospital in 2016–2020. Separate analyses including and excluding implant costs were carried out. Multiple regression was performed to establish the independent effect of robotic assistance on facility costs. Due to longer operative time, RA-UKA subjects had higher personnel costs and total facility costs ($2270 vs $1854). Controlling for demographics and comorbidities, robotic assistance was associated with an increase in personnel costs of $399.25, reduction in supply costs of $55.03, and increase in total facility costs of $344.27 per case. However, after factoring in implant costs, robotic assistance was associated with a reduction in total facility costs of $235.87 per case. However, further research is required to establish if RA-UKA can improve clinical results and create value in arthroplasty [6].

17.2.4 Accordance Between Femoral Component Position and Contact Stresses on the Polyethylene Insert Could Be a Contributing Factor of Long-Run Survival of UKA

In 2022 Dobelle et al. stated that UKA was a procedure with low morbidity and fast recovery [4]. Anatomic implants or robotic-assisted UKA had been proposed to improve results with precise positioning. Femoral component position (FCP) relative to the tibial insert could be a factor influencing the contact stresses. Dobelle et al. assessed the impact of the FCP relative to the tibial insert on clinical results and stress distribution after M-UKA. Sixty-two fixed-bearing M-UKAs were assessed at a minimum two-year follow-up using the Knee

Society Score. Postoperative radiological assessment carried out on frontal X-rays classified the FCP relative to the tibial insert into the following: group M (medial), group C (central), and group L (lateral). A finite element model was developed to assess the biomechanical impacts of the FCP relative to the tibial component. The postoperative radiological assessment demonstrated 9 cases in group M, 46 cases in group C, and 7 cases in group L. The maximum knee flexion angle and the 2-year postoperative "symptom" and "patient satisfaction" scores of the Knee Society Score were significantly higher in group C. Compared with central positioning, a shift along the mediolateral axis led to a displacement of the contact pressure center. The conclusion was that the FCP relative to the tibial insert might increase subject outcomes at a minimum follow-up of 2 years after fixed-bearing M-UKA. Accordance between FCP and contact stresses on the polyethylene insert could be a contributing factor of long-run survival of UKA [4].

17.2.5 Mid-Run Survivorship and PROMs of Robotic-Assisted Lateral UKA

Heckmann et al. assessed mid-run survivorship and PROMs of robotic-assisted lateral UKA (RA-L-UKA) [7]. A retrospective case series was performed on all RA-L-UKAs carried out by a single surgeon between 2013 and 2019. Subject demographics, surgical variables, and Kozinn and Scott criteria were collected. Implant survivorship was calculated utilizing the Kaplan-Meier method with all-cause reoperation and conversion to TKA as endpoints. Participating subjects were evaluated for patient satisfaction and the Forgotten Joint Score-12 (FJS). Correlations between subject demographics and subject outcome scores were studied. In total, 120 L-UKAs were recognized, 84 of which met inclusion criteria, with a mean follow-up of 4 years. Five-year survivorship was 92.9% with all-cause reoperation as the endpoint and 100% with conversion to TKA as the endpoint. One

participant was converted to TKA after the 5-year mark, resulting in a 6-year survival for conversion to TKA of 88.9%. Average Forgotten Joint Score-12 score was 82.7/100, and patient satisfaction 4.7/5. Mean coronal plane correction was 2.5° toward the mechanical axis. Neither final postoperative alignment nor failure to meet classic Kozinn and Scott criteria for UKA resulted in differences in PROMs. This study showed high mid-run survivorship and excellent PROMs with RA-L-UKA. RA-L-UKA was a viable treatment alternative for isolated lateral compartment OA even in subjects who did not meet classic indications [7].

17.2.6 Comparative Studies

Yeroushalmi et al. investigated the mid-run cost-effectiveness of RA-UKA compared with C-UKA in the United States [2]. A cost-effectiveness analysis utilizing a four-state Markov model was carried out utilizing information from the 2018 National Joint Registry of England and Wales and a retrospective multicenter, cohort study on a cohort of 65-year-old subjects having experienced RA-UKA. The main outcome was cost per revision avoided and sensitivity analyses were conducted to assess the influence of utilizing different model assumptions on the outcomes. The Markov model illustrated that the benefit derived from RA-UKA versus C-UKA was beneficial from a payer's perspective. The estimated incremental cost-effectiveness ratio was $14,737 per revision avoided in a facility seeing 100 subjects a year. Case volume was demonstrated to be the primary variable impacting cost-effectiveness, with the value of RA-UKA directly increasing with higher case volumes. Cost-effectiveness analyses showed that the utilization of RA-UKA was an effective option to C-UKA in subjects with single-compartment knee OA. While this report could benefit from longer follow-up clinical studies to demonstrate the benefits of RA-UKAs beyond the current 2 years' time horizon, RA-UKAs remained cost-effective, even after investigating several different assumptions [2].

In a study with level 2 of evidence, Haffar et al. compared surgeon physiologic stress and ergonomics during RA-UKA and conventional UKA (C-UKA) [5]. Cardiorespiratory and postural information from a single surgeon was recorded during 30 UKAs, (15 RA-UKAs, 15 C-UKAs). Heart rate (HR), HR variability, respiratory rate (RR), minute ventilation, and calorie expenditure were utilized to measure surgical strain. Intraoperative ergonomics were evaluated by measuring flexion/extension/rotation of the neck and lumbar spine and shoulder abduction/adduction. Mean operative time was 32 minutes for C-UKA and 45.9 minutes for RA-UKA. Mean neck flexion was -23.4° for RA-UKA and -49.1° for C-UKA, while mean lumbar flexion was -20.3° for RA-UKA and -0.4° for C-UKA. Mean lumbar flexion was similar; however, a significantly greater percentage of time was spent in lumbar flexion >20° during C-UKA. Bilateral shoulder abduction was substantially higher for RA-UKA. Mean calorie expenditure was 154 calories for RA-UKA and 89.1 calories for C-UKA. Mean HR was also higher for RA-UKA (88.7 vs. 84.7). HR variability was slightly lower for RA-UKA (12.4) than for C-UKA (13.4), although this did not reach statistical significance. No difference in RR or minute ventilation was found. RA-UKA resulted in less neck flexion but increased shoulder abduction, heart rate, and energy expenditure. The theoretical ergonomic and physiologic advantages of robotic assistance utilizing a handheld sculpting device were not observed in this study [5].

17.3 Robotic-Assisted TKA

17.3.1 Clinical Results and PROMs

In 2022 Jo et al. reported patient and clinical outcomes following RA-TKA at multiple institutions with a minimum two-year follow-up [10]. This was a multicenter registry study from October 2016 to June 2021 that included 861 primary RA-TKA subjects who completed at least one pre- and postoperative PROM questionnaire, including FJS, Knee Injury and Osteoarthritis Outcomes Score (KOOS) for Joint Replacement (KOOS JR), and pain out of 100 points. The mean age was 67 years (35 to 86), 452 were men (53%), mean body mass index (BMI) was 31.5 kg/m² (19 to 58), and 553 (64%) were cemented and 308 (36%) cementless implants. There were significant improvements in PROMs over time between preoperative, 1- to 2-year, and >2-year follow-up, with a mean FJS of 17.5, 70.2, and 76.7; mean KOOS JR of 51.6, 85.1, and 87.9; and mean pain scores of 65.7, 13, and 11.3, respectively. There were eight superficial infections (0.9%) and four revisions (0.5%). RA-TKA showed consistent clinical outcomes across multiple institutions with excellent PROMs that continued to improve over time. With the ability to accomplish target alignment in the coronal, axial, and sagittal planes and provide intraoperative real-time data to obtain balanced gaps, RA-TKA showed excellent clinical results and PROMs [10].

17.3.2 Comparative Studies

In a study with level 1 of evidence reported in 2022 by Vaidya et al., it was hypothesized that mechanical axis alignment of lower extremity, postoperative joint line restoration, and femoral and tibial component alignment is more precise with the new handheld semi-active RA-TKA [8]. From April 2019 to March 2020, 60 subjects with unilateral knee OA who experienced TKAs were included in a prospective randomized controlled study. Computer-generated randomization was utilized. The study included 48 women and 12 men. Preoperative and postoperative radiographic measurements were performed and compared between the two groups. There was a significant difference between the two groups with respect to mechanical axis deviation, joint line deviation, and coronal alignment of femoral and tibial prosthesis. Mechanical axis deviation >3° was seen in eight cases (28.5%) in the -TKA group compared to one case (3.1%) in RA-TKA. Joint line deviation of 3.5 mm was noted in the C-TKA group as compared to 0.9 mm in the RA-TKA group which was statistically significant. However, whether this difference of 2.6 mm of joint line elevation between C-TKA and RA-TKA led to any difference in clinical result in terms of knee kinematics and knee flexion requires to be analyzed with further studies. Clinically reestablishing a normal joint line is important for improved knee function following primary TKA. No significant difference was found in femoral component rotation on postoperative computed tomography (CT) scan. The imageless, handheld semiautonomous robotic system for TKA was highly precise with respect to component positioning in coronal plane and mechanical alignment as compared to C-TKA. Joint line was elevated in C-TKA but was precisely restored utilizing the RA-TKA which might result in better patellofemoral kinematics [8].

RA-TKA has shown improved alignment and outcome scores when compared with C-TKA; however, few studies have compared differences in the same patient. In 2022 Ali et al. evaluated clinical results of 36 subjects who experienced a primary RA-TKA and had experienced a prior contralateral C-TKA [11]. All surgeries were carried out by a single surgeon at the same hospital. Subjects were evaluated for differences in hospital length of stay (LOS), improvement in pre- versus postoperative range of motion (ROM), KOOS, and WOMAC scores. Student's *t*-test and Fisher's exact test were utilized to detect significant differences. Patient demographics showed a mean age of 64.5, 24 females (67%), and mean body mass index (BMI) of 35.1. The average follow-up time was 2.9 years for C-TKA and 1.3 years for RA-TKA. Hospital LOS was decreased by 5.5 h for RA-TKA. Total postoperative WOMAC score was not statistically different between RA-TKA and C-TKA; however, pain and stiffness components were statistically improved in RA-TKA, respectively. KOOS was higher in RA-TKA, which approached statistical significance. Knee flexion improved significantly in both groups. There was a significant difference in pre- versus postoperative ROM at 3, 6, and 12 months follow-up after RA-TKA in comparison to C-TKA. There were no postoperative adverse events. Subjects who experienced RA-TKA showed early improvement at 1-year follow-up in pain, stiffness, and knee flexion when compared with their prior contralateral C-TKA. There was a significant reduction in postoperative hospital length of stay (LOS) by 5.5 h in the RA-TKA group. Limitations included a small sample size and differences in follow-up times between RA-TKA and C-TKA [11].

RA-TKA might improve the accuracy of bone preparation and component alignment when compared to the conventional surgical approach; however, the detailed cost analysis of RA-TKA is lacking. Steffens et al. compared in-hospital costs between RA-TKA and computer-navigated TKA (CN-TKA) [12]. Subjects experiencing primary TKA between October 2018 and June 2019 were included. Subject demographics, surgical results, and in-hospital cost variables including staff, critical care, emergency department, diagnostic, prosthesis, operating room, ward, and other related costs until the discharge to the community were collected. Differences across in-hospital costs between RA-TKA and CN-TKA were compared utilizing independent Student's t-tests. Of the 258 primary TKAs, 181 (70.2%) were CN-TKAs and 77 (29.8%) RA-TKAs. Surgical time and operating time were both significantly shorter in CN-TKA, while RA-TKA cases were more likely to be discharged directly home without extended in-patient rehabilitation. When removing the capital costs of surgical equipment and maintenance, there was no difference in total in-hospital cost between CN-TKA ($19,512.3) and RA-TKA ($18,347.1). When these capital costs were included, the mean in-hospital cost of RA-TKA was $21,507.6 compared to $19,659.7 for CN-TKA. The total in-hospital cost, during the implementation period of RA-TKA, was comparable with CN-TKA. RA-TKA was significantly more expensive when the upfront cost of the robotic system and maintenance costs were included. Longer-term cost benefit of RA-TKA should be investigated in future studies [12].

Rajan et al. studied the cost-effectiveness of RA-TKA versus C-TKA in subjects with knee OA [13]. A Markov model simulated the lifetime results of TKA of subjects at an average age of 60 years. Costs of RA-TKA included a preoperative CT scan and the costs for acquisition and use of robotic equipment (average $706,250). Rajan et al. utilized three institutional case volumes to generate average per-case robotic costs: low volume (10 cases, $71,025 per case), mid volume (100 cases, $7463 per case), and high volume (200 cases, $3931 per case). Systematic reviews were utilized to establish early ($\leq$1 year) and late (>1 year) revision percentages after RA-TKA (0.3 and 0.6%, respectively) and C-TKA (0.78% and 1.5%, respectively). Outcomes were total costs and health outcomes measured in quality-adjusted life-years (QALYs). Costs and QALYs were organized into incremental cost-effectiveness ratios (ICERs). A procedure was considered cost-effective if its ICER fell below willingness-to-pay (WTP) thresholds of $50,000 and $100,000/QALY. Sensitivity analyses assessed the impact of data uncertainty. RA-TKA produced 13.55 QALYs versus 13.29 QALYs for C-TKA. Total costs per case for RA-TKA were $92,823 (low volume), $29,261 (mid volume), and $25,730 (high volume) compared with $25,113 for conventional. The ICERs for RA-TKAs were $256,055/QALY (low volume), $15,685/QALY (mid volume), and $2331/QALY (high volume). ICERs for mid- and high-volume institutions were below WTP. The average number needed to treat was >42 and > 24 RA-TKAs for cost-effectiveness at the $50,000 and $100,000/QALY WTP. RA-TKAs endured cost-effective when yearly revision rates <1.6% and quality of life values were > 0.85. With lower annualized percentage rates and higher postoperative quality of life, RA-TKAs possibly offer improved health result, especially when yearly institutional case volume > 24 cases per year. Continued prospective analysis will be essential to prove the value of this new technology [13].

Data on the clinical impact of CN-YTKA and RA-TKA are mixed. Wang et al. described contemporary use tendencies in CN-TKA, RA-TKA, and C-TKA and to evaluate for differences in postoperative adverse events and opioid consumption by procedure type [14]. A national database was queried to identify primary, elective TKA subjects from 2015 to 2020. Tendencies in procedural use percentages were evaluated. Differences in 90-day postoperative adverse events and inpatient opioid consumption were evaluated. Multivariate regression analyses were carried out to account for potential confounders. Of the 847,496 subjects included, 49,317 (5.82%) and 24,460 (2.89%) experienced CN-TKA and RA-TKA, respectively. CN-TKA use increased from 5.64% (2015) to 6.41% (2020) and RA-TKA use increased from 0.84% (2015) to 5.89% (2020). After adjusting for confounders, CN-TKA was associated with lower periprosthetic joint infection, pulmonary embolism, and acute respiratory failure risk compared to C-TKA. RA-TKA was associated with lower deep vein thrombosis, myocardial infarction, and pulmonary embolism risk than C-TKA. Lower postoperative day 1 opioid usage was found with CN-TKA and RA-TKA than C-TKA. Lower postoperative day 0 opioid consumption was also observed in RA-TKA. From 2015 to 2020, there was a relative 13.7% and 601.2% increase in CN-TKAs and RA-TKAs, respectively. This tendency was associated with reductions in hospitalization duration, postoperative adverse events, and opioid consumption. This information supports the safety of RA-TKA and CN-TKA compared to C-TKA. However, further research into the specific indications for these technology-assisted TKAs is required [14].

Li et al. compared the radiologic and clinical results of HURWA (Beijing HURWA-Robot Medical Technology Co. Ltd., China) RA-TKA to those of C-TKA [15]. A total of 150 subjects were randomized into two groups – 73 and 77 subjects experienced RA-TKA and C-TKA, respectively. Preoperative and postoperative WOMAC score, Hospital for Special Surgery (HSS) score, 36-item Short Form Health Survey (SF-36) score, KSS, and ROM were attained and compared between these two groups. The preoperative and postoperative hip-knee-ankle (HKA) angle and the rate of HKA $\leq$ 3° in the two groups were also compared. The postoperative mean HKA angle was 1.801° of varus for the RA-TKA group and 3.017° of varus for the C-TKA group; these values were significantly different. The alignment rates for mechanical axis lower than 3° in the RA-TKA group and the C-TKA group were 81.2% and 63.5%, respectively. Subjects who experienced RA-TKA or C-TKA had similarly improved knee flexion and functional recovery reflected by WOMAC score, HSS score, SF-36 score, and KSS. HURWA RA-TKA was safe and effective, resulting in better alignment for mechanical axis than C-TKA. The improvement in knee flexion and functional recovery after HURWA RA-TKA were similar to those after C-TKA. However, longer follow-up is required to establish whether the improved alignment of mechanical axis will produce better long-run clinical results [15].

Excellent durability with C-TKA has been reported, but substantial percentages of dissatisfaction remain. RA-TKA was introduced to improve clinical results, but associated costs have not been well analyzed. Cotter et al. compared 90-day episode-of-care (EOC) costs for C-TKA and RA-TKA [16]. A retrospective review of an institutional database from 4/2015 to 9/2017 identified consecutive C-TKAs and RA-TKAs utilizing a single implant system carried out by one surgeon. The TKA platform became available at the surgeon's institution in October 2016. Before this date, all TKAs were carried out with the C-TKA technique. After this date, all TKAs were carried out utilizing robotic assistance without exception. Sequential cases were included for both C-TKA and RA-TKA with no subjects excluded. Clinical and financial information were obtained from medical and billing records. Ninety-day EOC costs were compared. One hundred and thirty-nine C-TKAs and 147 RA-TKAs were identified. No significant differences in subject characteristics were found. Total intraoperative costs were higher ($10,295.17 vs. 9998.78) and inpatient costs were lower ($3893.90 vs. 5587.40) comparing RA-TKA and C-TKA. LOS was reduced by 25% (1.2 vs. 1.6 days, respectively) and prescribed opioids were reduced by 57% (984.2 versus 2240.4 morphine milligram equivalents, respectively) comparing RA-TKA with C-TKA. Ninety-day EOC costs were $2090.70 lower for RA-TKA than for C-TKA ($15,629.94 vs. 17,720.64, respectively). The higher intraoperative costs associated with RA-TKA were offset by greater savings in post-

operative costs for the 90-day EOC compared with C-TKA. RA-TKA showed improved value compared with C-TKA based on significantly lower average 90-day EOC costs and superior quality exemplified by reduced LOS, less postoperative opioid requirements, and reduced post-discharge resource utilization [16].

In 2022 Tompkins et al. compared the differences in cost and quality measures between C-TKA and RA-TKA [9]. All C-TKAs and RA-TKAs carried out between January 1, 2017, and December 31, 2019, by six high-volume surgeons in each group were retrospectively reviewed. Groups were propensity score matched. Operative time, length of stay (LOS), total direct cost, 90-day adverse events, use of post-acute services, and 30-day readmissions were studied. After one-to-one matching, 2392 C-TKAs and 2392 RA-TKAs were studied. In-room/out-of-room operating time was longer for RA-TKA (139 minutes) than for C-TKA (107 minutes), as was procedure time (RA-TKA 78 minutes; C-TKA 70 minutes). Median LOS was equal for C-TKA and RA-TKA (33 hours). Total cost per case was greater for RA-TKA ($11,615) than C-TKA ($8674). Home health care was used more commonly after RA-TKA (38%) than C-TKA (29%). There was no significant difference in 90-day adverse event percentages. Thirty-day readmissions happened more often after C-TKA (4.9%) than RA-TKA (1.2%). RA-TKA was a longer and costlier procedure than C-TKA for experienced surgeons, without clinically significant differences in LOS or adverse events. Home health care was used more often after RA-TKA, but fewer readmissions happened after RA-TKA. Longer-term follow-up and functional outcome studies are needed to establish if the greater cost of RTKA is offset by lower revision percentages and/or improved functional outcomes [9].

Although RA-TKA has demonstrated improved knee alignment and diminished radiographic outliers, there remains debate on functional outcomes and PROMs. In a study with level 3 of evidence published in 2022, Mancino et al. compared the 1-year clinical results of a new imageless robotically assisted technique

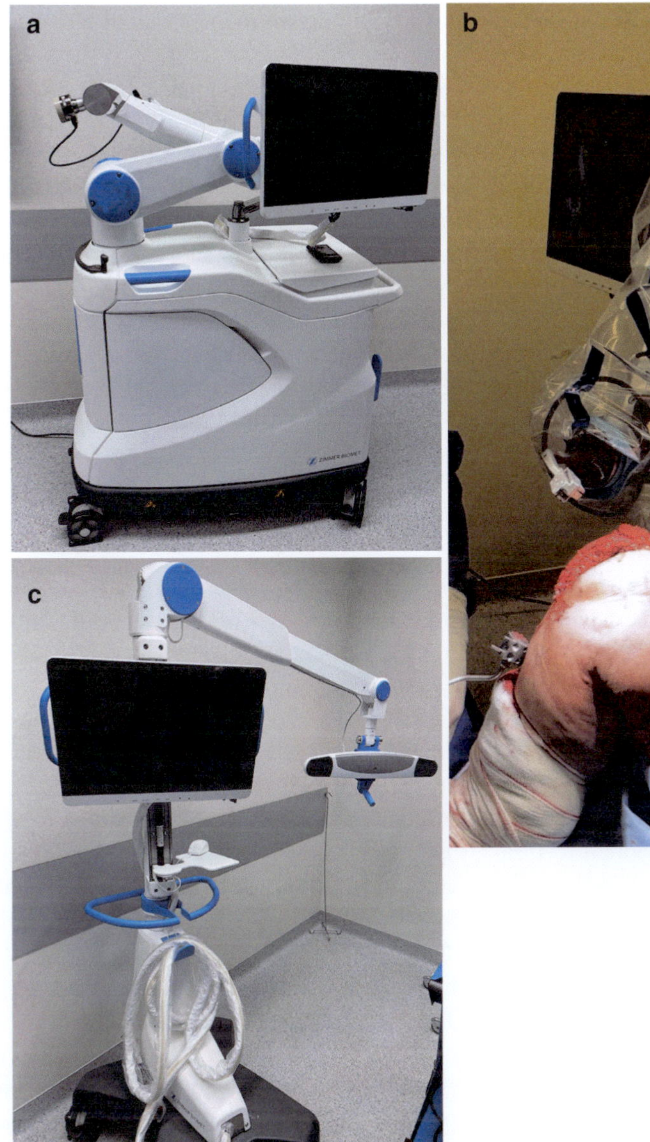
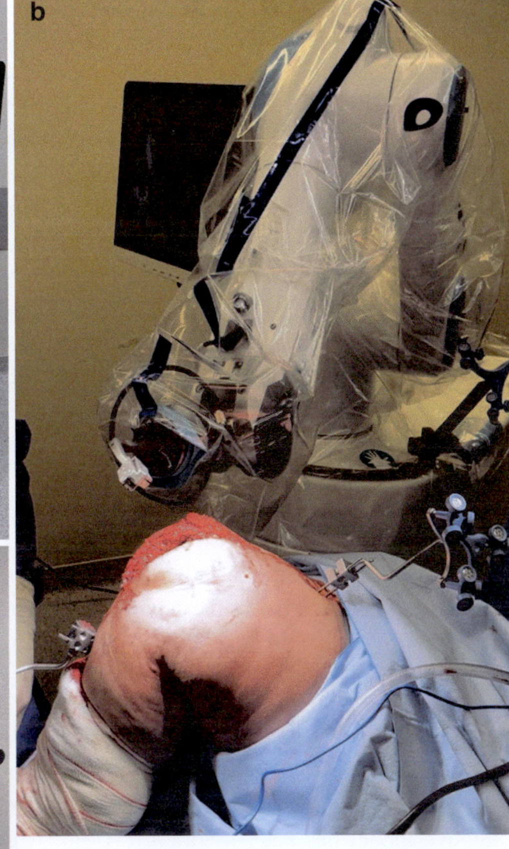

Fig. 17.2 (a–c) ROSA robotic-assisted total knee arthroplasty (RA-TKA) (Zimmer Biomet, Warsaw, IN, USA): (a) ROSA robot arm, to be positioned next to the surgeon. (b) ROSA robot arm positioning the cutting guide. (c) ROSA robot camera and monitor to be positioned in front of the surgeon

(Robotic Surgical Assistant [ROSA] Knee System, Zimmer Biomet, Warsaw, IN, USA) with an imageless navigated procedure (N-TKA, iAssist Knee, Zimmer, Warsaw, IN) (Fig. 17.2) [17]. The study was a retrospective analysis of prospectively collected information that compared the functional results and PROMs of 50 imageless RA-TKA with 47 imageless N-TKA at 1-year follow-up. Baseline characteristics and intraoperative and postoperative data were collected including adverse events, revisions, KSS, Knee Injury and KOOS scores, and FJS-12. Radiographic analysis of preoperative and postoperative images evaluating hip-knee-ankle

(HKA) angle was carried out. There was no difference regarding baseline characteristics between the groups. Mean operative time was significantly longer in the RA-TKA group (122 min vs. 97 min). Significant differences were reported for the "Pain" (85 [RA-TKA] vs 79.1 [N-TKA]) subsection of the KOOS score. In addition, RA-TKA was associated with higher maximum ROM (119.4° vs. 107.1°) and better mean improvement of ROM by 11.67° (23.02° vs. 11.36°). No significant differences were found for other subsections of KOOS, KSS, FJS-12, adverse events, or lower extremity alignment at 1-year follow-up. Imageless RA-TKA was associated with longer surgical time, better pain perception, and improved ROM at 12-month follow-up compared with N-TKA. No significant differences were encountered on other PROMs, adverse event percentages, and radiographic results [17].

17.3.3 Predicting Robotic-Assisted TKA Operating Time

No predictive model has been reported to forecast operating time for TKA. The objectives of a study reported by Motesharei et al. in 2022 were to design and validate a predictive model to estimate operating time for RA-TKA based on demographic data and assess the added predictive power of computed tomography (CT) scan-based predictors and their impact on the precision of the predictive model [18]. A retrospective study was performed on 1061 TKAs carried out from January 2016 to December 2019 with an image-based robotic-assisted system. Demographic information included age, sex, height, and weight. The femoral and tibial mechanical axis and the osteophyte volume were estimated from CT scans. These inputs were utilized to develop a predictive model aimed to forecast operating time based on demographic information only and demographic and 3D subject anatomy information. The key factors for forecasting operating time were the surgeon and subject weight, followed by 12 anatomical parameters derived from CT scans. The predictive model based only on demographic information demonstrated that 90%

of forecasts were within 15 min of actual operating time, with 73% within 10 min. The predictive model including demographic information and CT scans demonstrated that 94% of predictions were within 15 minutes of actual operating time and 88% within 10 min. The primary factors for forecasting RA-TKA operating time were surgeon, subject weight, and osteophyte volume. This study showed that incorporating 3D subject-specific information can improve operating time forecasts models, which may lead to improved operating room planning and efficiency [18].

17.4 Complications of Robotic-Assisted Joint Arthroplasty

The use of robotic assistance in arthroplasty is increasing; however, the spectrum of complications potentially associated with this technology is not clear. Improved understanding of the causes of complications in robotic-assisted arthroplasty can prevent future incidents and enhance patient results. In 2022 Pagani et al. reviewed complication reports to the US Food and Drug Administration (FDA) Manufacturer and User Facility Device Experience database involving robotic-assisted total hip arthroplasty (THA), TKA, and UKA to establish causes of malfunction and related patient impact [19]. Overall, 263 complications reports were included. The most commonly reported complications were unexpected robotic arm movement for TKA (59/204, 28.9%) and retained registration checkpoint for THA (19/44, 43.2%). There were 99 reports of surgical delay with an average delay of 20 min. Thirty-one cases reported conversion to manual surgery. In total, 68 subject injuries were found, 7 of which needed surgical reintervention. Femoral notching (12/36, 33.3%) was the most frequent for TKA and retained registration checkpoint (19/28, 67.9%) was the most frequent for THA. Although rare, additional reported injuries included femoral, tibial, and acetabular fractures, medial collateral ligament laceration, additional retained foreign bodies, and an electrical burn. Despite the increasing use of robotic-assisted arthroplasty in the United States, numerous complications are possible and technical difficulties experienced intraoperatively can lead to prolonged surgical delays. The complications found in this study appear to indicate that robotic-assisted arthroplasty is generally safe with only a few reported instances of serious adverse events, the nature of which appears more related to suboptimal surgical technique than technology. Based on this data, Pagani et al. claimed that the practice of adding registration checkpoints and bone pins to the instrument count of all robotic-assisted total joint arthroplasty (RA-TJA) cases should be widely implemented to avoid unintended retained foreign objects [19].

17.5 Learning Curve Associated with Robotic-Assisted Knee Arthroplasty

In a study with level 3 of evidence published in 2022, Schopper et al. investigated the learning curve associated with robotic-assisted knee arthroplasty [20]. Their hypothesis was that the presence of an experienced surgeon flattens the learning curve and that there was no inflection point for the learning curve of the surgical team. Fifty-five cases consisting of 31 TKAs and 24 UKAs carried out by three surgeons during 2021 were prospectively analyzed. Single surgeon and team performance for operation time learning curve and inflection points were studied utilizing cumulative sum analysis (CUSUM). A downward trend line for individual surgeons and the team performance regarding the operation time learning curve was found. No inflexion point was encountered for the overall team performance regarding TKA and UKA. The surgeon that carried out all cases with the assistance of the experienced surgeon had significantly shorter surgical times than the surgeon that only occasionally received assistance from the experienced surgeon. The presence of an experienced surgeon in robotically assisted knee arthroplasty can flatten the learning curve of the surgical team formerly unexperienced in robotic-assisted systems. Manufacturers should provide expanded support during initial cases in centers without previous experience to robotic-assisted knee arthroplasty [20].

17.6 Conclusions

Robotic-assisted primary unicompartmental arthroplasty (RA-UKA) achieves excellent implant accuracy and clinical results in the short run. The dependability of intraoperative measurements of the frontal femorotibial axis by robotic-assisted systems is acceptable. Cost-effectiveness analyses have shown that the utilization of RA-UKA is an effective option to conventional UKA (CUKA) in individuals with single-compartment knee osteoarthritis (OA). With the ability to accomplish target alignment in the coronal, axial, and sagittal planes and provide intraoperative real-time data to obtain balanced gaps, RA-TKA has shown excellent clinical results and patient-reported outcome measures (PROMs). Individuals who experienced RA-TKA have shown early improvement at 1-year follow-up in pain, stiffness, and knee flexion when compared with their prior contralateral conventional total knee arthroplasty (C-TKA). There is a significant reduction in postoperative hospital length of stay (LOS) in the RA-TKA group. Computer-navigated TKA (CN-TKA) is associated with lower periprosthetic joint infection, pulmonary embolism, and acute respiratory failure risk compared to C-TKA. RA-TKA is associated with lower deep vein thrombosis, myocardial infarction, and pulmonary embolism risk than C-TKA. Lower postoperative day 1 opioid usage is found with CN-TKA and RA-TKA than C-TKA. Lower postoperative day 0 opioid consumption is also observed in RA-TKA. The complications of robotic-assisted arthroplasty appear to indicate that the procedure is generally safe with only a few reported instances of serious adverse events, the nature of which appears more related to suboptimal surgical technique than technology.

References

1. Deroche E, Naaim A, Lording T, Dumas R, Servien E, Cheze L, et al. Femorotibial alignment measured during robotic assisted knee surgery is reliable: radiologic and gait analysis. Arch Orthop Trauma Surg. 2022;142:1645–51.

2. Yeroushalmi D, Feng J, Nherera L, Trueman P, Schwarzkopf R. Early economic analysis of robotic-assisted unicondylar knee arthroplasty may be cost effective in patients with end-stage osteoarthritis. J Knee Surg. 2022;35:39–46.
3. St Mart JP, Goh EL, Goudie E, Crawford R, English H, Donnelly W. Clinical and radiological outcomes of robotic-assisted unicompartmental knee arthroplasty: early lessons from the first 100 consecutive knees in 85 patients. Knee. 2022;34:195–205.
4. Dobelle E, Aza A, Avellan S, Taillebot V, Ollivier M, Argenson JN. Implantation of the femoral component relative to the tibial component in medial unicompartmental knee arthroplasty: a clinical, radiological, and biomechanical study. J Arthroplast. 2022;37(6S):S82–7.
5. Haffar A, Krueger CA, Goh GS, Lonner JH. UKA with a handheld robotic device results in greater surgeon physiological stress than conventional instrumentation. Knee Surg Sports Traumatol Arthrosc; 2022. https://doi.org/10.1007/s00167-022-06908-5. Online ahead of print.
6. Goh GS, Haffar A, Tarabichi S, Courtney PM, Krueger CA, Lonner JH. Robotic-assisted versus manual unicompartmental knee arthroplasty: a time-driven activity-based cost analysis. J Arthroplast. 2022;37:1023–8.
7. Heckmann ND, Antonios JK, Chen XT, Kang HP, Chung BC, Piple AS, et al. Midterm survivorship of robotic-assisted lateral unicompartmental knee arthroplasty. J Arthroplast. 2022;37:831–6.
8. Vaidya NV, Deshpande AN, Panjwani T, Patil R, Jaysingani T, Patil P. Robotic-assisted TKA leads to a better prosthesis alignment and a better joint line restoration as compared to conventional TKA: a prospective randomized controlled trial. Knee Surg Sports Traumatol Arthrosc. 2022;30:621–6.
9. Tompkins GS, Sypher KS, Li HF, Griffin TM, Duwelius PJ. Robotic versus manual total knee arthroplasty in high volume surgeons: a comparison of cost and quality metrics. J Arthroplast. 2022;37(8S):S782–9.
10. Joo PY, Chen AF, Richards J, Law TY, Taylor K, Marchand K, et al. Clinical results and patient-reported outcomes following robotic-assisted primary total knee arthroplasty: a multicentre study. Bone Jt Open. 2022;3:589–95.
11. Ali M, Kamson A, Yoo C, Singh I, Ferguson C, Dahl R. Early superior clinical outcomes in robotic-assisted TKA compared to conventional TKA in the same patient: a comparative analysis. J Knee Surg. 2022; https://doi.org/10.1055/s-0042-1743232. Online ahead of print.
12. Steffens D, Karunaratne S, McBride K, Gupta S, Horsley M, Fritsch B. Implementation of robotic-assisted total knee arthroplasty in the public health system: a comparative cost analysis. Int Orthop. 2022;46:481–8.
13. Rajan PV, Khlopas A, Klika A, Molloy R, Krebs V, Piuzzi NS. The cost-effectiveness of robotic-assisted versus manual total knee arthroplasty: a Markov model-based evaluation. J Am Acad Orthop Surg. 2022;30:168–76.
14. Wang JC, Piple AS, Hill WJ, Chen MS, Gettleman BS, Richardson M, et al. Computer-navigated and robotic-assisted total knee arthroplasty: increasing in popularity without increasing complications J Arthroplast 2022;S0883-5403(22)00677-5.
15. Li Z, Chen X, Wang X, Zhang B, Wang W, Fan Y, Yan J, et al. HURWA robotic-assisted total knee arthroplasty improves component positioning and alignment - a prospective randomized and multicenter study. J Orthop Translat. 2022;33:31–40.
16. Cotter EJ, Wang J, Illgen RL. Comparative cost analysis of robotic-assisted and jig-based manual primary total Knee arthroplasty. J Knee Surg. 2022;35:176–84.
17. Mancino F, Rossi SMP, Sangaletti R, Lucenti L, Terragnoli F, Benazzo F. A new robotically assisted technique can improve outcomes of total knee arthroplasty comparing to an imageless navigation system. Arch Orthop Trauma Surg. 2022; https://doi.org/10.1007/s00402-022-04560-9. Online ahead of print.
18. Motesharei A, Batailler C, De Massari D, Vincent G, Chen AF, Lustig S. Predicting robotic-assisted total knee arthroplasty operating time: benefits of machine-learning and 3D patient-specific data. Bone Jt Open. 2022;3:383–9.
19. Pagani NR, Menendez ME, Moverman MA, Puzzitiello RN, Gordon MR. Adverse events associated with robotic-assisted joint arthroplasty: an analysis of the US Food and Drug Administration MAUDE database00003. J Arthroplast. 2022;37:1526–33.
20. Schopper C, Proier P, Luger M, Gotterbarm T, Klasan A. The learning curve in robotic assisted knee arthroplasty is flattened by the presence of a surgeon experienced with robotic assisted surgery. Knee Surg Sports Traumatol Arthrosc. 2022:1–8. https://doi.org/10.1007/s00167-022-07048-6. Online ahead of print.

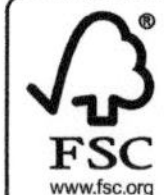
FSC
www.fsc.org
MIX
Papier aus verantwortungsvollen Quellen
Paper from responsible sources
FSC® C105338